Overcoming Depression

Overcoming Depression

THIRD EDITION

Demitri F. Papolos, M.D., and Janice Papolos

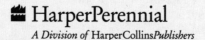 HarperPerennial
A Division of HarperCollins*Publishers*

HarperCollins books may be purchased for educational, business, or sales promotional use. For information please write: Special Markets Department, HarperCollins Publishers, Inc., 10 East 53rd Street, New York, NY 10022.

Designed by C. Linda Dingler

Library of Congress Cataloging-in-Publication Data

Papolos, Demitri F.
    Overcoming depression / Demitri F. Papolos and Janice Papolos. —
3rd ed.
        p.   cm.
    Includes bibliographical references and index.
    ISBN 0-06-092782-8
    1. Depression, Mental—Popular works. 2. Manic-depressive illness—Popular works.   I. Papolos, Janice. II. Title.
RC537.P36   1997
616.85'27—dc20   96-33534

03 02 01 00 99 RRD 20 19 18 17 16 15 14 13 12 11

For Alexander

CONTENTS

PREFACE TO
THE THIRD EDITION

It's hard to believe that ten years has passed since *Overcoming Depression* first appeared on bookshelves. This decade has been a literal explosion in our knowledge about depression and manic-depression, particularly in the fields of molecular biology, genetics, epidemiology, clinical research, and psychopharmacology. Although we noted many changes in the revised edition of 1992, the field continues to develop at so rapid a pace that a book such as this is never really finished. When HarperCollins asked us to do a tenth anniversary edition, we were delighted to have another opportunity to return to the manuscript, detail some of the newer developments, and bring the book and our readers up-to-date. Let us outline some of the changes we've made in the third edition of *Overcoming Depression*.

In 1992, we noted the ascendancy of Prozac, as well as a novel antidepressant, Wellbutrin, for the treatment of depression. Zoloft, Paxil, Effexor, and Serzone were introduced soon after and each has taken its place in the psychiatric armamentarium. Information about each of these newer drugs has been included in Chapter 5, The Somatic Therapies. But, as avidly as these new medications have been embraced by physicians and patients (and with good reason), the drugs—like the tricyclic antidepressants—have been observed to accelerate cycle frequency and/or induce hypomania, mania, or mixed states in patients with bipolar disorder, and we have added references to this important clinical phenomenon here and throughout the manuscript. Also, it has been discovered that these newer antidepressants can inhibit certain liver enzymes and so produce higher levels of other commonly coadministered drugs. A chart that advises patients which drugs may be problematic when prescribed with one of these antidepressants is included on page 171.

We have always felt strongly that women with mood disorders and their partners should have as much information as possible about the use of psychotropic medications during pregnancy. Until recently, existing data about the use of lithium during the first trimester of pregnancy pointed toward the drug as a probable cause of heart anomalies in newborns. But results of an extensive literature study now show that much of the information about the teratogenic effects of lithium was based on skewed statistical reporting. The risks seem to be less than originally feared. A discussion of these findings and new treatment recommendations to psychiatrists for lithium use in women with bipolar disorder as well as the encouraging results of studies of women who took Prozac during their first trimester has been added to Chapter 8: Mood Disorders and Pregnancy.

Chapter 8 also contains a new section on the comorbidity of substance abuse and mood disorders. Although earlier editions of this book noted the association between alcoholism and depressive disorders, only recently have researchers focused their efforts on determining the true incidence of this association. In this chapter we discuss the latest studies, which increasingly point to undiagnosed mood disorder—in particular bipolar disorder—as possible causative factors in the development and perpetuation of substance abuse in the general population.

The genetics chapter has also undergone some revision. Originally we described the discovery of a possible genetic marker for manic-depressive illness in the Old Order Amish in Lancaster, Pennsylvania. In the ensuing years, however, the complexity of these conditions and the likelihood that many genes influence their development have become more apparent, and we have tried to give the reader an expanded glimpse of more recent developments. We have added the newest linkage findings among the Amish pedigrees as well as those published by other researchers and have included an intriguing report that points to a strong association between bipolar disorder and a genetic condition caused by the deletion of a small swatch of DNA on chromosome 22.

Readers familiar with this book will also notice significant differences in Chapter 12, Underwriting the Illness: The World of Insurance. For a sea change has taken place in the delivery of health care in this country. Within a few short years, managed care has become the predominant force in the private sector and is quickly moving into the public sector as well. We summarize the reasons for its omnipresence in the marketplace, and its intricacies and new vocabulary, and we note our concerns and guarded hopes for this new system.

We would again like to acknowledge Ross J. Baldessarini, M.D., of the Harvard Medical School, who was a guiding force from the beginning. Solomon Baredes, M.D.; Richard Brown; John Clark; Johnine Cummings, M.S.W.; Robin Dea, M.D.; Gianni Faedda, M.D.; Rosalie Greenberg, M.D.; Laura Lee Hall, Ph.D.; Theresa Harney; William Kuster; Mehde Kazmi, M.D.; Robert T. Malazin, M.D.; Thomas R. Margenau; Pat Milone, R.Ph.; John Plewes, M.D.; Jody Rapport; Mark Sampieri, R.Ph.; Andrew P. Schyuler, M.D.; E. Fuller Torrey, M.D.; and Myrna Weissman, Ph.D, also responded graciously to our requests for information, and we are very grateful to all of them for their advice and assistance.

A special thank-you to Kristen Auclair, our fine editor, who was extremely supportive throughout the revision, and to Carol Cohen, who first championed this book and has continued to shepherd it through its decade of life.

Demitri F. Papolos, M.D.
Janice Papolos
Westport, Connecticut, 1996

PREFACE TO
THE FIRST EDITION

Although mood disorders have always been a part of human experience, the past 10 to 15 years have seen such advances in their treatment that people no longer have to struggle through crippling sieges of depression or uncontrollable mania. With proper diagnosis and treatment, mood swings can be prevented or diminished in severity. In fact, so many advances have been made in such a short period of time that a lag in communication has developed—people aren't aware that psychiatry has a new understanding of recurrent mood disorders and that available treatments can dramatically improve the quality of their lives. An update is in order.

In the pages that follow, we explore the nature and course of depression and mania and describe the medications used in their treatment—the benefits as well as the complications. We summarize and explore the current scientific concepts of the underlying causes of mood disorders: first, because they're interesting and important, and second, because they are the scaffolding for the research that should result in new and more sophisticated treatment in the future. While the research findings presented throughout the book were culled from the major scientific and clinical journals in the fields of psychiatry and the basic sciences, we have made an effort to make this information accessible to the layperson without oversimplifying or overstating the present state of knowledge. We tried not to let the ascendant biomedical model of psychiatry become an opportunity to gloss over the difficult psychological and social issues pertinent to mood disorders. These conditions involve periodic disturbances in mood, concentration, sleep, activity, appetite, and behavior and they profoundly affect an individual's functioning, social relations, life-course, and self-esteem. Major sections of this book are devoted to exploring what happens to a person who suffers recurrent episodes of depression or mania, as well as the impact of these illnesses on family members. In these sections we outline ways in which everyone concerned might better cope with the problems the episodes present.

In order to broaden the scope of the book and provide a three-dimensional picture of the realities of these disorders and of a patient's interactions with the mental health profession, we devised a rather extensive questionnaire and distributed it nationally through the manic-depressive support groups. Many people responded with moving and informative accounts of their experiences during cycles of illness. They told us their concerns and problems and urged us to convey to others the methods they had found to cope with these disorders.

Knowledge is a great balancer, and informed individuals can and do respond more constructively to the problems of illness. It is our intention to aid in the early recognition of depression and manic-depression, to reinforce and supplement the information given by the consulting psychiatrist or physician, and to clear away some of the mysteries from the field of psychiatry and its treatment of the major mood disorders. We want to let people know what to expect so that they can better assess their treatment and act in their own best interest. It is our hope, then, that this book will be a resource that will make living with the illness easier for all concerned.

Demitri F. Papolos, M.D.
Janice Papolos
New York City, 1987

ACKNOWLEDGMENTS

Throughout the writing of this book, we were privileged to have the special counsel of Ross J. Baldessarini, M.D. He put his enormous store of experience and knowledge at our disposal, and his attention to the manuscript contributed countless improvements.

We would also like to acknowledge the other professionals who responded generously to our requests for information and assistance. They are: Olivia H. Baker, R.N., Miron Baron, M.D., Judith Berenson, M.S.W., Judith Bernz, Wade Berrettini, M.D., Joseph Biederman, M.D., Vernon R. Bruette, Debra M. Cassel, Johnine Cummings, M.S.W., Linda E. Franz, L.C.S.W., Gary Goldsmith, Rosalie Greenberg, M.D., Marian C. Harkavy, Teresa Harney, Artie Houston, Stephen B. Kahn, Esq., Thomas Kranjac, M.D., Dulcie E. Lewis, R.N., Elizabeth Mackintosh, Ph.D., David Moltz, M.D., Eric J. Neutzel, M.D., Grace Oettinger, O.T., William Parsons, Ph.D., Said Saber, Ph.D., Richard Satkin, Maggie Schie, Bruce J. Schwartz, M.D., Delores Segal, Scott Sherrill, Esq., Andrew E. Skodol, M.D., Jorge L. Tapia, D.D.S., Kenneth G. Terkelsen, M.D., Maryellen Walsh and Marilyn Weiss.

Special thanks are owed to the many members of the manic-depressive support groups across the nation who answered our questionnaire. Their voices have added an immediate and vital perspective to these pages.

Pam Bernstein, our agent and friend, encouraged this project from the start, and Carol Cohen's keen eye and intelligent editing brought clarity to the manuscript and kept us on course.

Finally, we wish to acknowledge the people who were most directly involved with the evolution of this volume, and who offered us crucial and unfailing support: Rose B. Albicocco, Laurie Scandurra Ball, Rosalie Snyder Bate, Richard L. Hauger, M.D., Herb M. Lachman, M.D., Mervyn M. Peskin, M.D., Stephen P. Reibel, M.D., Barbara L. Sand, Barbara Solomon, Herman M. van Praag, M.D., Ph.D., and Kevin Walz.

The purpose of this book is to make you aware of psychiatry's progress in the study and treatment of the major mood disorders. Proper diagnosis and the treatment of depression and manic-depression require an expert. You should consult only with a highly qualified physician about questions specific to yourself.

All names, characteristics, backgrounds, and other details about the people described in the case examples in this book have been changed.

ONE

ABOUT THE ILLNESS

1

THE PERSONAL EXPERIENCE

When we first told friends and people outside the psychiatric field that we were writing a book on depression and manic-depression, we expected polite but lukewarm interest. That wasn't what happened. Instead, one person after another confided to us: "I've had experience with it; my mother and brother are bipolar"; "My grandmother and younger sister were just put on lithium"; and "My adopted son suffers from recurrent depression. . . . I don't know if his real parents had it." These people were stating what clinicians have always observed: depression and manic-depression are very common illnesses and tend to concentrate in families.

Mood disorders are the "common cold" of major psychiatric illnesses, and more than 20 million Americans will suffer an episode of depression or mania during their lifetimes. One in five families will directly feel their impact. Those who have manic-depression will veer from periods of superactivity, manic elation, and grandiose schemes to periods of despondency, immobility, guilt, and inability to experience pleasure or even to think normally. The people who experience these highs and lows have what psychiatrists now call *bipolar disorder.* Those who suffer recurrent severe depression without the highs are said to have *unipolar* or nonbipolar major depression. The psychiatric profession groups these mood disturbances under the rubric *major affective disorders.* At first glance the term "affec-

tive" doesn't send the mind traveling, but it's a word philoso-
phers and psychologists have traditionally used for emotion or
one's "spirits."

Whatever these disorders are called—affective, manic-
depressive illness, recurrent mood disorders, unipolar or bipolar depression—they've been affecting humankind throughout
the centuries. Some very familiar individuals figure among the
victims: King Saul of the Bible (who needed David's music to
soothe his despondency), King George III (the last English king
to rule the American colonies), Abraham Lincoln, Winston
Churchill, and Theodore Roosevelt. The writers and poets
Johann Goethe, Honoré de Balzac, Leo Tolstoy, Virginia Woolf,
Ernest Hemingway, Robert Lowell, and Anne Sexton suffered
mood swings, as did the composers George Frederick Handel,
Robert Schumann, Hugo Wolf, Hector Berlioz, and Gustav
Mahler. These people are well known and respected, so it may
be that the illness fuels a certain kind of drive and creativity.
However, a study of their lives would also reveal searing
anguish, shattered relationships, psychosis, and even suicide.

Mood changes are hallmarks of the human experience, and
mood has a powerful evolutionary value: it regulates our disposition to action and behavior, and keeps us involved in life and yet
relatively safe. However, those who are too pessimistic may not
realize their potential; someone who is depressed will step back
from life and not participate. On the other hand, a person with
too optimistic a mood may also place himself or herself at risk;
someone experiencing a manic episode can get carried away
with an exalted sense of power and self-importance and act
impulsively or recklessly. An immoderate mood disposition can
cause life to be fragmented, disorganized, painful, and potentially
dangerous.

Mood also has a strong influence on the way someone
feels about himself. When depressed, he or she often dwells on
exaggerated memories of losses or failures, or focuses on the
morbid and negative aspects of life to the exclusion of all else.

Negative thoughts or perceptions about oneself can erode self-esteem, resulting in an unrealistic sense of worthlessness and the feeling of being a burden to others. A person may experience persistent feelings of sadness and emptiness, become tearful for no apparent reason, or become irritable and hostile.

The depressed person may be slowed down, lack energy, and have fewer ideas. Decisions seem nearly impossible to make, and everyday tasks and challenges become intimidating. Some severe types of depression may include irrational, psychotic, or delusional symptoms. Since these episodes may last for several months or longer, one's morale or self-esteem can become seriously impaired. Prolonged periods of depression can lead to the wish to die and to thoughts of killing oneself.

In contrast to this bleak picture, the person experiencing the "highs" of manic-depression often describes feeling better than at any other time in his life. He cannot understand why anyone would call his experience abnormal or part of an illness. The rate of thinking is markedly increased; one thought after another bursts into consciousness demanding expression. During a manic episode, a person feels more excited, has surges of energy, and describes feeling more active, creative, intelligent, and sexual than he ever thought possible. Sleep seems unnecessary, and he's ready to "take on the world." It is not unusual for a person in a manic state to decide to try to write the great American novel or to embark on audacious and risky business ventures.

The seemingly boundless energy and enthusiasm that are often a part of the manic swing can be infectious at first. Those witnessing a person charged with exuberance and confidence are often quite intrigued. Mania is not a state to be envied, however. Decisions made during a manic high are typically reckless and impulsive. Spending sprees and sexual indiscretions are common, and some people experiencing the disorder find the excess energy and excitement unbearable. They may turn to alcohol or drugs to calm the agitation or irritability. As the manic throttle is pushed, the person becomes more argumentative, intrusive, and insistent about getting his own way. Others around him then become confused, angry, and alarmed.

While some people experience a more controlled state of mania with elation and excessive activity called *hypomania,* others lose contact with reality as their thinking becomes fragmented, disorganized, and delusional. The person may envision himself as the savior of the world, or he may experience paranoia and respond to others with extreme irritability and anger. In this psychotic stage, the disorder can be confused with schizophrenia. Eventually the manic episode runs its course, though, and the person may be plunged into the depths of depression—surrounded by the shards of his life, career, and relationships.

The person who experiences out-and-out manic episodes alternating with periods of depression is referred to as having *bipolar I* disorder. The person who suffers very mild hypomanic periods as well as severe depression is said to have *bipolar II* disorder. There are also some people who experience only the manic highs and little or no depression, and they are referred to as having *unipolar mania.*

The onset of the first episode of an affective disorder may not always be obvious. Some people have brief, mild episodes infrequently and do not seek treatment or even know that they are ill. Since we all experience periods of sadness, disappointment, and grief, it is difficult to know when a depressed mood becomes a medical condition. While there continues to be debate about this question, it may be useful to conceptualize the state of depression as developing along a continuum from mild to severe.

When a person experiences some major disappointment in a career or relationship, the loss is usually followed by a few days of sadness, withdrawal, sleep disturbance, and anxiety, but it is not long before the normal mood is reestablished and the person regroups and goes on with life. When, however, the depressed mood persists, the isolation from others continues, and the individual loses a sense of pleasure and meaning in life and begins to develop physical symptoms such as loss of appetite, a marked interruption in the regular sleep cycle, and a marked decrease in the ordinary level of activity, these signs signal the onset of a *clinical depression.* The person has moved across the boundaries that demarcate normal mood fluctuations to a medical condition. (It should be noted that the clinical syndrome of depression can present itself without any noticeable precipitants such as loss or disappointment.)

Typically, episodes of illness are time-limited: they come and go, last from several weeks to several months, and are followed by periods of relatively normal mood and behavior. Untreated, the average depressive episode lasts about four months, and the average manic episode about three months. Periods of depression, however, can last for twelve months or more without remitting.

Not all people who experience a major depression will suffer a recurrence, but psychiatrists are beginning to realize that depression is more recurrent and chronic than originally thought.

Dr. Jules Angst in Zurich found that 70 to 80 percent of patients with an initial episode of major depression experienced recurrence; and data from the U.S. Catchment Area study revealed that patients who have had at least three or more episodes will have an 80 percent chance of relapse within a three-year span of time; that rate rises to 90 percent or higher after 5 years. The lifetime average for depressive episodes is 5 to 7, but as many as 40 episodes have been reported.

Bipolar illness is typically a recurrent or episodic disorder: a 1973 study examined nearly 400 patients who had an episode of manic-depressive illness, and only 2 failed to have a recurrence. Without treatment, the frequency and severity of the illness tend to increase over the years, but usually reach an eventual plateau.

The unipolar form of mood disorder (depression) is more common than the bipolar, and it is estimated that two-thirds of the individuals who experience a mood disorder have depressions only. However, 10 to 15 percent of the people who first experience one or more depressive episodes go on to experience a hypomanic or manic episode and thus are reclassified as bipolar. It is not unusual for a relative to have the unipolar form of the disorder and a descendant to have the bipolar form, or vice versa.

Manic and depressive episodes present themselves differently in different persons, but there are two basic types of episode:

1. Periods of depression are characterized by:
   - depressed or irritable or anxious mood
   - poor appetite and weight loss, or the opposite, increased appetite and weight gain
   - sleep disturbance: sleeping too little, or sleeping too much in an irregular pattern
   - loss of energy: excessive fatigue or tiredness
   - change in activity level, either increased or decreased
   - loss of interest or pleasure in usual activities
   - decreased sexual drive
   - physical aches and pains (including headaches, stomachaches, and lower back pain)
   - diminished ability to think or concentrate
   - feelings of worthlessness or excessive guilt that may reach grossly unreasonable or delusional proportions
   - other psychotic and delusional thinking
   - recurrent thoughts of death or self-harm, wishing to be dead or contemplating or attempting suicide
2. Periods of hypomania or the more severe state of mania are characterized by:
   - persistently "high" (euphoric) or irritable (dysphoric) or agitated moods

- marked shifts in mood
- decreased need for sleep
- appetite disturbance
- increased activity, sociability, or sexual drive
- pressured, rapid speech
- racing thoughts, rapidly changing thought patterns that may be hard for others to follow
- loss of self-control and judgment
- excessive spending, reckless and impulsive behavior
- grandiose thinking about oneself, inflated ideas about one's capabilities
- paranoid, or other delusional and psychotic thinking (in the manic state)

It's a discomforting, unhappy menu of symptoms with much potential for misery and shame. This can be compounded by a lack of understanding of what actually is going on inside—on the part of both the patient and those closest to him or her. When someone doesn't understand that he is in the throes of a depression, he is likely to ascribe the symptoms to erroneous causes, thereby delaying medical treatment. Not only is he confused, he also doesn't have an adequate explanation for those who are witnessing the changes, and the situation is ripe for myth, misunderstanding, and distortion. Over and over again you hear families say: "I thought he was an alcoholic with big ideas"; "We thought she was just lazy and wouldn't get out of bed"; and, "How can she be unhappy? She has so much to be grateful for in life. Why can't she pull herself up and get going?" What they don't realize is that these illnesses are insidious, and once they take hold, the victim is without the power to lighten or temper his or her mood or symptoms.

If someone had cancer and were promised a cure in a far-away clinic, nothing would stop that individual from getting on a plane to seek out that cure. But Dick Cavett put his finger on the very thing that separates depression from any other illness.

When speaking of his own experience with a severe depression, he said: "What's really diabolical about it is that if there were a pill over there, 10 feet from me, that you could guarantee would lift me out of it, it would be too much trouble to go get it."

Tragically, only 1 in 3 people suffering from a major mood disorder seeks help, and only 1 in 10 seeks help from a psychiatrist trained to diagnose severe psychiatric disorders and treat them medically. Today, thanks to lithium and other anticonvulsant and antidepressant medications, these disorders are eminently treatable. It is estimated that over 80 percent of people suffering from depression and manic-depression can achieve substantial relief from their crippling symptoms. Stigma and a lack of knowledge as well as the often insidious nature of these disorders are a lethal combination.

It is crucial that people recognize the symptoms and understand the nature of these severe, recurring illnesses. But a list of symptoms alone is not sufficiently telling—it does not capture the human experience. Therefore, we've used patients' accounts and descriptions from literature to allow a more intimate look into these variable mood states.

WHAT DOES IT FEEL LIKE TO BE DEPRESSED?

A person who enters a depressive episode often describes his mood as sad, hopeless, down in the dumps, irritable, and black. There is, however, another dimension to the depression experienced by a significant number of people—an anxious, restless, anguished feeling. Some people seem to be trapped in an agitated state of arousal as Robert Burton describes in his 1621 *Anatomy of Melancholy:* "They are in great pain and horror of mind, distraction of soul, restless, full of continual fears, cares, torment, anxieties, they can neither drink, eat, nor sleep for them, take no rest, neither at bed nor yet at board."

Many patients report a change in their thought patterns,

in both the rate and content of thoughts. There is a paucity of ideas and a loss of the natural capacity to imagine a future. When the mind is laid barren of thought, the imagination cannot make the necessary leap into the future, and the individual experiences himself as out of time and isolated from the ongoing current of life. He cannot reconnect. One person described it this way:

> The most awful thing was that I realized my days had been composed of little moments of anticipated pleasure: that first cup of coffee in the very early morning, the inner thoughts that made me chuckle, a browse through a bookstore, the satisfaction of a job or chore completed. . . . Now these moments failed to hold the crest of pleasure— everything was flat and gray. Life seemed locked away from me and I was filled with unspeakable dread.

One young woman who was forced to leave college after her freshman year explained how terrified she was by the sense of inner strangeness and isolation she felt during her first encounter with depression:

> When I came home I was in a severe state of depression and anxiety, and my family was at a complete loss. I felt very isolated, unable to communicate. I felt I had let them down incredibly and I had this tremendous guilt.
> But I couldn't talk to them. I felt like my brain wasn't functioning. I had a hard time just carrying on a conversation. The depression was really scary, because I felt that some incredible, horrible thing had happened to me, but there were no signs on the outside. I couldn't explain to people that inside I was completely different. I felt estranged, bizarre, weird. My thoughts were much slower. It was terrifying to be in college and sit through a whole lecture and be unable to remember a word of what the professor had said. Or, I'd sit down and read the textbook and I couldn't absorb any of it. I felt like some bizarre trick

of fate, that something terribly wrong had happened to me on the inside, but nobody would understand.

It is common for people in the throes of a depression to feel that the world is drained of color—that everything is stale and empty, and that there is no "light at the end of the tunnel." Previously enjoyed activities hold no interest or pleasure for them, and they are said to have the clinical symptom known as *anhedonia.* The word doesn't in any way reveal the awfulness of the symptom. Author Maryellen Walsh describes what it's like to witness its appearance in a loved one:

> Joy, affection, desire, pride, humor are all drained away. What makes life worth living disappears slowly, relentlessly until nothing seems to be left. . . . Anhedonia creeps in and claims the person who once laughed with you, who once hugged you, who once loved to be first on the hill to catch the new powder snow. The lights go out one by one. It is the death of the spirit.

Major depression is more than an anguished mood or the loss of the capacity to experience pleasure. It is accompanied by severe disturbances in appetite and sleep patterns—the so-called biological or vegetative symptoms. Usually a person complains of having no appetite—food just doesn't taste good anymore. One man was able to pinpoint the onset of his depression when he recalled sitting at a table in a restaurant with friends listening to them rave over food he felt tasted like sawdust.

In the case of a severe depression, the person may lose a great deal of weight. Sometimes, as in an *atypical* depression, the opposite may occur: the person actually develops a craving for sweets and carbohydrates and begins to put on weight. (This type of depression is frequently associated with the bipolar form of the disorder.)

Some people notice a change in their sleep pattern before any other signs of depression appear. They may have trouble going to sleep at night (initial insomnia), wake up during the middle of the night and find it difficult to get back to sleep (middle insomnia), or find themselves awakening early, around 4:00 or 5:00 A.M., and are overtaken by anxious, guilty thoughts they cannot quell. The journalist Percy Knauth chronicled his battle with depression in *A Season in Hell* and had this to say about the sleep disturbance:

> As the lack of sleep wore me down, a sense of hopelessness enveloped me. I knew that nothing I did could change the situation. There was nothing I *could* do. I was convinced that I was laboring under some kind of curse so that any efforts of my own to fight this situation were foredoomed to failure.
>
> More realistically, I understood that the only tool I could fight with—my mind—was the very part of me that was affected. Can a legless man get up and walk even if he knows that only walking will save his life? My mind was going; how could I use it to extricate myself from my despair?
>
> With this hopelessness came the final stage in my loss of self-esteem: in my own eyes I became worthless. In long night sessions, I reviewed my life and saw everything that I had done wrong. Not even the most trivial detail escaped this deadly scrutiny. I remembered arguments I had had with my older children when they were very young, in my first marriage, and I realized what a poor excuse for a father I had been. I recalled the details of my divorce, and I understood precisely why my wife had left me for another man: I had never really filled the role of husband. Viewed in the merciless gloom of this early-morning self-analysis, even my work appeared to me to have been a fraud. At last I was being showed up for the hapless faker that I was, and this was my punishment.

Because there is no sense of the future in depression, the past, as Dr. Leston Havens says, "becomes fixed, immovable, bad, the place of irredeemable mistakes."

Although the majority of depressed people report some kind of insomnia, approximately 15 to 30 percent feel the need to sleep excessively (hypersomnia) and never feel rested, even after 12 or 14 hours of sleep. In addition to the mood, appetite, and sleep disturbances of depression, people may experience bodily pains such as headaches, backaches, constipation, or stomach problems. Sexual appetite, as one man described it, is "the first to go . . . you don't even remember what it felt like."

There may be a variation in the intensity of symptoms that a patient feels at different times of the day, typically referred to as a diurnal variation of mood. For some, the mornings are an agony with some relief occurring in the afternoon. For others, like the author William Styron, the days of depression had a different rhythm:

> Afternoons were the worst, beginning at about three o'clock, when I'd feel the horror, like some poisonous fogbank, roll in upon my mind, forcing me into bed. There I would lie as long as six hours, stuporous and virtually paralyzed, gazing at the ceiling and waiting for that moment of evening when, mysteriously the crucifixion would ease up just enough to allow me to force down some food and then, like an automaton, seek an hour or two of sleep again.

Changes that occur in a depressed patient's activity and mental processes are described as *psychomotor agitation* or *retardation*. Thought and action are either sped up or very slowed down. Some individuals experiencing depression can't sit still: they pace, wring their hands, and pull at their hair or clothing. Others seem suspended in slow motion, so drained of energy that the capacity to initiate activity is all but extinguished. One woman used the analogy: "It's like trying to function wearing a 200-pound body suit. My brain feels submerged in oil."

Speech, like everything else, is deadened, and the person may speak in a low, monotonous voice with long pauses before answering. In *The Loony-Bin Trip,* Kate Millet mourns this loss of language:

> During depression the world disappears. Language itself. One has nothing to say. Nothing. No small talk, no anecdotes. Nothing can be risked on the board of talk. Because the inner voice is so urgent in its own discourse: How shall I live? How shall I manage in the future? Why should I go on? There is nothing ahead, my powers are failing, I am aging. I do not want to continue into the future as I see it. . . . And so, on the little surface of life, these deeper questions being so peremptory, there is nothing to advance by way of conversation. One's real state of mind is a source of shame. So one is necessarily silent about it, leaving nothing else for subject matter. Therefore, one listens, bullied by others' talk, that very talk an invasion. Yet one needs to have something said, something has to fly across a restaurant table, even if it's the interminable description of a conference one didn't attend and cares nothing about. Since one's field of interest is now very small. Oneself. In danger.

She goes on to say:

> The loss of language is so crucial, such a bereavement. Language does not really go away, it goes inward. Downward. Shriveling in the process, becoming repetitious, as when one facing great peril repeats the same protective formulas. Yet one mourns language, sociability, camaraderie, needing it now more than ever. And how necessary it becomes just as one observes its superficiality; the wavering of friends, the coldness of strangers, the essential uncaring of life itself, its monstrosity. And in the

face of this evil—not even to have words to protect one from the vacuum. To grow mute as well as hopeless.

The capacity to participate in life, interact with others, take pride in past accomplishments, and initiate or complete everyday tasks—the means by which one maintains a sense of worth, effectiveness, or value—seems forever lost in depression. The emotion of sadness can become so pervasive, so compelling, that it eclipses any consideration of past achievement or success. Like Percy Knauth, the depressed person may wrestle constantly with punitive thoughts and self-accusations. He or she may magnify minor failings or transgressions, experience excessive guilt, and feel that some terrible punishment is deserved. The person may even believe that he does not deserve to be helped:

> The power that overcame me did so with a peculiar thoroughness. It was unknowable and untouchable and it worked by robbing me of all self-esteem. Every horrible feeling that had ever been buried inside my psyche now surfaced and distilled into a self-image of pure loathing. I was worthless, and any momentary energies I would occasionally muster and that might have enabled me to seek help were twisted by this power into relentless thoughts of self-destruction.

The sense of worthlessness and guilt may reach delusional proportions. A person in a psychotic depression may be convinced that he is being persecuted and is to be held accountable for some imagined wrongdoing, or that a life-threatening disease is wracking his body when all the evidence is to the contrary. These delusional ideas are held with absolute and unshakable conviction—virtually all efforts to convince a person of their unreality are unsuccessful.

Some patients may experience what are called *nihilistic delusions*—they are convinced that the world is going to end by Armageddon or holocaust. These delusions reflect the patient's overwhelming sense of helplessness and hopelessness. Hallucinations, especially of voices, may also be present in such psychotic forms of depressions. They usually are related to the content of a particular delusion. For instance, if the delusion is of being persecuted, the voices are often berating, or derogatory and blaming or threatening. If the delusion is nihilistic, the voice or voices may threaten doom and destruction.

Clearly, a host of terrible symptoms can be manifested during a depressive episode, but most subside as the episode remits. However, the illness is not over when the symptoms clear. A person's confidence in himself, his relationships, and his future may be shaken seriously by the experience. His career or job advancement may have been jeopardized, and he may have resorted to alcohol or drugs to help numb the unbearable feelings. He may recover only to find that he is now dependent on these substances. In the worst of all possible scenarios, the person may not survive the depression. The appalling feelings of hopelessness and worthlessness can lead to suicide. He or she may become obsessed with finding a way out of the misery. Van Wyck Brooks, in his book also called *A Season in Hell,* describes it thus:

> I had always been possessed by this idea or that, usually the notion of the book I happened to be writing, which I pursued like a beagle with his nose to the ground; and I was possessed now with a fantasy of suicide that filled my mind as the full moon fills the sky. It was a fixed idea. I could not expel this fantasy that shimmered in my brain and I saw every knife as something with which to cut one's throat and every high building as something to jump from. A belt was a garotte for me, a rope existed to hang oneself with, the top of the door was merely a bracket for the rope, every rusty musket had its predestined use for me.

In his powerful book *Darkness Visible,* William Styron describes the depressed person's need to escape the torture that engulfs all life:

> What I had begun to discover is that, mysteriously and in ways that are totally remote from normal experience, the gray drizzle of horror induced by depression takes on the quality of physical pain. But it is not an immediately identifiable pain, like that of a broken limb. It may be more accurate to say that despair, owing to some evil trick played upon the sick brain by the inhabiting psyche, comes to resemble the diabolical discomfort of being imprisoned in a fiercely overheated room. And because no breeze stirs this cauldron, because there is no escape from this smothering confinement, it is entirely natural that the victim begins to think ceaselessly of oblivion.

Approximately 15 percent of untreated or inadequately treated patients with a mood disorder commit suicide. (Paradoxically, many complete the plans just as the depression is lifting and they become more energized and active.)

In the following passage from Patricia Bosworth's superb biography of the photographer Diane Arbus, Diane's mother, Gertrude Nemerov, recalls her own depression and the one that caused her daughter to end her life:

> All I know is that I had everything in life that a woman wants and I was miserable. I didn't know why. I simply could not communicate with my family. I felt my husband and my children didn't love me and I couldn't love them. I stopped functioning. I was like a zombie. My friend May Miller had to take me shopping and help me try on clothes. I wasn't able to take them off the hangers I felt so weak.
>
> That night I remember putting on my prettiest evening gown and we went up to the dining room. I forced myself to laugh and act as if I was having a mar-

velous time—inside I was absolutely choked. Panicked. *Because I could not define my depression. . . .*

I felt no better and remained depressed the entire summer and into the fall. Then slowly, very slowly, I came out of it. I don't quite know how. A year went by and I was all right again. I was exhausted. I felt as if I'd recovered from a hideous disease and had finally healed.

I tell you this because Diane, I think, was concerned for me; she observed me during those painful months. We never talked about what was troubling me, of course, but years later when she contracted hepatitis and had to go into the hospital, she fell into a ghastly, unending depression that went on for three years—until her death. Periodically she would call me on the phone in Florida and cry, "Mommy—Mommy—tell me the story of your depression and how you got over it." And although I had no real answer—no solution—I would repeat my story and it seemed to reassure her. That if I had gotten well, so could she.

WHAT DOES IT FEEL LIKE TO BE MANIC?

A person experiencing hypomania, or the first stage of a manic episode, feels imbued with energy, optimism, and self-confidence. Ideas and conversation flow easily and the mood is euphoric, expansive, and often infectious. One woman explained that she felt a "kinship with the effervescence of Dom Perignon." People who are hypomanic seem enthralled with themselves and the universe; they are captivated by their own sense of power and virtuosity. Many people describe feelings of being reborn— as if they are for the first time recognizing their true potential. As one individual put it:

I experienced a sudden feeling of creative release before my illness, was convinced that I was rapidly attaining the height of my intellectual powers, and that for the first time in my life, I would be able to function up to the level of my ability in this direction. . . . I also had a sense of discovery, creative excitement, and intense, at times mystical inspiration in intervals where there was relief from fear. . . . My capacities for aesthetic appreciation and heightened sensory receptiveness, for vivid grasp of the qualities of living, and for imaginative empathy were very keen at this time.

People in the manic state are caught up with the ideas that pour into their minds. Association after association occurs to them, and their speech can be full of jokes, plays on words, and amusing irrelevancies. The following poem, written in a few moments by a woman while in a hypomanic state, illustrates the punning and infectious humor:

God Is a Herbivore

Thyme passes, mixed with long grasses of herbs in the
    field.
Rosemary weeps into meadow sweeps
While curry is favored by the sun in its heaven.
The glinting scythe cuts the mustard twice
And the sage is ignored on its rock near the shore.
Hash is itself—high by being.
The law says shallots shall not—so they shan't.
    But . . .
The coriander meanders, the cumin seeds come
While a saffron canary eats juniper berry
Ignoring the open sesame seeds on the ground.

Sometimes a person in a manic state chooses words not because they are logical, but because they sound alike or rhyme. These kinds of associations are called clang associations. The eighteenth-century English poet Christopher Smart wrote his poem "Jubilate Agno" ("Rejoice in the Lamb") while manic and in an insane asylum. A section of it reads:

For the instruments are by their rhimes,
For the shawm rhimes are lawn fawn and the like.
For the shawm rhimes are moon boon and the like
For the harp rhimes are sing ring and the like
For the harp rhimes are ring string and the like.
For the cymbal rhimes are bell well and the like.
For the cymbal rhimes are toll soul and the like.

Speech during a manic episode is very striking. There is a push of words, they are spoken rapidly, and the voice is loud and intense. There is an insistent, nonstoppable quality to it— it brooks no interruption from others—and is called *pressure of speech.* During the more muted hypomanic state, the enthusiasm and intensity conveyed can be compelling and even engaging to others. But eventually the conversation comes undone. As the hypomanic state escalates closer to mania, the person's thoughts begin to race, and he leaps from topic to topic. One thought cannot be completed before another grabs his attention. The rules of logic that would normally govern a person's verbal production are unhinged in the manic state and there is a scattershot quality to the phrases. This *flight of ideas,* as it is called, is described by one patient thus:

> My trouble is that I've got too many thoughts. You might think about something, let's say that ashtray, and just think, oh! yes, that's for putting my cigarette in, but I would think of it and then I would think of a dozen different things connected with it at the same time.

Another patient explained it this way:

> My thoughts get all jumbled up. I start thinking or talking about something but I never get there. Instead I wander off in the wrong direction and get caught up with all sorts of different things that may be connected with the things I

want to say but in a way I can't explain. People listening to me get more lost than I do.

Speech is not the only thing that revs up in the manic state. There is a great increase in activity, an urge to get going. A person may pace up and down, move about constantly, or plan sudden, exotic trips. There is a decreased need for sleep, and the individual may go to bed for only short periods of time and awaken full of energy, or go for days with no rest at all. Ernest Hemingway once went through a 42-day period where he slept only two-and-a-half hours a night.

Appetite may be increased, and frequently the taste is for bizarre things, as this patient reveals:

> I have often in manic states eaten ordinary cabbage leaves or new brussels sprouts picked straight off the plants with such relish that they appeared to me the greatest delicacies—a kind of manna from Heaven. Even common grass tastes excellent, while real delicacies like strawberries or raspberries give ecstatic sensations appropriate to a veritable food for the gods.

Many patients speak of a heightening of all the senses, especially the way they perceive colors and light:

> The first thing I note is the peculiar appearances of the lights—the ordinary electric lights in the ward. They are not exactly brighter, but deeper, more intense, perhaps a trifle more ruddy than usual. Moreover, if I relax the focusing of my eyes, which I can do very much more easily than in normal circumstances, a bright star-like phenomenon emanates from the lights, ultimately forming a maze or iridescent patterns of all colours of the rainbow, which reminds me vaguely of the Aurora Borealis.
>
> Connected with these vivid impressions is a rather curious feeling behind the eyeballs, rather as though a vast electric motor were pulsing away there.

This patient also describes a sensation that often occurs early in a manic phase: a kind of oceanic feeling, a desire to merge or be at one with the universe:

> One night I woke up and started feeling good again. I felt I could do more with my time, that anything was possible. I felt alive and vital, full of energy. My senses seemed alive, colors were very bright, they hit me harder. Things appeared clear-cut, I noticed things I had never noticed before. There was a feeling of exhilaration, a sense of union with the whole world.
>
> Time slowed down, much more experience could be crowded into a brief time span. Sexually I felt awakened, competent, responsive. I seemed to notice symmetry and harmony, and I wanted to experience everything. I could concentrate on a speck of something and just stare at it. A whole new world opened up, and I felt more secure than ever before.

One patient noted that she loved "the sunrise, the sunsets, people, life"; another said he felt like hugging people he passed in the street. There is a compelling desire to be involved and interact with people and the environment. Often this mood prompts the person to call friends at all hours of the night and regale them with details of the new and exciting projects he is planning. The poet Robert Lowell wrote to the Nobel laureate T. S. Eliot after a manic episode:

> I want to apologize to you for plaguing you with so many telephone calls last November and December. When the "enthusiasm" is coming on me it is accompanied by a feverish reaching to my friends.

Accompanying this increased sociability is an increased sexual drive (hypersexuality). It is not uncommon for the person to "fall in love" and impetuously pursue a love affair or a string of affairs, possibly jeopardizing an established relationship or marriage.

During these periods of manic elation, people are suffused with a sense of specialness and purpose. They are so overly optimistic and their mission is so compelling that they lose the sense that their actions have consequences. For them, there is no day of reckoning. Buying sprees are a common feature of manic episodes, and it is not unusual for the person to go out and purchase outlandish things. One respected businessman left his office in Hong Kong one afternoon, went shopping, and wrote a purchase order for 400 rickshas. Months later they arrived at a New York port, and he couldn't fathom what had possessed him to buy them. A young woman from Chicago wrote to us that in one week she bought $27,000 worth of clothes and furs. After spending her money, she decided to organize things at work. "I ordered a $100,000 computer that we didn't need and couldn't afford," she revealed. "One day I decided our firm needed a little more space, so I decided to buy the Xerox building."

Unfortunately, the upbeat, indefatiguable quality of the mood cannot be maintained. Within minutes the euphoria can dissolve into irritability and anger. During such periods, a person might talk exuberantly and outline all his current plans and thoughts. The listener may be fixed in rapt attention, unprepared for the sudden shift of tone and intention. Abruptly, and without provocation, the mood may turn irritable or hostile. The patient can become belligerent and suspicious, and launch into an angry and effusive tirade.

These dramatic shifts of mood and behavior, termed *labile affect*, are characteristic of the manic state and often leave others perplexed and baffled. If the hostile outburst is directed toward the listener (as it usually is), he or she may experience this symptomatic behavior as a personal attack, become alienated, and withdraw.

A telling account of one man's switch from depression

into mania is presented in *Mood Disorders: Toward a New Psychobiology* by Drs. Peter Whybrow, Hagop Akiskal, and William McKinney. Here, a young man chronicles the characteristic lability of mood as well as the changes in perception and thinking that occur in these states:

It was in the spring that I first began to be plagued by sleeplessness for which I sought medical advice and was given at various times Elavil and Librium (I think). I was drinking, not heavily but steadily, both socially and in order to help the sleeping problem. It also served to break the boredom of my job. For the first time I felt it was becoming unmanageable. I disliked the sycophancy demanded of the workers—disliked is not strong enough here—I despised any expression of authority, whether it applied to me or not. I was becoming angry over little things, feeling I could run the place better, more efficiently, more humanely. Everything seemed static, futile, even though I was earning a reasonable wage and intended to leave for Europe within weeks.

Retrospectively I suspect I was a little depressed. I know I was anxious about not sleeping, as I kept telling people about it, wanting to acquaint them with my difficulties. Then during the week or two before departing for Europe, my mood lightened quite suddenly. Things seemed almost humorous at the office and my colleagues like so many robots. I believe I was increasingly anxious to get everything under way, growing tense waiting to be in Europe and relying on more than the prescribed dose of Elavil in order to gain some calm. One evening after having only two glasses of beer (I remember the amount precisely), I sat on the corner of a street downtown and found myself laughing and crying simultaneously. I was struck by the ludicrous nature of the simple actions performed by other people: looking both ways before crossing the road, for instance. People tended to ignore me, and this made the entire situation all the more comical. I began to feel a great sense of energy and a wish to move. I began to defy the traffic, running in and out (I had a sense of fear, but also power which seemed to allow me to take enormous risks). The whole street seemed brilliantly lit, as though from an arc lamp, and I felt wonderful and yelled epithets at the motorists, who stopped and screamed at me.

Also my increased strength was not imaginary. After I got back to my apartment, I smashed down the kitchen door, although it was locked and although I had the keys with me. I simply kept butting it with my shoulder until I tore it from its hinges. I didn't sleep much, if at all, that night, feeling a great pressure and a sense of elation. I decided to leave for Europe immediately rather than in a week's time as planned and indeed did so only two days later.

The laughing episode did not return, but I went to Europe with a good deal of energy and buoyancy. I was not there long (a week or two) when I became irascible and difficult to live with. (I had met a girl on the plane and we were touring together.) I felt that she didn't appreciate me, either for my sexual prowess or for my wit. Anyway, I felt I had an idea for a novel and it was imperative for me to return home to line up a publisher.

I think I remember these episodes in retrospect with more coherence than they had at the time. Some things are just lost. I remember being shocked later, for example, how much money I had spent, even though my stay in Europe had been but a few days. On my return I was trying to write, something I had always wanted to do.

The work I produced was appalling, however—fragmented, no discipline, sporadic, and uneven. I felt "other worldly" and under pressure, aware that something must give but convinced I was a genius. There were also short periods of calm, an overwhelming sense of euphoria that was rather nice really, almost mystical. But my emotions weren't all happy, they seemed to fluctuate tremendously: self pity, hatred (I was probably capable of doing physical injury), a diffuse and general love, abject helplessness, hopelessness, and guilt. These last three began to predominate, even though for a time it seemed that whenever I hit a record "low" some bright and incredible idea came to offer hope temporarily. But decline from each of these plateaus left me deeper in despair, with less capacity to halt the downward trend even temporarily. My inability to confront people reached a pitch. There was a sinking of all my faculties.

Most people who have the disorder experience the mood and behavioral changes we have been describing. Some, however, proceed so far as to become psychotic. Those who do may experience paranoia, hear voices, or (less often) see visions, as well as express bizarre or delusional thinking sometimes considered to belong to the realm of schizophrenia. (Indeed, even today, patients seen at this stage of mania are often misdiagnosed as schizophrenic. The difficult diagnostic distinction between these disorders is explored in the next chapter.)

Some manic patients suffer grandiose delusions: they may become convinced that some special force has empowered them to save the world from catastrophe, or that they have a special relationship to God or some national or international figure. Others exhibit more paranoid persecutory features and feel that they are being watched, controlled, or attacked. A man who loaded his family into a car and raced through several states to warn the Commissioners of Public Works that the Communists were poisoning the reservoirs was experiencing a delusion that was both paranoid and grandiose: America was being attacked; only he could save the country from disaster.

The PGA champion golfer Bert Yancey suffered a manic episode while traveling to Japan. His story, told retrospectively with a touch of humor, illustrates the grandiosity and paranoid patterns of thought. When the ordinary constraints of logic dissolve, songs, statues, and even the name of a popular musical group take on a multitude of personal meanings:

I had just left Hawaii on the way to Japan where I was to promote golf clubs and do seminars and make videos for instruction. Somewhere on my way to Japan, there was a six-hour time change. Something began to happen. I began to think that I was not only a professional golfer, but I was some sort of messiah that would rise out of the PGA of America and make the world safe for democracy. I would eliminate all Communism from the Oriental world. It was my job to do that.

I was lying on the bed in the Hilton Hotel when I got a sort of a feeling listening to the Armed Forces Radio station. The song "Take a Walk, Take a Walk" was playing and that was a direction to me alone to get up and move. It was time to make this facade real, to begin to convert these nations to democracy. And Arnold Palmer was going to pay my expenses!

I started to walk. It was 2:00 in the morning, and I went out across the street. I didn't know where I was going, but I was praying for direction. I walked up these steps toward a glass-enclosed Japanese shrine that was guarded by the statue of a samurai warrior, and I winked at him. I swear he winked back.

There was a surge of mania. I was reaching for the support of the Japanese and Oriental ancestry and everybody was behind me now. And I came down into the streets of Tokyo and I ran into the singing group the Temptations. Now, no self-respecting messiah could ignore the name of this group, so I approached them and said: "You're the devil and I'm here to take you on."

The Temptations were not in the mood to hear me say this or to talk about democracy in the streets of Tokyo, and when I assumed a pose from the martial arts, one of the singers who really knew Karate, dropped me with a chop.

In the lobby of the hotel, I pushed over a large Christmas tree and went up to my room and tried to jump out of a locked window.

Another hallmark of psychosis, auditory hallucinations, is not an uncommon experience in severe mania or in psychotic depressions. The voices are experienced as real, and often have extraordinary influence over the individual. They may be heard only occasionally or continuously during an episode. There may be one voice or even several that carry on a conversation. The manic person may simply overhear the voices, or the voices may make direct statements to him. For instance, they may inform him of some dire consequences of his behavior or thoughts, or command allegiance or some action. Often the directive will be in concert with a delusional idea, as in the case of the patient who believed that the Communists were poisoning the water supplies. In his case, the voices gave him his itinerary by telling him which Commissioners of which states to approach and convincing him of the need for his intervention.

In the majority of cases, the hallucinated voices in mania are disturbing, accusatory, or derogatory, although at times they may be pleasant or even humorous:

> At first I'd had to strain to hear or understand them. They were soft and working with some pretty tricky codes. Snap-crackle-pops, the sound of the wind with blinking lights and horns for punctuation. I broke the code and somehow was able to internalize it to the point where it was just like hearing words. In the beginning it seemed mostly nonsense, but as things went along they made more and more sense. Once you hear the voices you realize that they have always been there. It's just a matter of being turned to them.

> The voices weren't much fun in the beginning. Part of it was simply my being uncomfortable about hearing voices no matter what they had to say, but the early voices were mostly bearers of bad news. Besides they didn't seem to like me much and there was no way I could talk back to them. Those were very one-sided conversations.

But later the voices could be very pleasant. They'd often be the voice of someone I loved, and even if they weren't, I could talk too, asking questions about this or that and getting reasonable answers. There were very important messages that had to get through somehow. More orthodox channels like the phone and mail had broken down.

Every day, millions of people throughout the world experience these signs and symptoms of mania and depression. However sobering these numbers may be, there is still much cause for optimism. Today, a person no longer has to be overwhelmed by the symptoms and the social problems that arise from depression and manic-depression. Acute episodes can be attenuated and lithium or other mood-stabilizing and antidepressant drugs prevent or moderate the recurrence of the episodes. Psychotherapy can help a patient contend with the confusion and other terrible feelings the illness engenders.

Accurate diagnosis is the starting point for the treatment of all illness, and the 1980s saw the improvement of diagnostic systems for mood disorders that ensure more specific treatment selection and more focused research. It is to this that we turn next.

2

DIAGNOSING
THE DISORDERS

If a person has a persistent cough with an accompanying fever, he or she will very likely see a doctor. The physician listens to the lungs with a stethoscope and, if crackling sounds at the base of the chest are detected, orders a chest X-ray. Should a shadow appear on the film, the doctor can order a sputum culture and often establish the precise organism that is producing the pneumonia. Moreover, the culture determines which antibiotic is prescribed. Equipment, lab tests, X-rays, and tangible points of reference that can be seen and measured are the building blocks upon which a diagnosis is made in most areas of medicine.

This is generally not the case with psychiatric disorders. There are no lab tests that undeniably pinpoint a diagnosis, symptoms of many disorders overlap, and each person experiencing an illness expresses it through the unique filter of mind and personality. The patient's report of symptoms, observable behavior, the clinical course of the disorder, and family history are the main instruments the psychiatrist has. And they are more subjective than objective. Yet it is vital to the patient's well-being that the correct diagnosis be made, since the proper diagnosis guides the treatment, provides the patient and family members with an informed idea of outcome, and facilitates professional communication and research efforts.

HISTORICAL ATTEMPTS AT DIAGNOSIS

Although the written description of mood disorders dates back 40 centuries to Pharaonic Egypt, it is only very recently that we've had a reliable, structured diagnostic system.

The diagnosis of mental disorders has been a problem historically. Since there were no scientific treatments, and no understanding of the causes, the physicians who attempted to deal with them were up against a host of handicaps. With very little to go on, and few treatments in all of medicine, the same treatments were applied to the array of mental problems. Although attempts were made to classify the illnesses, the lack of effective treatments made diagnosis rather academic.

In the 1950s, however, the discovery of antimanic and antidepressant medications galvanized the psychiatric community. "The right medication for the right patient" became the admirable and exciting mission, but the lack of an objective system for describing and grouping these patients was all too apparent. Psychiatry looked to a medical model, and the paterfamilias of this view was a German physician who lived and wrote in the late nineteenth and early twentieth centuries, Emil Kraepelin.

Kraepelin spent countless hours with the mentally ill, carefully noting their symptoms and the course of their illnesses. He felt that proper classification, diagnosis, and prognosis were extremely important, and he began to focus his attention on two groups of patients. Those who had symptoms of euphoria and an excess of energy at times, followed by periods of depression and a lack of energy, and who tended to recover, he labeled as having manic-depressive insanity. Those who exhibited bizarre symptoms such as hallucinations and delusions and who tended to become ill earlier in life and follow a deteriorating course, he labeled as having *dementia praecox* (or precocious dementia, to separate it from senility). Later this illness concept was renamed schizophrenia and broadened by Eugen Bleuler.

Kraepelin organized his clinical data and psychiatric observation in his very successful textbook *Psychiatrie: Ein Lehrbuch für Studierende und Aertze*. He laid the foundations for modern psychiatry by meticulously describing the symptoms of mental illness, chronicling case histories, and emphasizing the *course of illness* as a major distinction between dementia praecox and manic-depressive illness.

In the 1950s and 1960s, amid the vast changes taking place in psychiatric thought and delivery of care, a group at Washington University in St. Louis picked up the Kraepelinian mantle and began again to focus on diagnosis, rigorous classification, and the biological underpinnings of mental disorders. Although Sigmund Freud himself had felt that psychiatry would become more biological in the future, his psychodynamic approach to the mind had been dominant in the United States since the 1930s. The St. Louis group—led by Eli Robins, Samuel Guze, and George Winokur—began to push for a diagnostic framework for psychiatry that was squarely within a medical model and that concentrated its efforts on a distinct classification system based on objective criteria. The more that psychiatric research could accomplish and the more data that could be generated thanks to new techniques in neuroscience, the more vital it became that a psychiatrist in California who cited a case of manic-depressive illness or schizophrenia be understood by a colleague in West Virginia or Germany.

But this was not the case. Two international studies whose results were made public during the 1970s—the International Pilot Study of Schizophrenia (the IPSS) and the US–UK Study—identified the lack of consensus about diagnosis within the profession. The IPSS was spearheaded by some British psychiatrists who wanted to study the symptoms of schizophrenia in different countries. They used standardized interviewing and evaluating methods and diagnosed patients in the United States, England, Taiwan, Colombia, the USSR, and other countries. Eventually it became clear that the physicians in the

Soviet Union and the United States diagnosed schizophrenia more often than those in any of the other countries.

The American psychiatric profession received an even sharper view of its diagnostic tendencies when Drs. Robert Kendell and John Cooper and several other British psychiatrists designed the US–UK Study to compare the diagnostic practices of American psychiatrists to those of the British. They videotaped diagnostic interviews with eight patients and then showed the tapes to psychiatrists throughout the British Isles and to psychiatrists from East Coast cities in the United States. There were glaring differences in the diagnostic practices of the two groups: again the American psychiatrists saw schizophrenia in the majority of the cases, whereas the British psychiatrists diagnosed personality or affective disorders.

This American tendency to be overgenerous with the schizophrenic label was a noticeable and knotty problem, and the "neoKraepelinians" of the St. Louis group decided to attack it head on. Under the direction of John Feighner, they developed a standardized set of definitions for 14 psychiatric illnesses and specified which symptoms and how many of them had to be present in order to make a particular diagnosis. These became known as the Feighner or "St. Louis" criteria, and as more research groups and clinicians began to see the logic of the idea and employ its methods, the American Psychiatric Association (APA) decided to overhaul its *Diagnostic and Statistical Manual* (one edition had been published in 1952 and a second in 1968). In June 1974, the APA appointed a task force under the leadership of Dr. Robert Spitzer of New York, and work began on what was to become known as the DSM-III.

The people involved had their work cut out for them. They set out to develop a classification system that would reflect the current state of knowledge about mental disorders, maximize its usefulness for both clinical practice and research studies, and ensure that the new nomenclature was as compatible as possible with the ICD-9—the ninth version of the *Inter-*

national Classification of Diseases, Injuries and Causes of Death developed by the World Health Organization.

There were meetings, hundreds of memos, telephone conversations, and more than 100 advisers; there were drafts and revisions of drafts. At a special convention, scores of experts from the biological, psychoanalytic, and behavioral schools of thought gave speeches and made their points about the definitions and diagnosis of mental disorders. Feelings ran hot and high as the arguments continued. But six years after the APA task force appointments, and after more than 800 clinical psychiatrists field tested the material in 212 psychiatric facilities with over 12 thousand patients, the APA published the DSM-III. So many copies were sold in the first year, 1980, that it was the best-selling nonfiction book after the Bible and the *Fannie Farmer Cookbook.* The demand caught the APA by surprise, but it powerfully emphasized the need for the DSM-III within the psychiatric community.

A BRIEF LOOK AT THE DSM-III

The DSM-III was not a catechism; it was a tentative working system of classification that was intended to undergo change and refinement as it kept pace with the new developments in psychiatry. Because the scientific underpinnings of psychiatric diagnosis are far from complete, DSM-III's contents were sometimes pushed by the winds of politics and personalities; still, its debut was groundbreaking and impressive. In its 494 pages it brought clarity and order to some 187 disorders, and it not only defined the disorders, but, taking its cue from the Feighner criteria, it also provided inclusion and exclusion criteria that enhanced diagnostic agreement among clinicians. (Because the DSM-I and II and the ICD-9 had not provided such precise guidelines, doctors were left to their own resources when it came to defining the content and boundaries of the diagnostic categories.) A revised edition of the DSM-III (dubbed the

DSM-IIIR) was published in 1987, and the DSM-IV, the latest revision, was published late in 1994.

In the DSM-IV, mood disorders are divided into depressive disorders and bipolar disorders. The criteria that must be met before the diagnosis of a major depressive episode can be made are as follows (our comments appear in italic):

Criteria for Major Depressive Episode

I. Five (or more) of the following symptoms have been present during the same 2-week period and represent a change from previous functioning; at least one of the symptoms is either (1) depressed mood or (2) loss of interest or pleasure.

NOTE: Do not include symptoms that are clearly due to a general medical condition, or mood-incongruent delusions or hallucinations.

A. depressed mood most of the day, nearly every day, as indicated by either subjective report (e.g., feels sad or empty) or observation made by others (e.g., appears tearful).

NOTE: In children and adolescents, can be irritable mood.

B. markedly diminished interest or pleasure in all, or almost all, activities most of the day, nearly every day (as indicated by either subjective account or observation made by others).

C. significant weight loss when not dieting or weight gain (e.g., a change of more than 5% of body weight in a month), or decrease or increase in appetite nearly every day.

NOTE: In children, consider failure to make expected weight gains.

D. insomnia or hypersomnia (*sleeping excessively*) nearly every day

E. psychomotor agitation or retardation nearly every day (observable by others, not merely subjective feelings of restlessness or being slowed down)

F. fatigue or loss of energy nearly every day

G. feelings of worthlessness or excessive or inappropriate guilt (which may be delusional) nearly every day (not merely self-reproach or guilt about being sick)

H. diminished ability to think or concentrate, or indecisiveness, nearly every day (either by subjective account or as observed by others)

I. recurrent thoughts of death (not just fear of dying), recurrent suicidal ideation without a specific plan, or a suicide attempt or a specific plan for committing suicide

II. The symptoms do not meet criteria for a Mixed State (*where a patient displays symptoms of mania and depression every day during at least a one-week period; see pages 47–49*).

III. The symptoms cause clinically significant distress or impairment in social, occupational, or other important areas of functioning.

IV. The symptoms are not due to the direct physiological effects of a substance (e.g., a drug of abuse, a medication) or a general medical condition (e.g., hypothyroidism).

V. The symptoms are not better accounted for by bereavement; i.e., after the loss of a loved one, the symptoms persist for longer than 2 months or are characterized by marked functional impairment, morbid preoccupation with worthlessness, suicidal ideation, psychotic symptoms, or psychomotor retardation.

The criteria that must be met before the diagnosis of a manic episode can be made are as follows:

Criteria for Manic Episode

I.   A distinct period of abnormally and persistently elevated, expansive, or irritable mood, lasting at least 1 week (or any duration if hospitalization is necessary).

II.   During the period of mood disturbance, three (or more) of the following symptoms have persisted (four if the mood is only irritable) and have been present to a significant degree:

A. inflated self-esteem or grandiosity

B. decreased need for sleep (e.g., feels rested after only 3 hours of sleep)

C. more talkative than usual or pressure to keep talking

D. flight of ideas or subjective experience that thoughts are racing

E. distractibility (i.e., attention too easily drawn to unimportant or irrelevant external stimuli)

F. increase in goal-directed activity (either socially, at work or school, or sexually) or psychomotor agitation

G. excessive involvement in pleasurable activities that have a high potential for painful consequences (e.g., engaging in unrestrained buying sprees, sexual indiscretions, or foolish business investments)

III.   The symptoms do not meet criteria for a Mixed State (*see pages 47–49*)

IV.   The mood disturbance is sufficiently severe to cause marked impairment in occupational functioning or in usual social activities or relationships with others, or to necessitate hospitalization to prevent harm to self or others, or there are psychotic features.

V.   The symptoms are not due to the direct physiological effects of a substance (e.g., a drug of abuse, a medication, or other treatment) or a general medical condition (e.g., hyperthyroidism).

NOTE: Manic-like episodes that are clearly caused by somatic antidepressant treatment (e.g., medication, electroconvulsive therapy, light therapy) should not count toward a diagnosis of Bipolar I Disorder.

As a number of the DSM-IV criteria caution, there are a variety of medical conditions that can mimic or masquerade as depression or mania. The following chart lists such conditions, which range from hormonal disorders and neurological syndromes to malignancies and diseases of the blood.

MEDICAL CONDITIONS THAT CAN MIMIC DEPRESSION OR MANIA

Hormonal and Metabolic Disorders

Hypothyroidism
Hyperthyroidism
Cushing's disease
Addison's disease
Wilson's disease
Diabetes
Hyperparathyroidism
Hypoglycemia

Infectious Diseases

Influenzas
Mononucleosis
Hepatitis
Viral pneumonias
AIDS
Syphilis

Cancers

Pancreatic
Central nervous system tumors

**MEDICAL CONDITIONS THAT CAN MIMIC
DEPRESSION OR MANIA** (cont.)

Autoimmune Disease

Systemic lupus erythematosus (and its treatment with steroids)

Neurological Disorders

Parkinson's disease
Alzheimer's disease or other dementia
Temporal lobe epilepsy
Multiple sclerosis
Huntington's chorea
Stroke

Blood Diseases

Iron deficiency anemia
Acute intermittent porphyria

Metal Intoxications

Thallium
Mercury
Manganese

Nutritional Disorders

Pellagra
Pernicious anemia

Other Diseases

Lyme disease
Chronic fatigue syndrome

Almost all of these medical conditions can be ruled in or out by physical examination coupled with appropriate clinical laboratory studies. Therefore, it is extremely important that the diagnosing physician take a personal patient and family medical history as well as request that the patient have a complete physical examination and selected blood tests, including thyroid function studies. Only then should a primary depressive or manic episode—one that is not secondary to or caused by a primary medical condition—be diagnosed.

BIPOLAR VS. UNIPOLAR DEPRESSION: MAKING THE CRITICAL DISTINCTION

All too often, bipolar disorders—particularly those that present with brief episodes of hypomania—are undetected during initial diagnostic evaluations. Since brief episodes of hypomania rarely prompt contact with a psychiatrist, whereas depressive episodes (which typically create greater impairment and pain) do, it is much more likely for the treating physician to diagnose and treat a major depression. Also, patients in the throes of a depression frequently do not remember any previous periods of elevated mood. And since they do not recall them, they are not forthcoming with a description of these high energy states, no matter what their duration. (The presence of atypical symptoms such as excessive sleeping, an increased craving for carbohydrates and sweets, along with a family history of bipolar disorder, should raise the suspicion that the patient may have a bipolar disorder.)

Overlooking the existence of high energy states (hypomania or mixed states) in the past can lead to an inappropriate treatment strategy: for instance, prescribing an antidepressant that may not only induce hypomania or mania, but also cause an acceleration of cycling (see pages 46–47).

Therefore, it behooves all treating physicians and patients

carefully to exclude the possibility of a bipolar diathesis (no matter how brief the high energy periods were) before instituting antidepressant treatment.

SCHIZOPHRENIA, MANIA, AND SCHIZOAFFECTIVE DISORDER: THE LACK OF CERTAINTY

DSM-III helped remove much confusion from the field of psychiatry, but it didn't clear up all diagnostic dilemmas. Even with the more rigorous criteria, there is still controversy about the diagnosis of patients who have psychotic symptoms. Are they schizophrenic, are they manic, do they have a severe depression with psychotic symptoms, or is their condition better described by the term *schizoaffective*—a hybrid category that overlaps the criteria for schizophrenia and major affective disorders?

As mentioned earlier, Kraepelin drew boundaries between manic-depressive psychosis and dementia praecox and emphasized the difference in the *course* of the illnesses as well as their form. In 1911, Eugen Bleuler, the Swiss physician, rechristened dementia praecox as schizophrenia and focused on its *symptoms.* He described a concept of schizophrenia with very elastic boundaries—so elastic, in fact, that they stretched to encompass a large portion of patients that Kraepelin would have called manic-depressive. Bleuler believed that schizophrenia was characterized by a disorder of the thought processes. Manic-depressive illness, on the other hand, was characterized by problems in mood.

In 1960 the German psychiatrist Kurt Schneider composed a list of symptoms that he felt strongly suggested a diagnosis of schizophrenia. He termed them "first-rank" symptoms, and they included auditory hallucinations, hallucinations of touch, the feeling that thoughts are being inserted into one's mind or that one's thoughts are being broadcast, and the feeling that all of one's actions are under the control of others. It became diagnostic tradition to assume that even short-lasting delusional, bizarre, and psychotic thinking established one firmly as a schizophrenic.

But is this so? Gabrielle Carlson and Frederick Goodwin of the National Institute of Mental Health reported in 1973 that there seemed to be three stages of mania. In the third, and most extreme, stage the patients experienced hallucinations, bizarre beliefs, and paranoia. Drs. Carlson and Goodwin felt that the patients would have been diagnosed as schizophrenic if they hadn't appeared clearly manic both earlier in the course and later as the episode was resolving.

Dr. Harrison Pope of Harvard Medical School's McLean Hospital in Belmont, Massachusetts, reviewed 20 studies that showed that the so-called schizophrenic symptoms (including visual and auditory hallucinations, thought broadcasting, and experience of influence) occur among 20 to 50 percent of patients with well-validated cases of manic-depressive illness. "The evidence," he writes, "suggests that the presence of cross-sectional 'schizophrenic' symptoms is of little differential diagnostic value. Such symptoms merely establish that the patient is psychotic, and are of little help in distinguishing whether the patient has manic-depressive illness or schizophrenia."

Dr. Pope and Dr. Joseph Lipinski teamed in 1977 to write what has become a seminal article in the psychiatric literature. Entitled "Diagnosis in Schizophrenia and Manic-Depressive Illness: A Reassessment of the Specificity of 'Schizophrenic' Symptoms in the Light of Current Research," it took rigorous issue with the traditional concept that psychosis and schizophrenia are synonymous. Whereas Bleuler stated that a diagnosis of manic-depressive illness should be made only by elimination of the diagnosis of schizophrenia (thus directing doctors to look for schizophrenic symptoms first), Pope and Lipinski and a growing number of other thoughtful clinical investigators who share their point of view make the argument that schizophrenia should be diagnosed only after exclusion of manic-depressive illness. Their tack is that the symptoms are not as important as the family history, the patient's functioning before the onset of illness, the course of the disorder, the response to treatment, and the eventual outcome. Since DSM-III "schizophrenics" rarely respond to lithium, and approximately 70 percent of manic-depressives do, a trial of lithium would be a valuable test.

The family history is an important clue, however. Genetic data suggest a low familial cross-over between affective disorders and schizophrenia: the illnesses tend to breed true. Thus, if the family history reveals manic-depression, depression, or alcoholism, it would appear highly unlikely that the patient is schizophrenic.

Schizophrenia is still overdiagnosed in young people. Historically the name dementia praecox—*early-occurring* dementia—emphasizes that schizophrenia affects people at a young age. This is true—three-quarters of all cases start in the 16 to 25 age group. Although affective disorders typically occur later in life, major affective illnesses are being recognized in young adults, adolescents, and even elementary school-aged children. Nevertheless, chances are that if a 15- to 19-year-old entering the hospital for the first time is manic and acutely psychotic, it is likely that he or she will be diagnosed schizophrenic.

Dr. Peter Joyce conducted a study at the Sunnyside Hospital in New Zealand and found that although the *mean* age of first hospitalization with an affective syndrome was 30.8 years, the most *common* age of onset was 15 to 19 years and that over 70 percent of these young people received an initial diagnosis of schizophrenia.

The problem is even more complicated. There are patients whose symptoms and poor response to lithium seem inconsistent with the diagnosis of bipolar illness. They seem to present a confusingly mixed group of symptoms that straddle the definitions of schizophrenia *and* mood disorders. For example, these patients' symptoms fulfill criteria for depression or mania but their hallucinations or delusions are not related to the disordered mood—they are "mood incongruent"—and thus are more characteristic of schizophrenia. Even after the resolution of the affective symptoms, these patients continue to have disturbances in thinking and perception.

The inadequate solution to this diagnostic problem was the creation of a controversial intermediate disease category called *schizoaffective disorder.* The DSM-IIIR admitted that its description of the disorder was not definitive but instructed psychiatrists to consider the category for "conditions that do not meet the criteria for either schizophrenia or a mood disorder, but that at one time have presented with both a schizophrenic and a mood disturbance, and, at another time, with psychotic symptoms but without mood symptoms."

DSM-IV returned schizoaffective disorder to the categories of schizophrenia and other psychotic disorders. The criteria were then further refined to include two subtypes—the bipolar type and the depressive type—and to require the existence of delusions or hallucinations for at least two weeks in the absence of prominent mood symptoms.

Some of the questions that fuel the controversy are: (1) Is schizoaffective disorder a variant of schizophrenia? (2) Is it a variant of affective disorders? (3) Is it a third independent psychosis, a transitional state between schizophrenia and affective psychosis? (4) Is it a combination (mixed form) of schizophrenia and affective psychosis? or (5) Is it a heterogeneous syndrome including different conditions?

Many psychiatrists would respond affirmatively to number (2)—schizoaffective disorder is a variant of affective disorders. In family studies of patients who meet criteria for schizoaffective bipolar type, there is a higher incidence of bipolar disorders, almost identical to that of the families of pure bipolar patients. Some treatment studies have indicated that clozapine in conjunction with mood stabilizing agents such as lithium, divalproex sodium, or carbamazepine are effective in the treatment of these conditions.

The truth is that at present no one really knows for sure. No doubt scientific developments in the years ahead will bring some clarity to many of these diagnostic dilemmas.

SUBTYPES OF AFFECTIVE DISORDERS

The chapter has for the most part focused on the rather classical manifestations of the affective disorders, but there are several subtypes of the illness that have been identified and that need to be discussed. The medications mentioned in this section are thoroughly described in Chapter 5.

Rapid Cycling

Patients who experience frequent continuous recurrences of depression and mania are said to have an uncommon type of bipolar illness called *rapid cycling*. Drs. Ronald Fieve and David Dunner coined the now widely accepted term "rapid cyclers" and defined the subtype for those who have four or more episodes of illness in a one-year period.

The phenomenon occurs in 10 to 20 percent of bipolar patients and is more common in women than men. Rapid cycling can arise at the onset of bipolar illness, but more typically occurs later in the course of the illness—often in middle age and, for women, at the time of menopause. In many cases, it is the use of antidepressant medications prescribed to treat the depressive phase of bipolar disorder that precipitates a hypomanic or manic episode. Often this is followed by an acceleration of cycle frequency. In such cases, the antidepressant should be withdrawn.

Patients who rapidly cycle are difficult to treat. They often respond poorly to lithium (lithium itself may cause an underactive thyroid, which can contribute to rapid cycling). Therefore, the anticonvulsant medications—carbamazepine (Tegretol) and divalproex sodium (Depakote)—are more effective in treating this form of bipolar disorder.

Although relatively uncommon, a form of autoimmune disease called Hashimoto's thyroiditis has been associated with rapid cycling. This is an illness in which an individual forms antibodies to his or her own thyroid gland. A blood test for the presence of these antibodies can rule out this immune disease as a contributor to rapid cycling.

There is a rare subtype of rapidly cycling patients who have an extremely accelerated rate of cycling with full bipolar episodes that occur within a one-week time frame, or even within a day. One woman reported experiencing brief 4- to 6-hour periods of mania or hypomania followed by severe depression within a 24-hour period. Such individuals often require combinations of mood stabilizers. Additionally, some case reports indicate that calcium channel blockers like nimodipine (Nimotop) and the atypical antipsychotic clozapine (Clozaril) may have a place in the treatment of this subgroup of patients.

Mixed States

Patients who simultaneously display significant symptoms of depression and mania are said to be in a *mixed state*. There are various theories as to the causes of the mixed state: one is that it is a transitional phase in which depression "switches" to mania and the patient becomes trapped in the switch state. This theory leaves much unexplained, but it is generally well accepted that patients who experience mixed states are more difficult to treat than those people who have manic episodes well separated from their depressive ones.

The following case history demonstrates a mixed state:

> F. L. was a 60-year-old woman who came to the hospital with all the signs and symptoms of a psychotic, agitated depression. This was her fourth episode during the last 21 years. For two of the episodes she had received

electroconvulsive therapy (ECT). For the third she had received an antidepressant medication and experienced improvement without remission. The remission finally occurred on its own a year later.

The present episode had begun with obsessive concerns about her invalid husband. She continually worried about mistakes she had made in her husband's diet and care and began to feel that death lurked everywhere. She became apprehensive, then agitated. She had trouble falling asleep and awoke early in the morning, her obsessive concerns whirling in her head. But throughout this typical melancholic picture ran another thread of delusional ideation. On occasion she would experience an upsurge of exhilaration and energy. She would begin to sing religious songs and, if others were around, preach to them vigorously and intrusively. She would then smile beatifically saying that she was suffused with the love of God because she and Jesus were saving the world. But through it all her facial expression looked depressed and she was always on the verge of tears. Family history showed paternal uncles who were gamblers and alcoholics; she had two sisters who had experienced typical agitated depressions.

Three weeks of treatment in the hospital with the antidepressant that had finally worked in the earlier episode ended her agitation and apprehension, but her religious talk and depressive mood continued. In the outpatient clinic it was decided that she was suffering the effects of a mixed manic-depressive state and she was started on lithium. After two weeks she was in remission and has remained symptom-free on maintenance lithium alone for three years.

Although the patient might have been thought to have a unipolar "agitated depression" with psychotic features, the presence of manic symptoms in the midst of severe depressive symptoms is a clue to recognizing the mixed state. F. L.'s grandiose, radiant, beatific religious delusions were out of tune with the patient's misery.

This case report is used to illustrate the appearance of a mixed bipolar state in a woman presenting with severe depression. She responded to treatment with lithium carbonate when other treatments failed.

However, recent controlled studies coordinated by the National Institute of Mental Health reported a poor response that patients with mixed manic episodes ordinarily have to imipramine or lithium, both in the initial phase of treatment and during maintenance treatment to prevent recurrence. That is, patients who were diagnosed with mixed manic-depressive states and were treated with lithium alone had a higher rate of recurrence than did the patients who had suffered "pure" manic episodes who were treated with the same drug regimens, and even higher rates of recurrence when imipramine was added.

These findings and others have brought into question the use of imipramine and other tricyclic antidepressants when treating patients with mixed bipolar states. Instead, some physicians recommend that such patients be treated primarily with lithium or with a mood-stabilizing anticonvulsant such as carbamazapine (Tegretol) or sodium valproate (Depakene, Depakote), in both the initial and long-term maintenance phases of treatment.

Cyclothymia

A milder manifestation of manic-depressive-like illness is *cyclothymia*. People who receive this diagnosis experience short and irregular cycles of depression and hypomania. The episodes are not of sufficient duration or severity to qualify as a major affective disorder as the cycles typically last for days, not weeks. The cycles often begin in the teens or early childhood, and the problem may appear to be a personality disorder or hyperactivity. The mood states can change so frequently that patients often remark that they awaken with a distinctly different mood than they had the day before.

Dr. Hagop Akiskal, the director of the International Mood Clinic at the University of California at San Diego, and his colleagues feel that cyclothymia has a two-phased course and that people with the disorder have certain identifiable problems in their behavior and relationships. These are summarized as follows:

Two-Phased Course

1. There is an increased need for sleep alternating with decreased need for sleep (although intermittent insomnia can also occur).
2. The self-esteem is shaky. It can alternate from a lack of self-confidence to a naive or grandiose overconfidence.
3. There are periods of mental confusion and apathy, alternating with periods of sharpened and creative thinking.
4. There is a marked unevenness in quantity and quality of productivity, often associated with unusual working hours.
5. There is uninhibited people-seeking (which may lead to excessive sexuality) alternating with introverted self-absorption.

Typical Behaviors

1. irritable, angry, and explosive outbursts that alienate others
2. episodic promiscuity; repeated failures of marriages or romances
3. frequent changes in careers, academic pursuits, and future plans
4. alcohol and drug abuse as a means of self-treatment or augmenting excitement
5. occasional financial extravagance

The family pedigree of people with cyclothymia is often "loaded" with all types of affective and "related" disorders, including depressive and manic-depressive illness, alcoholism, drug dependence, and suicide.

Approximately 60 percent of the patients diagnosed with cyclothymia respond to lithium. However, much remains to be explored about this bipolar subtype and its treatment.

Chronic Depression

Although a majority of patients have major depressive episodes that are separated by periods of normal functioning, 15 to 20 percent of patients do not recover fully from any given episode and have symptoms of depression that persist for at least two years. They are said to have *chronic depression.* The painful symptoms of the acute episode fade into an emotional aridity and these patients live without any positive feelings. Their mood is low, they lack energy, and their outlook on the future is generally bleak.

DSM-IV defines *dysthymia* as a depression in which a person is bothered most or all of the time during a two-year period by a depressive syndrome or symptoms of depression that are not of sufficient severity or duration to meet the criteria for a major depressive episode. The DSM-IV excludes from this category patients whose chronic depressive symptoms were preceded by a major depression. It is thought that a significant number of Americans suffer from dysthymia, which can begin early in life or have a late onset.

Unfortunately, not a lot is known about the classification and treatment of these milder disorders. This is perhaps because the people who suffer them don't end up in emergency rooms or hospitals and are thus rarely the subjects of research. Also, many psychiatrists have not commonly viewed these long-term depressive syndromes as mood disorders, but rather as personality disorders. Recently, investigators have begun to explore the use of antidepressants and different kinds of psychotherapies for these milder depressions. Early results from some of these studies indicate that drugs such as fluoxetine (Prozac) may be quite useful.

Patients with *double depression* are those who go a full two years in a low-grade state of depression—the dysthymia mentioned previously—but who then go on to have a major depressive episode. The period of time during which the major depressive episode is layered over the dysthymic symptoms is called double depression. Often the dysthymic symptoms continue even after the resolution of the major depressive episode, and there are high rates of relapse to recurrent major depressive episodes. In fact, the longer the patient remains chronically ill before recovering from the major depression, the greater the likelihood of relapse. For these reasons, patients with double depression should receive intensive treatment during and after recovery from the major depressive disorder.

There are severe deficiencies in our knowledge of how best to treat chronic depressions. More studies need to be conducted in order to assess the efficacy of antidepressants, lithium, electroconvulsive therapy, and psychotherapy. Such studies will surely lead to a better understanding of these disorders and further define their treatment.

SYNDROMES WITH FEATURES OF MOOD DISORDERS: ANOREXIA, BULIMIA, AND OBSESSIVE–COMPULSIVE DISORDER

Researchers, in investigating the symptoms, genetic patterns, neuroendocrine disturbances, and pharmacological responses of the eating disorders and obsessive–compulsive disorder, have found some similarities between them and the affective disorders. *Anorexia nervosa* is a disorder characterized by a disturbed body image, severe weight loss, and an intense fear of becoming obese that does not diminish as the weight loss progresses. *Bulimia* is a disorder characterized by binge eating, followed by attempts at purging the food consumed—either by vomiting or by laxative abuse. Both illnesses are classified as eating disorders by DSM-IV, but there are many unknowns surrounding the classification. For instance, some researchers consider bulimia to be a symptom of anorexia rather than a separate illness, as bulimic behavior has been noted in 16 to 47 percent of patients who have anorexia.

A significant percentage of patients with anorexia nervosa and bulimia also have symptoms of depression. They describe dysphoric moods, low self-esteem, hopelessness, suicidal thoughts and suffer from insomnia, weight loss, constipation, and reduced libido. Several studies found that 35 to 75 percent of bulimic individuals had a mood disorder during the acute stage of the illness, and follow-up studies examining patients 4 to 10 years after treatment found that approximately 44 percent were diagnosed as having a primary mood disorder. Data has also revealed that there is a higher rate of mood disorders in the first-degree relatives of patients with eating disorders than in those of normal controls.

Further evidence of the link between eating disorders and mood disorders is seen when certain laboratory tests—the dexamethasone suppression test (discussed on page 98) and the thyrotropin-releasing hormone test—are administered to anorectic and bulimic patients. These tests reveal a dysfunction in the neuroendocrine system in a significant number of patients with mood disorders and patients who have anorectic and bulimic features.

In the 1970s, investigators began to report some encouraging results when patients with anorexia and bulimia were treated with tricyclic antidepressants and MAO inhibitors, the medications used to treat depression. Today these drugs are known to be beneficial to some patients with anorexia, but even more so to patients with bulimia.

There is definitely evidence to suggest considerable overlap between the eating disorders and the affective disorders, but it is presently unclear whether eating disorders are a variant of mood disorders, or whether the symptoms of mood disturbance result from an eating disorder.

There may also be a relationship between mood disorders and *obsessive-compulsive disorder* (OCD). People suffering from this psychiatric illness have recurrent and intrusive thoughts that cause discomfort and anxiety and depression. The obsessive thoughts can be allayed only by some compulsive act. Anyone who locks up the house and goes back to make sure the stove is turned off so the house won't burn down has some idea what it's like to act compulsively on an obsessional thought. Most people can stop after the second check; the person with OCD, however, must repeat a compulsive action over and over, without knowing why and often with the understanding that it is senseless. Still, there is a sense of pressure and the anxiety is partially relieved by the action.

Many patients with OCD describe obsessions about dirt or contamination (of one's self or others), and it is not uncommon for their fear to have an element of disgust to it—often it is focused on urine, feces, or semen. A great many patients describe handwashing or showering rituals in which they wash their hands over 80 times a day or spend hours attempting to shower themselves clean.

There are several links between OCD and depression. Many of the symptoms, such as guilt, indecisiveness, low self-esteem, exhaustion, and sleep and hormonal disturbances, are common to both. Although OCD has traditionally been difficult to treat, the same class of drugs used to treat depression—the tricyclic antidepressants—has been found to reduce some of the obsessional symptoms. (A drug called clomipramine [Anafranil] has been found to be effective for this condition. In addition, a newer agent that enhances the serotonergic system—fluvoxamine [Luvox] has also been approved for the treatment of OCD.)

In the April 1986 issue of the *Journal of Clinical Psychiatry,* Drs. Steven Dilsaver and Kerrin White further confirmed the relationship between mood disorders and OCD when they reported on the family of a 17-year-old girl with a recurrent mood disorder. Not only did three generations of the family have major mood disorders, but the girl and her two brothers exhibited obsessive–compulsive behavior during episodes. Interestingly, the 17-year-old and three of her cousins suffered from bulimia also, and she and quite a few of her relatives suffered from panic attacks. This pedigree implicates associations between bipolar disorder, bulimia, panic attacks, and obsessive-compulsive disorder. The authors of the article suggest that such a pedigree study offers a potentially powerful method for determining whether there is an association between these various types of disorders.

3

THE SEARCH FOR
GENETIC MARKERS

As we mentioned at the opening of this book, rarely does a person speak of only one family member with depression or manic-depression. More often there are two or more relatives affected, as these illnesses tend to concentrate in families. Familial tendencies suggest a genetic transmission, but since genetic theories don't survive on hints and suggestions, intense scientific inquiry has lately been focused in this direction. The next few years should yield some heady information about the genetics of mood disorders, but right now researchers are looking for a gene and its location and a possible mode of transmission. They are searching hard for a genetic marker that would identify those who are at risk.

Current research indicates only that the vulnerability to these disorders is "passed down" (inherited) in families—the way a physical illness such as diabetes shows up in a family pedigree. Family studies continue to show that the relatives of people who have manic-depression or depression have a significantly higher rate of these disorders—perhaps two to three times higher—than occurs in the general population. But how does a scientist disentangle the subtle strands of heredity from those of environmental influences? Is the problem one of nature or of nurture? To solve this puzzle the researchers turned to two classic investigative techniques in genetic research: twin studies and adoption studies.

Twins are particularly rich territory for the geneticist. Identical twins develop from a single fertilized egg and thus are genetic carbon copies of each other; fraternal twins develop in the womb together, but from two separate fertilized eggs (like any sibling pair, they share only 50 percent of their genes). If a trait is 100 percent genetically determined and one partner of an identical pair develops a disorder, then the other twin will develop it also. Their "concordance rate" or rate of similarity would be 100 percent. If, then, the concordance rate of identical twins is higher than the concordance rate of fraternal twins for the same disorder, researchers begin to assume that there is an underlying genetic component.

The results of seven twin studies conducted in the United States, England, Germany, Norway, and Denmark pegged the combined concordance rates for identical twins with affective disorders at 76 percent and found that 19 percent of the fraternal twins were concordant for affective disorders. These results support the general case for a genetic factor in affective disorders, but they still fail to tease apart the skeins of heredity and environment. This is because nearly all of the twin pairs were raised together in the same homes and it is known that a twin's behavior has a major influence on his or her partner.

Adoption studies attempt to separate more precisely the influences of heredity and environment. A summary of all the reports in the psychiatric literature of identical twins raised apart from their partners revealed that 8 of 12 pairs, or 67 percent, were concordant for unipolar and bipolar illness. This established that the intrapair concordance rate for twins raised apart was approximately the same as for twins reared together. Again the data attested to a genetic component. On the other hand, it also suggested that the disorder is not wholly genetic (approximately 33 percent of the identical twins were *not* concordant for the illness). Some environmental or social factors must interact in some way with the genetic trait.

A report published in 1977 by Drs. Julien Mendlewicz and

John Rainer described a study they had conducted in Belgium. They looked at the biological and adopting parents of adopted adults who had been diagnosed as manic-depressive. They also examined three comparison groups: the parents of nonadopted adult manic-depressives, the biological and adoptive parents of normal adults, and the biological parents of adults with polio. The parents of the patients with polio were included in order to determine whether or not a chronic disabling disorder in a child may induce depression in his parents.

Rainer and Mendlewicz found that there was a greater degree of affective illness in parents biologically related to the manic-depressive adoptees than in parents who adopted and raised these same individuals. Nature was indeed having its say over nurture, at least to a certain degree. This study bolstered previous research implicating genetic factors in bipolar illness, but that's about all that can be concluded from the "observed-from-the-outside" type of data that adoption and twin studies offer. More specific information will have to be coaxed from the genes themselves.

THE AMISH: A NATURAL LABORATORY
FOR THE STUDY OF AFFECTIVE DISORDERS

Another approach used to mine information about affective disorders is to examine multigenerational pedigrees of very large affected families. Dr. Janice Egeland of the University of Miami School of Medicine has been conducting an important and imaginative study, here in this country, with the Old Order Amish of Lancaster County, Pennsylvania, a group of people who dress in plain clothes and live much as they did when they came to America in the eighteenth century. The Old Order Amish are an ultra-conservative religious sect with many settlements throughout the United States. This project, now in its eighteenth year, continues to reveal some intriguing things about affective disorders—both genetically and epidemiologically.

In many ways the Amish community provides a natural laboratory for all genetic research. They are a well-defined, closed population numbering some 12 thousand people, with little migration into or out of the community. They can trace their ancestry back to 30 progenitors, and they maintain extensive genealogic records. The community encourages a high birth rate, so a researcher can study large families. It is also important that this community prohibits the use of alcohol and drugs, substances known to complicate diagnostic assessment. Finally, the Amish were extremely cooperative with Dr. Egeland because of a long-standing, trusting relationship. Without a doubt, this is an outstanding milieu in which to conduct an affective disorders study. (It should be noted that the Amish have no more mental illness than the rest of the population, but the social values mentioned above do make illnesses easier to diagnose.)

Dr. Egeland and her research staff began to look closely at several large, multigenerational families with a significant number of members who suffered from bipolar disorder. Originally they were researching the question of whether mood disorders tend to occur with other known genetic markers such as color blindness or certain blood types.

It is estimated that there are over 100,000 genes, and the locations of about 6,000 are currently known. Researchers did know, however, where the genes for color blindness and certain blood types resided, and they assumed that if the gene for an affective disorder was near one of the known genetic markers, the two traits would be inherited together. Studies of this kind are called linkage studies.

No linkage could be established in the preliminary Amish studies. The case could not be made that the gene for bipolar disorder traveled in the company of those known genetic markers. It was fortunate, therefore, that at that point molecular biologists developed a remarkable technique of gene probing using recombinant DNA that allowed investigators to continue the linkage studies.

This new method of getting genetic markers came about when scientists discovered that they could produce DNA in the laboratory. (DNA is the stuff chromosomes are made of.) Each chromosome has a unique sequence of "rungs," known as bases, and a gene is a short segment of the ladder-like DNA. These researchers found that if they came up with a piece of manufactured DNA that happened to match a segment of the natural DNA, the two pieces would stick together. Probing with the synthetic DNA, they discovered that chromosomes are studded with interesting variations. Each variation is unique to a particular point on a specific chromosome in an individual's cells. These variations have been named restriction-fragment-length polymorphisms (RFLPs); geneticists refer to them affectionately as "riflips."

By using the RFLP probes, geneticists are mapping the human genetic structure. They are searching the blood cells of families who have certain inherited diseases. If a specific variation is present primarily in people who have bipolar disorder, it may be assumed that the RFLP is close to a gene that may play a part in the illness's manifesting itself. In other words, if a marker—an RFLP—can be found that shows that it segregates with the disorder, that would mean that the gene for that disorder is located in the DNA close to that particular marker.

In order to conduct these genetic linkage studies, large families are needed. The search was on again since Dr. Egeland and her colleagues realized that they could apply the new molecular genetic techniques by establishing cell lines for Amish families. The large families and stable population of the Amish have made it possible for them to find enough ill and well family members to begin tracking the fate of the RFLP landmarks through three generations. In 1983, Dr. Egeland collected blood samples from 51 subjects and established permanent cell lines for one large pedigree—Pedigree #110—at the Coriell Institute for Medical Research in Camden, New Jersey. The DNA from those cells is then available for repeated genetic probing. The goal is to link the gene that carries the code for the illness to a trackable landmark from which it rarely gets separated.

The laboratories of Drs. David Housman and Daniela Gerhard at the Massachusetts Institute of Technology and Kenneth Kidd and David Pauls at Yale University have been typing individuals in Pedigree #110 for RFLPs over the past several years and performing genetic linkage analyses on a number of markers.

It is hoped that we're not far away from a breakthrough in the area of mood disorders. In 1979, when the first blood samples were drawn, only one RFLP was known to exist in humans. By 1983 over 400 RFLPs had been described. The discovery of new probes mapped to specific chromosomes has continued at an unprecedented rate. At present over 5,000 RFLPs have been reported, and new ones are pinpointed every week.

These rapid and continuous advances provide a very strong impetus toward the identification by genetic linkage of the site of a major genetic locus for bipolar disorder. Dr. Egeland and her coworker Dr. David Pauls of Yale University have been working to address the question of the mode of inheritance in families of patients with bipolar disorder. From an analysis of 32 such Amish families, they have developed strong evidence of a single, dominant gene for predisposition to the illness. The evidence that a dominant gene contributes to expression of the illness further inspired the search for a linked marker.

Drs. Gerhard and Housman began to focus their attention on the short arm of chromosome 11, and preliminary evidence strongly supported the possibility of a genetic marker for that region. In fact, the more they analyzed the blood samples, the stronger the case became that there was linkage to the marker on this chromosome. In 1987, the Egeland team announced in the British scientific journal *Nature* the provocative evidence that a "susceptibility" gene for bipolar affective disorder was

Pedigree #110

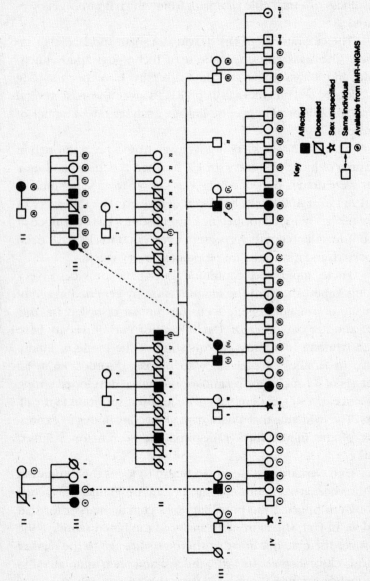

Key
- Affected
- Deceased
- Sex unspecified
- Same individual
- Available from IMR-NIGMS

Reprinted with permission from the Coriell Institute for Medical Research.

located on the short arm of chromosome 11 in a large family of Old Order Amish. Because of the profound implications of this finding, the international news media gave it very broad coverage: camera units were dispatched to the Pennsylvania countryside and hundreds of articles appeared in newspapers and magazines around the world.

With every interview, Dr. Egeland presented a tempered view. She explained that, although the findings and the statistical analysis were convincing, replications would have to be done to confirm the study and extend it to other populations, and that only time would tell the whole story.

Dr. Egeland continued on with her work, adding 40 new subjects to the original 81. But while the new subjects definitely seemed to have an inherited form of manic-depressive illness, the case could not be made for a gene on chromosome 11. More disappointment hovered over this vast project as two members of the original pedigree became mentally ill and one of these was found not to carry the marker on chromosome 11. The once-tight linkage began to unravel; the ratio of the odds for linkage (the LOD score) plummeted.

Janice Egeland said that watching the data weaken was a little like the experience of manic-depression itself. When speaking at the 1990 Albert Einstein Conference on the Genetics of Affective Disorders in New York she said: "There was the euphoria and the ecstasy when we thought we had made a significant step in trying to track down a gene for this common and terrible illness, and then, wham . . . LOD scores drop when you don't expect them to drop and you're down in depression. It's a real rollercoaster ride."

How is the scientific community as well as the public to understand these results? It could be that there are at least two genes in the Amish population and that the marital link on the lateral extension studied later introduced a new, not yet accounted for, gene. Also, the patient who suffered a serious depression but did not have the expected marker developed the symptoms quite late in life and in the context of a stressful life event. It's possible that the depressive syndrome in this individual was brought about by predominantly psychological stressors; it was a "situational" depression, not a genetic one. This observation raises an enigmatic question: does one need to have a specific genetic abnormality to develop a depressive syndrome? In this instance and at this juncture in history, while there appears to be a significant genetic component to the risk for depression, it is by no means certain that a gene or genes are necessary or sufficient to produce unipolar or bipolar depression in all circumstances. The difficulties with linkage studies in behavioral disorders—even with the advent of the powerful tools of molecular biology—are becoming apparent.

Dr. Egeland's 18-year gathering of information remains solid, however, and the "immortalized" cell lines are still in storage. Recently, Dr. Edward Ginns of the NIMH and his colleagues collaborated with the Egeland team and looked at the DNA of these cells and those of a further extension of the Amish families. They established positive LOD scores on chromosomes 6, 13, and 15, and reported these findings in the April 1996 issue of *Nature Genetics.*

Two other studies appeared in this issue reporting linkage to other chromosomes in families of different ethnic backgrounds. Dr. Nelson Freimer and his research group screened the members of two large Costa Rican families vulnerable to manic-depression and found linkage to chromosome 18.* Dr. Douglas Blackburn of Edinburgh University linked manic-depressive illness with genes on the short arm of chromosome 4.

Years ago, two independent association studies by Dr. Julien Mendlewicz of the Free University in Brussels and Dr.

---

*This is the third group to find linkage to chromosome 18. In 1984, Dr. Wade Berrettini of Thomas Jefferson University in Philadelphia and his colleagues at the NIMH linked the disorder to 18, as did Johns Hopkins researchers led by Dr. Colin Stine in 1995. However, these three linkage reports on chromosome 18 encompass nearly the entire chromosome.

Miron Baron at the New York State Psychiatric Institute in New York City linked the illness to the X chromosome.

So does this mean that there are many different genes contributing to manic-depression? There is no definitive answer at this time, but researchers harbor different opinions. Some believe that manic-depression results from a combination of many different genes, each with some small effect. Others believe that manic-depressive illness arises from only a few genes, and that the large number of positive linkages reported represent false positive results that could be attributed to study populations simply too small for accurate statistical analysis. In any case, replication of any of these linkage findings will require large numbers of affected families—perhaps ten times as many as have already been studied. This is a daunting task.

A different approach being employed by a team at the Albert Einstein College of Medicine involves a unique population of children and young adults who have been diagnosed with a disorder known as Velo-cardio-facial syndrome (VCFS). This syndrome was characterized by Dr. Robert Shprintzen in 1978 and these patients suffer a variety of anomalies: nasal speech (usually with cleft palate), cardiac problems, learning disabilities, and a characteristic facial appearance that includes a vertically long face, large nose, small ears with overfolded helices, narrow "squinting" eyes, and flat facial expression.

Unexpectedly, a very high percentage of the 26 patients in the initial study led by Dr. Demitri Papolos were diagnosed with bipolar spectrum disorder. And there appeared to be a relationship between age and syndrome. In childhood, the patients frequently suffered marked separation anxiety, were easily startled by loud noises, and were commonly diagnosed with attention deficit disorder with hyperactivity; during latency and early adolescence, bipolar II disorder was often diagnosed. Older patients, in late adolescence, were diagnosed with bipolar I disorder, and finally, patients interviewed as adults met criteria for schizoaffective disorder, manic subtype.

What has excited the researchers involved in this study is that they know which specific region of a well-mapped chromosome is deleted in individuals born with this syndrome—the eleventh quadrant of chromosome 22 (identified among geneticists as 22q11). For the first time, bipolar syndrome disorders have been linked to a molecular target. Could one or more of the genes that keep mood relatively stable be missing from this quadrant of the chromosome?

But this study had revealed another intriguing finding. Each human being has 22 pairs of chromosomes, as well as the two sex chromosomes—either two Xs or an X and a Y. While studying possible candidate genes in the most commonly deleted area of chromosome 22q11 in the DNA of VCFS patients, the Albert Einstein researcher Dr. Herbert Lachman analyzed a common variation of the catecholmethyltranseferase (COMT) gene, which produces an enzyme that breaks down two neurotransmitters, dopamine and norepinephrine. This common variation of the COMT gene was found to produce a form of the enzyme with a level of activity reduced four-fold from that of the most common form of the gene. The investigators then decided to look on the undeleted chromosome 22. They found that 100 percent of the VCFS patients who had this variation were diagnosed with the rapid-cycling form of bipolar disorder.

What could this mean? If the COMT gene is deleted in the eleventh quadrant on the first chromosome 22 and is present in a slightly altered variation of the gene that produces significantly less COMT, then perhaps the low level in these individuals causes a greater vulnerability to switch rapidly from one mood state to another. Could the level of the COMT enzyme be a factor involved in the evolution of a rapid-cycling disorder? Could an alteration in the most common form of the gene be a factor in the development of bipolar disorder?

The researchers at Einstein are attempting to answer these questions. Replication studies in the VCFS population will be necessary to confirm these findings, and if confirmation is obtained, an analysis of the COMT gene in rapid-cycling individuals within the general population will be an important next step.

Even if a major gene locus is found, environmental and other genetic influences do modify the expression of the illness. There is significant clinical variation in the illness and there may be more than one major gene locus found among patients with other varying forms of the disorder.

A number of extremely promising potentials can be expected if this gene or genes are found. Diagnosis would become more accurate, and the face of genetic counseling would be changed. We would gain information on how the gene and the environment interact. We would also have a better idea which nongenetic factors are related to the onset and course of the disorder. Finally, the information should help to determine the specific biochemical defect and origin of the disorder. Since genes control and regulate the production of enzymes and biologically important proteins, a problem at the level at which genetic information is translated could alter the structure and function of a protein, an enzyme, a neurotransmitter, or a receptor site (see the next chapter). This vulnerability within the central nervous system may underlie the sequence of events that results in manic or depressive symptoms. Identifying the gene and what it codes for would be a revolutionary breakthrough in understanding the functional changes that accompany manic-depressive illness. From there, the future might bring better drugs and medical treatments. Reaching these potentials is predicated on first locating a genetic marker.

THE EPIDEMIOLOGY OF MOOD DISORDERS

The Amish studies will undoubtedly tell us much about genetics, but they have already yielded some surprising data in the field of epidemiology (the branch of medical science that studies the incidence and distribution of disease in communities and whole countries). Previous epidemiological studies on the general population reported anywhere from a 10:1 to a 3:1 ratio of unipolar depression to bipolar depression. But Dr. Egeland found an equal 1:1 ratio in the families she studied. In her opinion, past studies based on hospital records tended to miss the hypomanic and even manic features that preceded or followed a serious depressive episode. Therefore, many people who were diagnosed during a depressive episode and recorded in studies as unipolar might actually have had bipolar illness. Of course, new studies in the general population will have to be conducted to confirm or refute a higher frequency of bipolar illness.

Dr. Egeland discovered another nonconforming ratio, this one involving the comparison of men to women with the disorder. The universal sex ratio for bipolar and unipolar disorders combined shows a preponderance of women—usually 2:1. This ratio reflects the reported 3:1 female to male ratio for major depression and the approximately equal—1:1—rate for bipolar disorder. The Amish study varies from the traditional statistic because it came away with a much closer female to male ratio of 1:1 for major affective disorders. Dr. Egeland notes the importance of several factors for this finding, explaining that the Amish culture prohibits the use of alcohol and drugs—substances that might mask the expression of affective disorders. It is suspected that many men self-treat the symptoms of an affective disorder with alcohol or drugs and thus find themselves added to the epidemiological roll calls of alcoholics or drug abusers. Since alcohol and drugs are culturally prohibited to the Amish, the unmasked symptoms of a primary affective disorder will manifest themselves—they will not be obscured—and a proper diagnosis can be made. Also, since crime and sociopathy are practically unknown among the Amish, none of the men are lost to the epidemiological study due to imprisonment. Everyone in the community is accounted for, and any manifestation of mental illness is usually observed and attended.

Future reports from southeastern Pennsylvania will no doubt do much to expand our knowledge of the causes and course of mood disorders.

GENETIC COUNSELING

So, in the meantime, what would help identify those at risk for the disorder as well as calm many fears about it? The answer is, genetic counseling. In various areas of the country there are doctors in the field of genetic research who can examine a family's history, explain the risk estimates and alleviate the anxieties a family lives with.

Actually, more and more people in this country are availing themselves of the services and science of genetic counselors: pregnant women who have amniocentesis routinely have a genetic counseling session, and people with diabetes and their families often talk with counselors. In the affective disorders field, even while we wait for further clarification of the nature of inheritance or possible genetic markers, the counselor can still explain the empirical risk estimates. These are percentages culled from the pooled results of large family studies that show the rate at which any given mental disorder occurs in each of the different classes of relatives of an affected patient. While these estimates are not totally accurate, they are at least informative. Until further progress is made on the molecular biology or psychosocial fronts, they're the best figures available.

We asked Dr. Miron Baron how families react to the knowledge that an affective disorder seems to have a genetic basis, and how they react specifically to genetic counseling. "Most people are relieved," he answered. "The information puts an end to self-blame and guilt. Often, in the fearful playground of the mind, people tend to exaggerate the risk factors, and counseling helps inject reality into the situation and puts things in perspective. As a matter of fact, sessions like this allow the families to vent a lot of concern and confront some of their anxieties. Genetic counseling shows a family how to retain a quiet attentiveness but go on with the business of living."

Most counseling is done in one to two sessions, and it is important that all family members come. In this way all can contribute personal recollections about relatives and themselves, and the counselor can be sure everyone understands the disorder and the statistical and medical information.

The counselor questions the family as to the number and order of relatives, parental age, ethnic background, possible occurrence of stillbirths or deaths, and lists the ages, sex, and health of living brothers, sisters, and children. Grandparents, aunts, uncles, and cousins are noted also. Then the counselor draws up a pedigree and gets an idea of the patterns of recurrence. One factor that must be considered in the determination of risk is that the *spouses* of people who have an affective disorder also have a relatively high rate of affective illness (approximately 20 to 30 percent). This may be because of the phenomenon of *assortative mating*—the tendency of people to choose marriage partners who are temperamentally similar to themselves. There is no real explanation for this at present, although some researchers hypothesize that people with the same disorder may have personality traits or similar life histories that may attract them to each other. If both parents are indeed ill, however, the risk to the children increases significantly.

A client has the right to expect that a genetic counselor will be emotionally supportive, sensitive and tactful, noncoercive, and competent. The counselor should speak in terms a layperson can understand and yet offer up-to-date information about genetic, biological, and epidemiological research in the field of affective disorders.

Psychiatrists who specialize in genetic counseling are not

common across the country. For the most part they are found at large medical or research centers and at university teaching hospitals. A psychiatrist may be able to recommend a counselor, or you can call the department of psychiatry at one of the centers just mentioned and ask for a recommendation.

Before we close this chapter, we'd like to point out one more time that while manic-depression and depression are familial disorders and seem to have an underlying genetic component, other factors that have yet to be identified modify or possibly mask their occurrence. No one is doomed by a visit to a genetic counselor—a session usually does more to alleviate than agitate. It can also stave off a great deal of future suffering. For example, if people know that they have a genetic background and perhaps a predisposition to develop an affective disorder, they may take better care of themselves and seek help earlier. This limits the damage an episode can cause and helps prevent a chronic course from developing.

The search for a genetic marker for bipolar disorder is a collaborative effort that involves clinicians in the field, molecular geneticists and, most important, families. The cooperation of concerned families is helping science to get to the bottom of so many of the disorders that affect humankind. Never forget that you are indeed a part of the whole, a valued and vital part of the ongoing search for the causes of the affective disorders.

4

WHAT CAUSES
THESE DISORDERS?

We want to warn you at the outset that this chapter will require concentration as it contains some of the most recent scientific information about mood disorders. Our object, however, is not to strain eyes or tax minds, but to outline how much new knowledge is accumulating from research efforts, and how many new research and therapeutic efforts are being prompted by this new knowledge.

The progress made in the study of the mood disorders during the past decade is unmatched by that in any other area of psychiatric research. These advances have been especially visible in the areas of clinical diagnosis, epidemiology, sociology, and psychology of depression and mania, as well as in the areas of genetics and molecular biology.

Equally impressive advances have been made in the neurosciences. Researchers can measure the brain's electrical impulses and determine some of its chemical components and interactions. Modern technology now allows us to peer beneath the bony vault of the skull and visualize the brain with diagnostic tools such as positron emission tomography (PET) and nuclear magnetic resonance imaging (MRI).

Our knowledge about these disorders has expanded exponentially, and our understanding should continue to grow. Yet, with all these recent advances, there is still no answer to the question: what causes these disorders?

Genetic, biological, and psychological studies provide clues, but clues only. There is a plethora of findings and a number of theories that are guiding the research efforts, but few of the findings have achieved the status of fact and none of the theories provides a broad enough framework to encompass the findings. However, there is good reason to believe that genetic, psychological, and other environmental forces operate in varying degrees to influence the development and course of affective disorders.

In this chapter, we explore this research and outline a few of the hypotheses constructed around the clues. The starting point for this discussion is the nerve cell and its means of sending messages via neurotransmitters. We will trace the neurotransmitter signal from the cell membrane and beyond to second messenger pathways that reach within the cell nucleus to the DNA archive, and explore some of the current ideas about lithium's effect on gene expression. We'll examine an interesting animal model of depression, learned helplessness, which provides the opportunity to examine the interplay between environmental stressors and the genetic susceptibility that produces depression. Then we'll look at the endocrine system and the hormone cortisol, which plays a critical role in the individual's response to stress and which has been found to be abnormally elevated in many patients suffering with depression. Next, we'll explore studies that reveal a relationship between stressful events, such as separation and loss, and the biological changes that accompany those events. Circadian rhythms, the 24-hour schedules of bodily activity that seem to be disregulated in depression and mania, will be discussed. And finally, we'll describe the kindling-sensitization hypothesis, a model that attempts to account for many of the features of affective illness, including the possible predisposition provided by early stressful experiences, as well as the pattern of cyclicity typical of these disorders. We begin with the brain's architecture and the mechanisms by which the brain communicates with itself, the body, and the world around it.

INSIDE THE BRAIN:
THE LIMBIC-DIENCEPHALIC COMPLEX

The human brain is the most complex structure on earth. Its three-and-a-half pounds of gray and white matter, compressed into a structure no larger than a grapefruit, sits above our bony spines. Packed into this space are perhaps 100 billion brain cells. It is said that the number of possible interconnections between the cells is greater than the number of atoms in the universe.

Near the center of the brain is the area on which most affective disorder researchers focus—the *limbic-diencephalic system*. This is composed of the limbic system, the hypothalamus, and the brainstem (including the reticular activating system, the locus coeruleus and raphe nuclei). The limbic system, as the mediator of human feelings, receives and regulates information of an emotional nature, and governs sexual desire, other appetitive and consummatory behaviors, and the self-protective mechanism of fight or flight.

By far the most important structure of the limbic system is the four-gram, walnut-sized hypothalamus. This "brain" within the brain regulates a host of human processes, including appetite, thirst, sleep, sexual desire, and body temperature, and it activates the reaction of the organism to stress, as well as the *timing* of many other basic functions on an hour-by-hour or daily basis. The hypothalamus also controls the master gland of the brain: the pituitary.

The hippocampus and the amygdala are the other major centers of the limbic system. They are both involved with memory formation, but they are also known to gauge emotional reactions such as elation, excitement, anxiety, agitation, rage, and aggression, as well as modulate the capacity to start and stop behaviors associated with these emotions.

The limbic forebrain provides a key integrating system for selectively modulating emotion and responses to sensations. Its

The Limbic-Diencephalic System

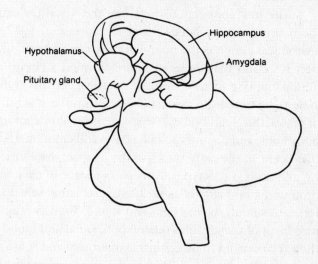

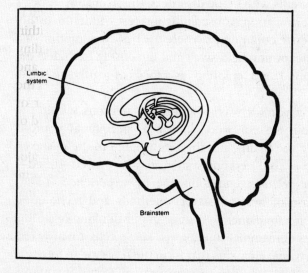

unique location within the forward part of the brain enables it to correlate and integrate every form of internal and external perception.

The interconnections between these various centers led the neuroanatomist James Papez to propose in 1937 that this anatomical circuit is the neuronal substrate of emotion. To support his claim that these structures formed a circuit that permitted emotion to arise through neuronal activity in the limbic system, he noted the association between the essential lesions of rabies, the Negri bodies, which are most abundant in the hippocampus, and the intense behavioral and emotional symptoms that occur in the early stages of the disease: insomnia, irritability, and restlessness typically usher in a stage of excitement and profound mood lability as well as excruciating sensitivity to all forms of stimuli such as light and sound. We may readily recognize in all of these rabies-related behavioral and mood changes their relationship to mechanisms of arousal and sensory awareness as well as their similarity to the signs and symptoms experienced by patients with mood disorders. Unfortunately, Papez's provocative formulation aroused little interest within the orthodox neuroscience community, where the basic assumption of a brain/mind dichotomy held sway and effectively excluded the problem of "mind" and "emotion" as a focus of legitimate scientific inquiry.

For many years it was assumed that neurons within the central nervous system were similar to peripheral neurons (those outside the brain), and this contributed to the mistaken view that the central nervous system was hardwired—fixed—and therefore relatively unmodifiable by experience. Today, largely because of new laboratory methods and techniques, there has been a fundamental change in our thinking regarding the properties of mammalian neurons. These cells are now recognized as dynamic elements that form the basis for an intricate connective system, which is responsive to all forms of environmental input. We now know that dramatic and enduring alterations in the effectiveness of connections between networks of neurons can result from such experiences as neonatal handling, sensory deprivation, and learning.

Recent advances in the neurosciences are gradually revealing the central nervous system to look more and more like an interactive network of oscillating nuclei (centers) that exchange information across spatial and temporal boundaries that are modifiable by experience. This understanding should eventually lead to a new way of viewing the relationship between social and biological processes in the generations to come.

Intercellular Communication

For an organism to survive and function effectively, its component cells must act in a coordinated fashion. Such coordination necessitates the transfer of information between cells in widely separated areas of the organism. In most higher animals, there are two major pathways of intercellular communication: the endocrine system and the nervous system. In the endocrine system, specialized cells secrete hormones, which are carried by the bloodstream to distant parts of the body and influence the activity of specifically responsive target cells.

A neuron, the basic cell of the nervous system, consists of a cell body, a long, thin tube jutting from the cell body (the axon), and a set of shorter fibers (dendrites) that branch and reach out to receive impulses from other nerve cells. A nerve impulse travels electrically down the axon until it cannot continue farther because of a tiny gap—the synaptic cleft—that separates it from other cell fibers. Little sacs or vesicles at the end of the axon spill out chemical transmitter molecules that ferry the impulse across the gap and attach to the cell membrane on the other side. Each of these chemicals, or neurotransmitters, has a certain shape and seeks out a molecule, or *receptor,* on the adjacent cell membrane into which it fits—like a key and its complementary keyhole. Depending on the type of transmitter, and the type of reception it gets from the receptive cells on the other nerve cell, the chemical will either excite the next cell to fire and continue the communication or inhibit it (in this case the message is "there is no message"). These neurotransmitters include amines such as *serotonin, norepinephrine, acetylcholine,* and *dopamine;* amino acids; glutamic acid, GABA; and peptides such as substance P, neuropeptide Y, and endorphins.

The synaptic cleft is about 20 millionths of a millimeter wide, and it takes less than $\frac{1}{5000}$ of a second for the neurotransmitter to leap the gap and arrive on the opposite shore. Each nerve cell evaluates all of the excitatory and inhibitory neurotransmitter inputs and decides whether or not to generate the impulse. Then the transmitter molecule responds to the constant vibration and motion going on around it and pulls off the receptor site. Back in the synaptic cleft, its future lies in one of two directions: either it will be "inactivated"—split into smaller molecules by an enzyme such as monoamine oxidase, acetylcholinesterase, or a peptidase—or, in a process known as "reuptake," it will be sponged up into the presynaptic nerve terminal from which it had been originally released. These two processes clear the site for the arrival of the next chemical messenger.

Two neurotransmitters have most often been implicated in depression and mania: norepinephrine and serotonin. The small cluster of norepinephrine nerve cells originates in an area of the brainstem called the *locus coeruleus* ("blue area") and projects up through the midbrain and extends throughout the cerebral cortex. The serotonin system begins in an area in the midbrain and brain stem called the *raphe nuclei* and projects its nerve pathways to the thalamus and to the gray matter of the cerebral cortex. This pathway is also involved with large parts of the limbic system and hypothalamus. These two neurotransmitter networks reach many parts of the brain that are responsible for a variety of functions disturbed in depression and mania, namely mood, sleep, appetite, and sexual activity.

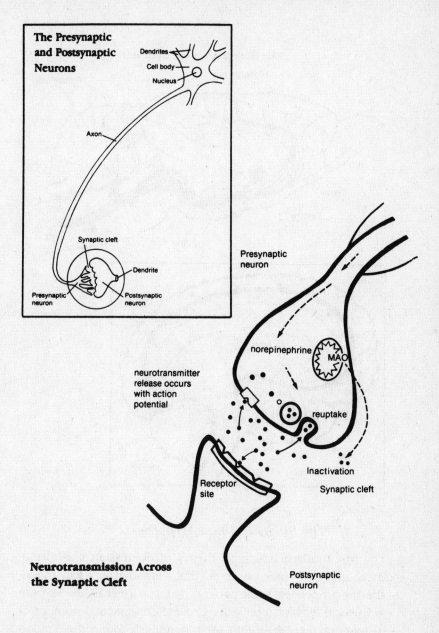

The Presynaptic and Postsynaptic Neurons

Dendrites
Cell body
Nucleus

Axon

Synaptic cleft
Dendrite
Presynaptic neuron
Postsynaptic neuron

Presynaptic neuron

norepinephrine
MAO

neurotransmitter release occurs with action potential

reuptake

Receptor site

Inactivation
Synaptic cleft

Neurotransmission Across the Synaptic Cleft

Postsynaptic neuron

The Norepinephrine System

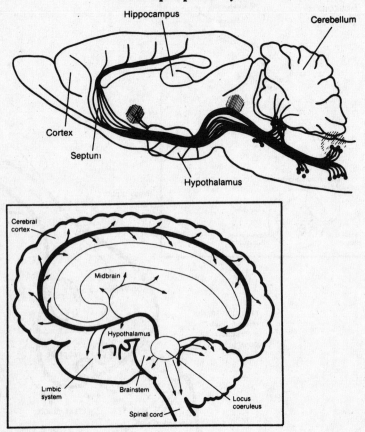

The Biogenic Amine Hypothesis

The first modern biological theory of depression was formu-lated after scientists observed that certain drugs had mood-altering properties. Some patients taking a drug called *reserpine* to lower their blood pressure became depressed; a number of patients taking *iproniazid* for tuberculosis found their mood

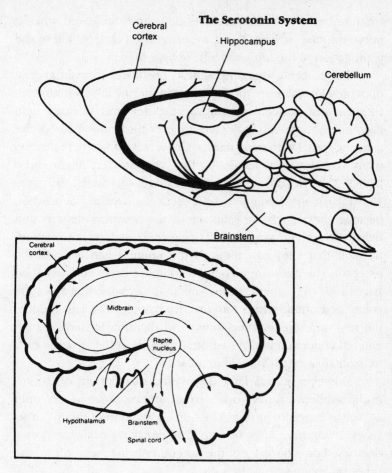

The Serotonin System

improving. When researchers explored what these drugs were doing at the level of the nerve cells, they found that reserpine caused norepinephrine to leak out of the storage vesicles, whereupon it was destroyed by the monoamine oxidase enzymes. Thus, there were too few molecules of norepinephrine to support neurotransmission. Iproniazid, on the other hand, inhibits the enzyme monoamine oxidase, which breaks down norepinephrine and serotonin. This inhibition increases the number of neurotransmitters that can be released when a nerve impulse arrives. These events at the cell level led to the formulation of the *biogenic amine hypothesis*.

The biogenic amine hypothesis postulates that in the state of depression there are too few norepinephrine or serotonin neurotransmitter molecules being synthesized and released, and therefore not enough molecules to ferry the impulse across the synaptic cleft. Depression results. Conversely, it was held that too many transmitter molecules in the synaptic cleft might cause mania. The tricyclic antidepressant drugs (discussed on pages 152–158) were thought to be effective in treating depression because they block the reuptake of the neurotransmitters and help keep their concentration at a high enough level in the synaptic cleft that they can transmit the impulse and activate the receptor. The monoamine oxidase inhibitor drugs (discussed on pages 158–163) inhibit the enzyme in the synapse that splits the amine neurotransmitters into inactive by-products. This reduces the neurotransmitter breakdown and therefore ensures a high enough concentration of neurotransmitters in the synaptic cleft to maintain a steady flow of impulses.

However, it was later discovered that certain of the tricyclic antidepressants worked to prevent reuptake of serotonin as well as norepinephrine. Thus, an elaboration of the hypothesis evolved: there must be two different types of depression— one based on a disorder of the norepinephrine metabolism, the other involving serotonin.

These theories came under fire as well. New, "atypical" antidepressants such as mianserin failed to inhibit significantly the reuptake of serotonin or norepinephrine and yet produced an antidepressant effect. Also, studies of amphetamines and cocaine—drugs known to prevent reuptake of these transmitters—indicated that these drugs were not useful in the treatment of severe depression. And, finally, it was observed that the antidepressants blocked reuptake or raised the level of the transmitters in the synaptic cleft within minutes or hours of a single dose, and yet the therapeutic response to these drugs took more than two to three weeks to manifest itself. There were holes in the theory.

Perhaps it was a change not just in the absolute number or levels of these neurotransmitters that led to depression or mania, but in the capacity for them to be received and act at receptor sites across the synaptic cleft. The simplistic notion of "too few" or "too many" neurotransmitter molecules did not explain the problem and began to give way to the more complex idea of a finely tuned system of checks and balances—a dynamic interaction of receptor responsiveness, release, and firing rate. The focus of inquiry began to encompass yet another level of organization.

Researchers then began to look at changes in *receptor sensitivity* as an important factor in the therapeutic effects of antidepressants. A receptor can be defined as a signal discriminator capable of specifically and sensitively receiving signals from outside the cell. With repeated antidepressant treatment, two types of receptor binding sites that accept the norepinephrine molecule appear to become less sensitive or less abundant: a percentage of the alpha 2 and beta receptors seem to sink back into the cell membrane and become temporarily inaccessible to the neurotransmitters. It has been proposed that these changes—which occur only after several days to weeks—parallel the clinical actions of antidepressants, whose therapeutic effects are typically delayed for two or more weeks. By determining through animal studies the number of receptor sites available to a given neurotransmitter, one can deduce whether "supersensitivity" (usually reflected in an increased number of receptor binding sites) or "subsensitivity" (usually reflected in a decreased number of binding sites) occurs after treatment with medications. This so-called downregulation effect, where the binding sites become less abundant, has been reported after treatment with almost all antidepressant drugs tested as well as with electroconvulsive therapy (ECT). This change in alpha 2 receptors is thought to contribute to a compensatory release of norepinephrine in the nerve terminals that employ this neuro-transmitter.

Once a hormone or neurotransmitter has bound to its receptor, how does it convey its message to the interior of the cell? Early in evolution, single-celled organisms developed ways to recognize crucial signals in their environment and to get that information across the cell membrane to the nucleus of the cell. Several common information transfer systems are used by neurons to achieve this same purpose. In one type of system, the receptor remains within the cell. The signal, say a steroid hormone like cortisone, passes through the cell membrane to bind to its receptor, which then causes changes in the cell's genetic material and consequently changes the synthesis patterns of specific proteins. Other types of signal molecules, like the neurotransmitters norepinephrine or serotonin, are not able to penetrate the cell membrane. The receptors for these molecules are embedded in and span the membrane. When a neurotransmitter signal binds to the receptor on the outside of the cell, it changes the "physical" configuration of the receptor molecule in such a way as to trigger further reactions involving the portion of the receptor that is inside the cell. In other words, there is a signaling pathway that transmits the message carried by a neurotransmitter from the receptor in the membrane to the deep center of the cell where the genes reside.

G-Proteins and Second Messengers

A class of membrane-based proteins known as G-proteins are among the first to respond when a neuronal cell receives a nor-epinephrine signal. They're named G-proteins because in their active state the protein grasps a cell molecule known as GTP, or guanosine triphosphate. In this GTP-bound form, the G-protein activates the next step in a chain of events that leads eventually to a cellular response. Often the signal activates an enzyme like cyclic AMP (cAMP) in such a way that, by adding a phosphorus atom, it can change the level of activity of an enzyme or allow a protein to bind to the cell's DNA and thereby have a direct effect on the kinds or amounts of proteins that the cell manufactures.

So far we have described how certain neurotransmitters, by binding to a specific receptor, stimulate the production of enzymes such as cAMP or protein kinase C (PKC) within the cell that receives the neurotransmitter signal. The question remains: how does an activation of this pathway translate the message of the neurotransmitter into some physiological action?

It appears as if a group of phospholipid molecules that lend structure to the cell membrane, namely the phosphoinositides, play a central role in signal transmission for a wide variety of neurotransmitters and hormones. When cells are stimulated, a phospholipid with the tongue-twisting name of phosphatidylinositol-bis-phosphate (PIP2) is broken down into two compounds: diacylglycerol (DAG) and inositol triphosphate (IP3), both of which act as "second messengers" capable of igniting great changes within the cell. IP3 provokes the release of calcium from tiny storage pockets in the cytoplasm; the calcium then begins to trigger a number of enzymes. At the same time, diacylglycerol sparks the enzyme protein kinase C, which starts exciting yet another string of cellular enzymes. Eventually all this activity reaches the nucleus of the cell.

It is possible that lithium may exert its therapeutic effect in this crucial part of the signal transduction pathway. As we mentioned, this phosphotidylinositol cycle is a "second messenger" system that relays and amplifies signals from neurotransmitters, hormones, and other molecules. Lithium apparently inhibits or throttles down the activity of this pathway. Dr. Michael Berridge was the first to propose that lithium's antimanic and antidepressant effects worked on this cellular pathway. Subsequently, James Allison and William Sherman of the Washington Univer-

G–Protein Receptors

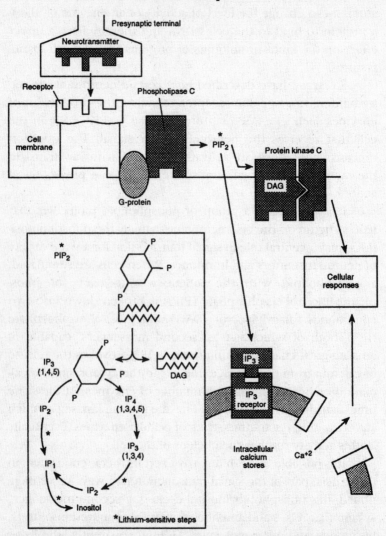

Schematic diagram of the polyphosphoinositide cycle. A neurotransmitter such as norepinephrine binds to its receptor which in turn activates a G-protein. The activated G-protein stimulates the enzyme phospholipase C (PLC) which breaks down phosphatidylinositol-bis-phosphate (PIP$_2$) into two molecules: diacylglycerol (DAG) and inositol triphosphate (IP$_3$). IP$_3$ mobilizes intracellular Ca^{+2}, and DAG activates protein kinase C. See inset for steps in the inositol pathway that are sensitive to lithium.

sity School of Medicine in St. Louis have found that the enzyme that removes the final phosphate group in this degradation pathway to form free inositol is inhibited by lithium ions. Paul Worley and Jay Baraban from Johns Hopkins have shown that when cells in a slice of the brain taken from the hippocampus are treated with low levels of lithium, their responses to neurotransmitters that cause either excitation and inhibition is dampened. Other investigators have suggested that the target of lithium's effect on cells may be via cyclic nucleotide metabolism. For example, in animals it has been reported that therapeutic concentrations of lithium inhibit the ordinary stimulation of adenylate cyclase (an enzyme that induces cyclic AMP). Sophia Avissar and colleagues from Israel have found that lithium blocks GTP binding induced by the neurotransmitter acetylcholine. Since this effect is a measure of the degree of activation of the important G-proteins, these investigators and others hypothesize that lithium reduces cAMP responsiveness via its inhibition of a G-protein that is known to regulate adenylate cyclase. Recently, researchers have turned their attention to the possibility that an effect of lithium at the level of gene expression may reveal insights into the molecular basis of bipolar disorder.

The Effect of Lithium Salts and ECT on Gene Transcription

Now we move even farther along the signaling pathway into the heart of the cell: the nucleus and the DNA it harbors. Transcription is the process by which genetic information is copied from DNA into RNA, which is then used to make the myriad proteins that make each cell very different from one another. For the elaborate transcription process to get under way, proteins known as transcription complexes must bind to the DNA near a target gene. The transcription complex determines when a gene will be transcribed. How well the DNA binding proteins promote or repress transcription depends on how many of these transcription complexes there are within the cell.

A transcription factor gene known as *c-fos* is involved in the transfer of membrane signals to the cell nucleus. Lithium has also been found to effect *c-fos* gene expression in neuronal cell lines, as well as rat hippocampal cells. In one set of studies, Dr. Herb Lachman and his colleagues at the Albert Einstein College of Medicine found that lithium enhanced *c-fos* gene expression in neuronal cells previously stimulated with the neurotransmitter acetylcholine. This direct effect of lithium on a protein involved in gene transcription raises the possibility that lithium may exert its therapeutic effect via some second messenger pathway that directly enhances or inhibits gene expression. Drs. Lachman and Demitri Papolos have proposed a cellular model for bipolar disorder that suggests that the genetic defect underlying bipolar disorder resides somewhere within this pathway.

LEARNED HELPLESSNESS: AN ANIMAL MODEL OF DEPRESSION

Understanding the molecular and genetic basis of mood disorders such as depression and manic-depression is hindered by the complexity and inaccessibility of the human central nervous system. A number of investigators have chosen, therefore, to focus on animal models that come close to reproducing the behavioral changes that occur in human depression, at the same time measuring the effects on the sensitivity of the receptors within selective areas of the brain. While many would debate the validity of extrapolating from animal models, if aspects of human depression can be reliably reproduced in animals and changes in brain function can be found to correspond with the depressed state, we might better understand the biochemical mechanisms and develop more specific antidepressant treatments.

Gene transcription and c–fos

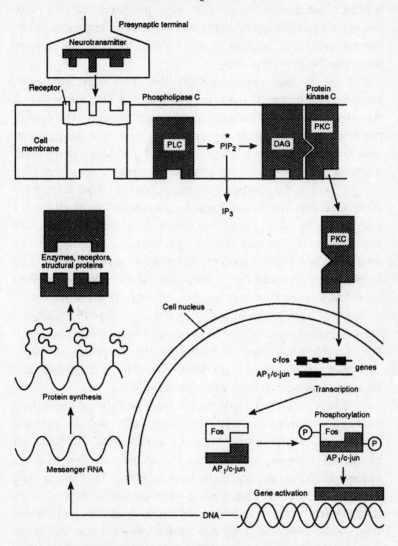

Diagram illustrates a pathway from neurotransmitter binding to gene activation. Once activated, protein kinase C (PKC) leads to an increase in c-fos gene expression. Fos protein combines with the product of the c-jun gene to form the AP₁ factor, which regulates a number of other genes. Lithium has been found to enhance protein kinase C mediated c-fos gene expression in neuronal cell lines. It also increases fos expression in animal hippocampal cells.

To establish the mechanism by which stressful conditions produce depression, it must be demonstrated that a neuro-chemical change occurs when stress-induced depression is observed, and the capability of that change to influence depression must be proven as well.

One of the animal models that has been explored, "learned helplessness," is an attempt to look at the link between stressful events and biological changes and provides the opportunity to examine the interplay between environmental stressors and the genetic susceptibility that produces depression within a neurobiological framework. The model was developed in 1967 when Dr. Martin Seligman observed that dogs who were first exposed to inescapable shocks had more difficulty learning to avoid an *escapable* shock than did dogs who had never before been exposed. (Unstressed animals figured out how to escape and did so easily.) The model was called "learned helplessness" because the researchers felt that the pre-exposed dogs had learned that they had no control over the situation.

Dr. Seligman found that the helpless animals exhibited behaviors that were similar to those seen in human depression. For example, they began to have difficulty sleeping and eating, they stopped grooming and taking care of themselves, and they showed signs of psychomotor retardation.

When Drs. Fritz Henn and Emmeline Edwards and their colleagues then at the State University of New York at Stony Brook induced depressive behavior in rats using the Seligman model of learned helplessness, some provocative findings emerged. The sensitivity of the beta receptors that receive the neurotransmitter norepinephrine were markedly altered in two discrete areas: the receptors were "upregulated," or more sensitive, in the hippocampus, and "downregulated," or less sensitive, in the hypothalamus. When they then treated another group of rats with antidepressants, the previously helpless "depressed" rats regained their capacity to escape the uncontrolled shock. They readily made the effort to push a lever that stopped the shock. Furthermore, this change developed within several weeks—the time frame that would be expected for a typical clinical response to antidepressant treatment. Moreover, the alterations in hippocampal and hypothalamic beta receptors observed during the period of learned helplessness had been reversed by the antidepressant treatment.

In a fascinating extension of this study, Dr. Henn and his colleagues induced depression in another group of rats, but treated them without medication. They made a behavioral intervention and "taught" the rats how to escape the shock. Actually, a medical student working in the lab knit the rats little sweaters with long sleeves over their front paws. Strings were attached to the sleeves and the researchers could pull the rats' paws up, marionette-like, and train them to push the lever that would stop the shock. With the rats no longer helpless, their symptoms of depression abated, and the beta receptor sites returned to their previous state. Dr. Henn and others have concluded from these studies that, just as neurochemistry affects behavior, changes in behavior affect neurochemistry.

Complementary findings have been found in the treatment of human depression. A brief psychotherapeutic treatment called *cognitive therapy* focuses on the thought processes of a depressed person, in particular the hopeless and helpless thinking, and by changing the negative thought patterns, has proved to be as effective as the antidepressant imipramine in treating the depression (see pages 204–205 for a description of cognitive therapy).

The percentage of rats that are vulnerable to helplessness is influenced by both environmental and genetic factors. For example, there is a regularly recurring seasonal sensitivity that results in a marked increase in the percentage of vulnerable rats to approximately 50 to 60 percent during the summer months. In addition, the actions of the hormone corticosterone also appears to play a role in the development of learned helplessness. Removing the adrenal glands (the primary source of corticosterone in the animal) increases the percentage of animals that develop the syndrome from 20 to 70 percent. Interestingly, the development of learned helplessness is also influenced by a strong genetic component. In experiments carried out in learned helpless rats taken to the tenth generation of a selection inbreeding colony, a strain emerged that exhibited a high frequency of learned helpless behavior in this escape-avoidance paradigm. These inbred rats exhibit many of the behavioral, neuroendocrine, and physiological changes—such as reduced appetite, motor activity, exploratory behavior, and sexual drive—found in patients with depression.

HORMONAL DYSFUNCTION IN DEPRESSION

For many years neurotransmitters were the focus of attention. More recently, the scope of investigations has widened to include changes in a number of important hormones. Most endocrine systems are controlled by the biogenic amines: norepinephrine, serotonin, and dopamine all play a part in the timing and regulation of the release of hormones, and the hormones themselves modulate the nerve cell activity of these neurotransmitters. Studies have shown that hormone secretion is influenced by neurotransmitters that are in *limbic centers* and, conversely, that alterations in neurotransmitter function affect hormone secretion.

The mood disorders seem to be the most likely psychiatric illnesses in which one might expect to find a basic hormonal disturbance beyond the simple stress response. The cardinal biological manifestations of these conditions consist of alterations in the hypothalamic centers that govern food intake, libido, circadian rhythms, and the synthesis and release of hypothalamic hormones into the systemic circulation. Indeed, one of the most consistent research findings in biological psychiatry is that patients with major depression often have increased levels of cortisol in the blood. Many of the clinical features of depression and mania suggest some dysfunction in the limbic-hypothalamic circuit. Changes in appetite, in sexual and aggressive drives, in sleep, and the often-described daily variation in the intensity of symptoms implicates a disturbance in the timing and variation of important rhythmic functions that are known to be under hypothalamic influence.

Mood changes occur in association with endocrine disorders. Clinicians have often noticed that people who suffer from diseases of the thyroid and adrenal glands have many symptoms similar to those seen in depressed and manic states. In some instances the behavioral manifestations are indistinguishable. Hyperthyroidism (increased thyroid function) can produce a syndrome that, on first examination, is similar to mania, including hyperactivity, pressured speech, sleeplessness, and so on. Hypothyroidism (decreased thyroid function) can present many of the features of major depression: fatigue, lethargy, and disrupted sleep cycles. In both cases, however, the functioning of the thyroid gland is abnormal and there are physical changes indicative of the gland's malfunction that do not occur in depression or mania. Both the physical and behavioral symptoms can be alleviated by correcting the hormonal imbalance.

Another hormonal disorder, Cushing's syndrome, is characterized by excessive cortisol secretion and can produce symptoms such as fatigue, change in appetite, and insomnia. These are all common symptoms of depression and are associated with a disturbance of the *hypothalamic-pituitary-adrenal axis.* The hypothalamic-pituitary-adrenal (HPA) axis is the endocrine system most extensively studied in affective illness.

Depression and the Neurobiology of Stress

The HPA axis first came under scrutiny about 60 years ago when Dr. Walter Cannon demonstrated that the neurotransmitter epinephrine was released in response to stress. He made this finding the basis of his hypothesis that this substance mobilized the organism for "fight or flight." Some years later, Dr. Hans Selye called attention to the response to stress of the adrenocortical hormone cortisol. While he was concerned chiefly with responses to physical stress, his observation that *psychological* stress could also stimulate cortisol secretion prompted a great deal of subsequent research.

The neuroendocrine system that regulates the release of cortisol helps the body remain flexible so that it can respond appropriately to changing environmental conditions—whether it be alterations in the day–night cycle, seasonal changes, stressful life events, or a sudden threat to survival. This system works to establish an intricate moment-to-moment balance by a series of feedback functions that are orchestrated through the hypothalamus, which is the central relay system for the endocrine and nervous systems. For example, if a person encounters a man with a knife in a darkened hallway, the eyes relay the threat to the brain, and the brain registers fear or anger, probably through the limbic system and its connection via various neurotransmitters to the hypothalamus. This emotional response to a stressful or dangerous event provokes a cascade of neurochemical responses. The fearful event is translated into chemical signals that move through a complex pathway, leading from hippocampal glucocorticoid receptors to the hypothalamus, which sends a message to the front lobe of the pituitary. The message is relayed by the release of *corticotropin-releasing factor* (CRF) from the hypothalamus. The hypothalamus sends the CRF to the pituitary via the private blood supply that connects them. When the pituitary receives the CRF messenger, it responds by pouring out *adrenocorticotropic hormone* (ACTH) into the bloodstream. ACTH, in turn, causes cortisol to be released into the bloodstream.

Within seconds, the ACTH molecule travels to the adrenal ("near the kidney") glands. Stimulated by the ACTH alarm, the adrenal glands pour out cortisol, which converts norepinephrine into epinephrine, and both hormone and neurotransmitter are released into the bloodstream. These substances ready the body for the "fight or flight" response: the heart pumps dramatically harder and faster, the lungs take in more oxygen, the liver releases sugar to provide more available energy, the muscles tense, the pupils of the eyes dilate, and the body begins to sweat so that it can cool itself in the event of violent activity.

This specific neurochemical cascade is clearly of evolutionary value. Even anticipation of threatening or novel events was found to stimulate the release of cortisol. Early animal experiments proved that psychological stress was a powerful stimulant of cortisol secretion, and attention soon turned to its effects in humans. Cortisol levels were measured in normal subjects exposed to experimental psychological stress, as well as in people whose real-life circumstances involved extreme emotional stress. It was discovered that anticipation of any frightening or complicated task, including parachute jumping, hospitalization, or landing an airplane, is a potent stimulant of cortisol. The degree of control that the individual could exert over the situation and the personal meaning of the challenge appeared to be important variables in determining the degree of response. (Recall the learned helplessness in rats.)

Adrenal steroids released into the circulatory system are able to reach the brain and influence central nervous system functions via hippocampal glucocorticoid receptors. Since hormone action is predominantly mediated by receptors, changes in receptor number, or affinity, can alter the degree to which a hormone is "heard" by the cell. Researchers Robert Sapolsky and Bruce McEwen, among others, have found that cortisol regulates its own receptors, particularly in the hippocampus, and does so together with at least two other humoral factors: vasopressin and ACTH. Moreover, glucocorticoid receptors appear to mediate a variety of physiological and neurochemical events, ranging from the shut-off of the adrenal stress response to the modulation of cyclic AMP formation stimulated by the

THE LIMBIC-HYPOTHALAMIC-PITUITARY-ADRENAL AXIS
("THE STRESS RESPONSE")

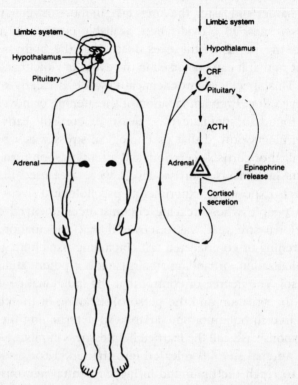

neurotransmitter norepinephrine. One example of adaptation influenced by cortisol elevation is the reduction in sensitivity to norepinephrine that results from repeated stress in the cerebral cortex. The brain changes as a result of the process of adaptation to repeated stress. Our ability to cope is influenced by the output of glucocorticoids. Thus the corticosteroid receptor, the primary site of adrenal steroid action, has become a focus of attention regarding the consequences of steroid response to stress.

Laboratory studies have found that the reduction of hippocampal glucocorticoid receptors brought about by repeated stress is correlated to a reduced capability of the animal to shut off an adrenal steroid stress response. For example, rats that are subjected to the stress of daily handling shortly after birth develop life-long changes in the number of hippocampal gluco-corticoid receptors and exhibit lower resting corticosterone levels, more rapid termination of stress-induced HPA activity, and greater corticosteroid feedback sensitivity relative to unhandled controls. Since glucocorticoid receptors regulate gene expression, it is likely that stressors experienced early in life produce their long-lasting effects on the HPA-axis via alter-ation in gene expression. Even transient stress may ultimately effect the neuron at the level of DNA, resulting in changes in the levels of transcription factors that direct new protein syn-thesis and synaptic excitability.

Things become somewhat more complicated because cor-tisol is not secreted only during stressful situations; it is also secreted episodically in a series of timed bursts throughout the day. These bursts of cortisol are synchronized with the 24-hour sleep–wake cycle and have both periodic (ultradian) and daily (circadian) variations. The sleep–wake alternation in humans is an example of a circadian rhythm, which requires about 24 hours to complete (circa = about, dia = a day). In most people, there is very little secretion of cortisol during the late evening. However, after about 2:00 A.M., a rapid rise occurs, with peak excretion between 5:00 and 9:00 in the morning.

In the 1970s, Dr. Edward Sacher, working at Columbia Pres-byterian Hospital in conjunction with Dr. Elliot Weitzman of the Albert Einstein College of Medicine in New York, began to look at the 24-hour profile of cortisol secretion. Their findings revealed two striking differences between depressed patients and nonde-pressed, healthy volunteers. In the depressed patients, the num-ber of daily episodes was increased, and the level of cortisol in the blood—both at the beginning and the end of the secretory episode—was much higher. Furthermore, in these depressed patients cortisol secretion continued unabated throughout both day and night. The ordinary boundaries of its daily rhythm were lost.

Following these discoveries, other abnormalities of the hypothalamic-pituitary-adrenal axis were reported. Researchers such as Dr. Bernard Carrol studied the functioning of the HPA axis by administering a synthetic cortisol, dexamethasone. Normally, the appearance of the increased level of the hormone in the bloodstream causes the hypothalamus to tell the pituitary that the level of cortisol is adequate and does not need to be replenished. However, in 40 to 60 percent of severely depressed patients, the feedback system does not function correctly: the message to stop sending out cortisol is not sent out and an oversupply of cortisol is maintained in the bloodstream. Both elevated blood cortisol levels and the dexamethasone suppression test (DST) become normal following recovery from an episode of depression.

It has been suggested that the persistence of dexamethasone nonsuppression after apparent clinical recovery may be associated with a high likelihood of relapse. Interestingly, J. P. Cosgriff and collegues from Christ-Church School of Medicine in New Zealand have reported that cortisol hypersecretion predicts early depressive relapse after recovery with electroconvulsive therapy. Although a number of hypotheses have been advanced in order to explain the cause of these defects and their potential relation to mood disorders, the causes and consequences are not yet fully understood.

Several research groups have developed and employed a "CRF stimulation test" to further examine the HPA axis in affective disorders. Dr. Phillip Gold and his coworkers reported that the ACTH response to CRF was blunted in depressed patients as compared to people who were not depressed. These studies are significant in that they point to a possible key role of CRF in the dysregulation phenomenon that is observed in major depression.

CRF has been found to have an interesting effect on the *locus coeruleus*—the area of the brain where norepinephrine cells originate. CRF, when applied directly to the locus coeruleus of awake animals, causes a rapid increase in the firing rate of noradrenergic cells. This sends waves of norepinephrine throughout the central nervous system and induces a state of heightened arousal and hypervigilance—a state commonly seen in human anxiety disorders and panic attacks. Both syndromes are increasingly found in association with major depression and are reported to occur more frequently in families of patients who have an affective disorder. This stimulatory effect of CRF on norepinephrine is another significant clue pointing to the delicate balance between the neurotransmitters, whose functions are known to be altered during depression, and the hormones that regulate the stress response. Gold and his colleagues have more recently found that the levels of CRF in the cerebrospinal fluid of patients with major depression correlate positively with indices of locus coeruleus activity, and they suggest the possibility of a functional connection between the activities of the locus coeruleus–norepinephrine and CRF hormone systems.

SEPARATION AND LOSS: PRECIPITANTS OF DEPRESSION?

Stressful events such as loss or separation have long been implicated as possible precipitants of or antecedents to depression. Indeed, the grief experienced during bereavement in many ways resembles major depression. Researchers have sought to define the relationship of separation events to the development of clinical depression. In these studies separation events are anything a person may experience as a "loss," whether it be the death of a loved one, separation by divorce, the loss of a job or one's status in the community, the loss of some goal, or even a promotion. While the studies are not unanimous, the majority suggest that for certain predisposed individuals, loss may be a trigger for depression.

The British psychoanalyst René Spitz was the first to describe the responses of institutionalized children who had suffered recent separations from their mothers (most of the mothers had been killed in the bombings of London during World War II). In response to the separation, these infants went through an initial stage of protest, becoming extremely restless, presumably attempting to attract attention and the return of the parent. This was followed by a period of despair, with weeping and diminished activity, and finally by a detachment phase in which the infants became severely withdrawn. Spitz labeled this entire reaction pattern *anaclitic depression.* (Anaclitic means "leaning on" and is a psychoanalytic term describing the infant's dependency on the mother for a sense of well-being.)

A very similar separation response has been observed in nonhuman primates. Infant monkeys respond to maternal separation by an initial stage of protest characterized by agitation, sleeplessness, distress calls and screaming, followed after one or two days by evident despair, accompanied by a decrease in general activity, feeding, play, grooming, social interaction, and by the assumption of a hunched posture and "sad" facial expression.

Studies of the HPA axis activity in such separated monkeys found separation to be accompanied by a rise of cortisol in the blood during the protest stage. The magnitude of the elevation has been found to predict the intensity of depressive responses during the despair phase. As was found in human depression, some separated monkeys also failed to suppress blood cortisol concentrations in response to dexamethasone.

In April of 1996, Dr. Charles Nemeroff of Emery University School of Medicine in Atlanta looked at the long-term effect of separation on the HPA axis. He and his colleagues separated 30 rat pups from their respective dams for six hours every day between the ages of six days and three weeks. A second control group of 24 rat pups were permitted to stay with their dams throughout the day.

Once the pups achieved adult size, they were subjected to a mild electrical foot shock. The maternally deprived rats over-reacted to the electrical shock biochemically. They were found to have ACTH levels that were 25 percent higher than those of the control rats. (Remember that the release of ACTH is prompted by CRF.)

Dr. Nemeroff and his colleagues concluded that the early stress of maternal deprivation rendered the rats more sensitive to stress as adults.

Some studies indicate that psychotically depressed individuals demonstrate increased secretion of CRF. Similarly, primates given CRF enter a "huddled-down" posture, a posture similar to that assumed by primates when separated from their peers. Again we see a hormonal dysregulation in the HPA axis that is seen with the depressive response, this time associated with separation or loss. Whether the evident overactivity of the HPA axis and the high outputs of cortisol in major depression are manifestations of an abnormal state, or are merely attempts to restore homeostasis *after the fact*—for example, after some stressful event—remains an open question.

A considerable extent of a human being's early life is sustained and safeguarded by members of the preceding generation—a phenomenon that resulted from the dramatic evolutionary developments that ensured the survival of our species. From the behavioral point of view, this has required the establishment of reliable means for intergenerational signaling whereby nourishment and care-giving can be provided for relatively helpless offspring, as well as a long apprenticeship necessary for learning particular behaviors that provide coping skills for novel situations. This requires a built-in flexibility allowing parts of the nervous system to develop as a result of experience. The limbic system is one part of the central nervous system that is assembled in larger as well as fine detail following birth. Therefore, the role of the limbic system in emotional expression can be shaped in association with infantile and early childhood experience. The consequence of this malleability during postnatal development enables the individual to adapt his or her behavioral and physical possibilities to a particular environment. The attachment of a baby to his or her parents may represent an experiential linkage between limbic development and the individual's capacity to attach meaning and emotion to biologically significant expression.

Let's summarize again. The limbic structures, and particularly the limbic system and its connections to the hypothalamus, are the sites for neurochemical events that orchestrate the stress response. Changes in the balance of neurotransmitters in the hypothalamus and in the levels of glucocorticoid receptors in the hippocampus, in turn, alter the release of important hormones. Ultimately they feed back upon the brain itself to influence neurotransmitters like serotonin, norepinephrine, and acetylcholine. The many disturbing signs and symptoms seen in depression and mania may reflect an imbalance in this complex system.

The information discussed so far has focused on cellular and regional areas within the central nervous system: the synapse and the pre- and postsynaptic membranes of the neuron, the effect of neurotransmitters and hormones on gene expression, the connections between hormone-secreting cells in the HPA axis and their importance in the regulation of the emotional response to stress, and, more directly, their relationship to neurotransmitters implicated in depression and mania. Simply knowing the map, however, does not necessarily provide us with a full knowledge of the territory. Moreover, large parts of the map remain to be charted.

CIRCADIAN RHYTHMS: TIME INSIDE OF SPACE

The timing of events within the central nervous system may be as important as spatial arrangements. Neurotransmitters must not only lock into their corresponding receptor keyhole, but they must also act with appropriate *timing*—in relationship to each other and to events occurring in the environment. The apparently stable functions of the brain and body are poised on the paradox of continuous but well-regulated change. Temperature, blood pressure, hormonal secretions, blood sugar, and dozens of other aspects of bodily activity continuously wax and wane according to varying schedules. These schedules occur approximately every 24 hours and are called *circadian rhythms.* Many of these rhythms are molded by the daily changes of the light–dark cycle.

All human beings have established sleep and activity cycles, as well as periods of hunger and satiety, but many other regular cycles take place below the level of conscious awareness, most notably the secretions of the endocrine system—hormones such as CRF, ACTH, cortisol, growth hormone, and melatonin. Interestingly, there are also regular, daily variations in the production of many neurotransmitters, including serotonin and norepinephrine, and possibly also in the numbers of receptor sites that receive these substances. There are times of day, of month, and of year from which a given biological activity is either necessarily restricted or in which it is most appropriately undertaken.

Why are scientists looking at chronobiological systems? For several reasons. If you examine the course of a mood disorder, you may find that each person has a pattern of recurrence: the cycles come and go, sometimes at the same time each year. For some, there appears to be a rhythmic, possibly seasonal process going on. Then there are variations in the symptoms that people with unipolar or bipolar disorders note during different times of the day. Many people suffering depression feel worse in the morning and find their spirits and energy lifting in the afternoon; others report feeling worse as the day goes on. Furthermore, the sleep cycles of people with mood disorders are disturbed. The syndrome of early-morning awakening—the person who complains of waking early in the morning and being unable to go back to sleep—is one of the classic symptoms of depression. Also, some people complain of sleeping too much, or, in cases of mania, there is suddenly almost no need for sleep. All of these disturbances are rhythmic and point to the possibility that mood disorders are temporal disorders in which the timing of biological rhythms is temporarily—but pathologically—altered.

The metaphor of alarm clocks hidden in the body, programming bodily processes to switch on and off, and then perhaps losing their function, is worth examining. For example, a look at the architecture of the normal sleep pattern and what happens to sleep rhythms when someone is depressed may make this idea clearer.

Normally, throughout the night a person experiences two kinds of sleep that alternate rhythmically. One is called rapid eye movement (REM) sleep, during which most dreaming takes place; the other (not too surprisingly) is called non-REM.

Non-REM sleep has a four-stage development plan as revealed by electroencephalogram (EEG) studies. Stage 1 is the light sleep that begins the night and from which a sleeper may be easily awakened. The brain waves are small and fast. After about half an hour, the sleeper slips deeper into sleep as Stages 2, 3, and 4 of non-REM sleep progress. EEGs of Stage 3 reveal larger and slower brain waves. State 4 brain waves are large, slow, and regular. This is the deepest period of sleep.

After approximately 90 minutes has passed, a brief period of REM sleep appears (the eyeballs can be observed moving rapidly beneath the eyelids), only to be followed by one of the non-REM stages. A pattern develops in which the REM and non-REM sleep phases alternate with each other, cycling back and forth in a remarkably periodic ebb and flow. Later on in the night, REM sleep asserts itself for longer periods of time. Apparently the sleep cycle oscillates on a 90-minute time frame, an example of another fundamental biological rhythm (an *ultradian* cycle that occurs more than once a day). For instance, the

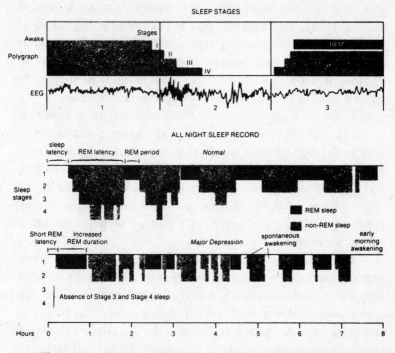

SLEEP STAGES

ALL NIGHT SLEEP RECORD

The top chart illustrates the four stages of sleep and the percentages of REM and nonREM sleep throughout the sleep cycle. The two charts beneath that compare the all-night sleep records of an individual with a normal sleep cycle with that of a patient with major depression. Note the depressed patient's shortened REM latency, the increased REM duration and the spontaneous and early-morning awakening.

first 90-minute cycle might consist of 85 minutes of non-REM sleep and 5 minutes of REM; by the time the fourth cycle rolls around, it might consist of 60 minutes of non-REM and 30 minutes of REM. This time cycle implies that sleep is controlled by a biological clock with a 90-minute period.

All-night EEG studies of depressed patients reveal several abnormalities. There are a marked absence of slow-wave sleep (Stages 3 and 4), an increased difficulty in falling asleep, and an increased number of spontaneous awakenings after sleep has been achieved. It is not difficult to arouse the depressed person from sleep. But perhaps most striking, depressed people go into their first period of REM sleep sooner than nondepressed people. There is a shortened period between the beginning of sleep and the first dreaming period. This is referred to as *REM latency*. It seems that people who are depressed have more REM sleep in the first third of the night and less REM sleep in the last third of the night than nondepressed individuals.

It has been discovered that the human circadian system is controlled by at least two coupled clocks or pacemakers: a strong one controlling body temperature, REM sleep, and cortisol secretion, and a weak one controlling the sleep–wake cycle and sleep-related hormone secretion. It is the relationship of one to the other and to outside time cues such as light or temperature that serves to establish a pattern of temporal order within the body.

Circadian clocks have been likened to cheap wristwatches that run consistently fast or slow and so must be reset frequently (ordinarily, daily environmental cues such as the appearance of dawn and dusk mold these clocks to the everchanging periods of light and dark). The pacemaker that controls the sleep–wake cycle is inherently flexible in order to adjust to the constantly changing length of the daily light period, determined by the position of the sun relative to the earth. A healthy individual who lives in a normal environment, with regular light or time cues to indicate the time of day, can adhere to the 24-hour day and adjust easily to the slow seasonal changes in the light–dark cycle. However, a number of studies that have examined circadian rhythms have noted that the rest-activity and temperature cycles of patients with affective disorders tended to desynchronize even though they were living lives with typical and regular daily schedules. Indeed, several current theories suggest that some form of circadian rhythm desynchronization may be responsible for the symptoms seen in affective disorders.

Let's look at this problem more closely. One of the "pacemakers" that drives a number of rhythms known to be impaired in states of depression and mania is localized in an area of the hypothalamus. It is called the *suprachiasmatic nucleus* (SCN), and it is a pair of small egg-shaped clusters of nerve cells that seem to be responsible for the periodic drinking, eating, and activity rhythms in animals (see the illustration).

The SCN acts like a central relay station exquisitely responsive to day–night changes. During the transition from twilight to dusk, nerve cells in the SCN increase their firing rate dramatically and stimulate the pineal gland to begin the transformation of serotonin to melatonin. The levels of this hormone show a marked circadian variation, rising at night and falling during the day.

A study by Dr. Lars Wetterberg found that depressed patients had a disturbance in the melatonin circadian pattern along with an abnormality of cortisol secretion. Dr. Julien Mendlewicz found that the normal nighttime increase in melatonin secretion was absent in three of four depressed patients studied, and that in patients with bipolar disorder, the melatonin rhythm was desynchronized. That this altered pattern persisted beyond the episode of illness has led to the speculation that the pattern of melatonin secretion may be a stable biological "trait" marker for bipolar disorder. Again, these findings have not achieved the status of fact and require further study.

More than 100 laboratories around the world are now investigating melatonin. Seasonal variations in human melatonin levels have been found with peaks in January and July and troughs in April and October. These findings have led some researchers to suggest a link between the seasonal variation in melatonin and the increased incidence of depression in spring and autumn.

A relationship between the change of seasons and alteration of mood has been observed since ancient times, and modern epidemiological studies show a seasonal variation in both depression and mania. Most studies agree that peak times for depression are in the spring and fall and that an excess of mania

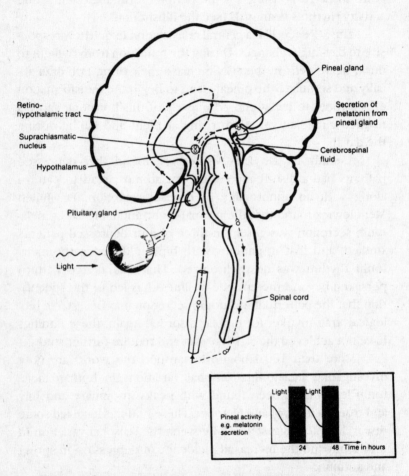

This drawing schematically illustrates the nerve pathways that transmit information about the levels of illumination in the daily light-dark cycle. The information travels from the retina through the retino-hypothalamic pathway to the suprachiasmatic nucleus (SCN), which then connects to the pineal gland via a circuitous pathway. The inset chart demonstrates the normal twenty-four-hour pattern of melatonin secretion from the pineal gland and its relationship to the light-dark cycle.

occurs most frequently in the spring, late summer, and early fall. The chart illustrates the dramatic seasonal fluctuation in suicide deaths with peaks in May and October.

Dr. Daniel Kripke of the University of California at San Diego has proposed that seasonal patterns of mania and depression might be expressions of vestigial seasonal behavioral rhythms—for example, breeding cycles. These behavioral rhythms are controlled by the neuroendocrine system, with the pineal gland and its hormone, melatonin, playing a key role. Desynchronization of biological rhythms around the spring and autumn equinox may be related to a seasonal susceptibility to affective illness.

Recently, scientists have begun to explore whether circadian rhythms can be shifted using brief pulses of light. Human circadian rhythms were once thought to be insensitive to light.

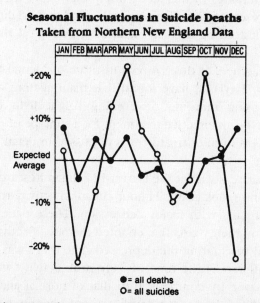

Seasonal Fluctuations in Suicide Deaths
Taken from Northern New England Data

●= all deaths
O= all suicides

Reprinted with permission from *Mood Disorders: Toward a New Psychobiology* by Peter C. Whybrow, M.D., Hagop S. Akiskal, M.D., and William T. McKinney, Jr., M.D. (New York: Plenum Press, 1984).

Scientists felt that synchronization to the 24-hour day was accomplished either through periodic social cues and/or the sleep–wake cycle. However investigators have found that bright artificial light can suppress human melatonin production. Sunlight, which is 20 to 200 times brighter than ordinary indoor light, also suppresses melatonin production. The demonstration of this intensity-dependent hormonal response has led to a renewed consideration of light as a possible synchronizer of the human circadian pacemaker. In a laboratory study, Dr. Charles Czeisler and his colleagues at Harvard University monitored the output of the circadian pacemaker of an elderly woman before and after exposure to four hours of bright light for seven consecutive evenings. The exposure to bright light in the evening delayed by six hours the rhythms of body temperature and cortisol secretion.

The findings of this study imply that exposure to bright light can reset the circadian pacemaker and that bright artificial light can indeed be used to manipulate biological rhythms in humans.

Researchers at the National Institute of Mental Health in Bethesda, Maryland, have found that manipulating biological rhythms using morning or evening bright light exposure appears to be an effective treatment for a subtype of mood disorders. (This form of treatment is discussed in detail on pages 220–224.)

A research team at the Harvard Mailman Research Center then began to look at the 24-hour circadian activity rhythms in elderly patients with major depression. These patients wore monitors on their wrists that counted the rate of activity, and it was found that during the depressed state there was an unexpected difference: the time of daily peak activity was significantly delayed by comparison to that of normal age-matched subjects. Also, the activity level in these patients was significantly higher than in nondepressed elderly subjects. Following antidepressant treatment and clinical recovery, these alterations returned to normal, suggesting that depressed elderly patients may have a pronounced chronobiological disturbance in activity level and rhythm and possibly other circadian processes.

To summarize, studies have raised the possibility that some diseases may be temporal disorders in which the timing of biological rhythms is pathologically altered. The disruption of timing functions within the central nervous system may contribute to or accompany—or perhaps even cause—mood disorders. Patients with manic-depression and depression have been shown to suffer from a variety of abnormal rhythm disturbances. Rhythms of activity, temperature, REM sleep, cortisol, and melatonin have been described. Thus, it is possible that manic and depressive symptoms arise from a lack of coordination between two or more circadian pacemakers and the rhythms that they control.

A chronobiological theory of affective illness, while by no means proven, is intriguing. As a model, it allows us to integrate the clinical symptoms of depression and mania, such as early morning awakening, diurnal variation in mood, and disturbances in activity, as well as features such as seasonality and cyclicity. In addition, it helps explain the abnormalities in the timing of secretion of various hormones, such as cortisol and melatonin. Research stemming from this theory may increase our understanding of the causes of affective disorders, and perhaps lead to new treatment approaches.

KINDLING AND BEHAVIORAL SENSITIZATION

An additional model that attempts to account for the pattern of cyclicity seen in affective illness is the kindling-sensitization hypothesis, proposed by Dr. Robert Post and his colleagues at the National Institute of Mental Health. According to this concept, once an initial affective episode has taken place, the susceptibility of the individual to further episodes increases so that successive episodes can be set off by less significant stressors. The kindling or sensitization of limbic areas may account for many of the features of affective illness, including the possible predisposition provided by early stressful experiences, the gradual worsening of affective episodes over time, the progressive acceleration in the frequency of cycling, and the gradual development of a tendency toward spontaneous relapses.

Repeated stimulation of an animal's limbic system with electrical current can eventually lead to the development of epileptic seizures and cause permanent changes in the organization of neuronal connections. This generation of a permanent epileptic predisposition in normal brain tissue is referred to as "kindling." An animal that is kindled, even if left unstimulated for many months, will respond with a seizure when subsequently stimulated. Additionally, a percentage of kindled animals have spontaneously recurring seizures, especially if placed in the setting in which the original electrical stimulation was given. Therefore, kindling can be environmentally conditioned. Similarly, exposure to a novel stimulus that stresses or arouses the central nervous system can produce an increased sensitivity on re-exposure to that same stimulus. An example of this phenomenon is seen in laboratory animals exposed to long-standing restraint stress. This behavioral stressor has been found greatly to enhance the ACTH response to future stress.

Because of the architecture of the hippocampus, and quite possibly because of the unique molecular characteristics of these connections, stimulation of fiber tracts in this brain region can induce an enhancement of neurotransmitter responses. The enhancement of both short-term responses and those lasting for longer periods of time has been described. Therefore, the stimulation of particular fiber tracts leading into the hippocampus, such as those from the septum (the primary relay station between the hippocampus and the hypothalamus), can lead to a kindled response. It is this mechanism that may account for the relationship between stressful events and the development of mood disorders and their propensity for spontaneous cycling.

The kindling-sensitization hypothesis would predict that early and aggressive treatment intervention should diminish the chances of subsequent episodes or at least reduce the likelihood of developing a more disabling form of the illness.

SUMMING UP

Our present information suggests some plausible hypotheses pointing to the operation of relatively specific social, psychological, biological, and environmental processes in the development of major mood disorders. The findings and hypotheses noted in this chapter are summarized as follows:

1. The limbic-diencephalic system near the center of the brain is the area that regulates information of an emotional nature and governs the "fight or flight" mechanism. The hypothalamus, which contains the suprachiasmatic nuclei (SCN), is a critical part of this system.

2. Two neurotransmitters have been most often implicated in depression and mania: norepinephrine and serotonin.

3. It is thought that antidepressants may change the level of receptor sensitivity to these neurotransmitters.

4. Neurotransmitters, by binding to specific receptors, stimulate the production of enzymes such as cyclic AMP or protein kinase C within the cell that receives the neurotransmitter signal. These second messenger molecules, through their effects on cellular metabolism, can cause a protein molecule to bind to the cell's DNA and thereby have a direct effect on the kinds or amounts of protein that the cell manufactures.

5. A group of membrane molecules, specifically the phosphoinositides, play a central role in this signal transduction process for a wide variety of neurotransmitters and

hormones. The phosphoinositide pathway has recently come under closer investigation as a place within nerve cells where lithium may exert its therapeutic effect.

6. Recently, investigators have turned their attention to the possibility that an effect of lithium at the level of gene expression may reveal insights into the molecular basis of bipolar and unipolar mood disorders.

7. Transcription, the process by which genetic information is copied from DNA into RNA, which is then used to make the myriad proteins that maintain cellular metabolism, may be affected by lithium salts.

8. Using techniques from molecular biology, studies have found that the expression of a particular transcription factor gene, *c-fos,* involved in the transfer of neurotransmitter signals to the cell nucleus, is affected by both ECT and lithium.

9. This direct effect of ECT and lithium on a protein involved in gene transcription raises the possibility that these treatments may exert their benefits via second messenger pathways that enhance or inhibit gene expression.

10. Because the understanding of the molecular and genetic basis of mood disorders is hindered by the complexity and inaccessibility of the human central nervous system, investigators have turned to the exploration of animal models that come close to reproducing the behavioral changes that are seen in human depression.

11. In one study, animals who were physically stressed by uncontrollable shocks developed "learned helplessness" and were unable to learn to escape controllable shocks. They exhibited behaviors similar to those seen in human depression (they began to have difficulty sleeping and eating, they stopped grooming and taking care of themselves, and so on). The sensitivity of norepinephrine receptors in their brains was markedly altered in the hypothalamus and the hippocampus. When other animals who

had such induced "learned helplessness" were treated with antidepressants, they regained their ability to escape the shock. The alterations in the receptor sensitivity observed after the period of "learned helplessness" was completely reversed by the antidepressant, as well as by behavioral interventions. Just as neurochemistry affects behavior, behavior affects neurochemistry.

12. Hormone secretion is influenced by neurotransmitters in limbic centers and, conversely, alterations in neurotransmitter function affect hormone secretion. The hypothalamic–pituitary–adrenal (HPA) axis controls the release of cortisol. Cortisol readies the body for "fight or flight." Depressed patients secrete more cortisol than nondepressed people. The HPA feedback system does not appear to be functioning correctly in depression, and an oversupply of cortisol is maintained in the bloodstream. Both elevated blood cortisol levels and the dexamethasone suppression test (DST) become normal following recovery from an episode of depression. All of these findings suggest hyperactivity of the HPA axis in depression.

13. Stressful events such as a loss or separation have long been implicated as possible precipitants of or antecedents to depression. The British psychoanalyst René Spitz described "anaclitic depression" in which children separated from their mothers in World War II went through an initial stage of protest in which they became extremely restless. This was followed by a period of despair, and finally a detachment phase in which they became severely withdrawn. A very similar separation response has been observed in nonhuman primates. Studies of the HPA axis in separated monkeys found separation to be accompanied by a rise of cortisol in the blood during the protest stage. The magnitude of the elevation has been found to predict the intensity of depressive responses during the despair stage. Similar to the findings in human depression,

some separated monkeys also failed to suppress blood cortisol concentrations in response to the dexamethasone suppression test. Again we see a hormonal dysregulation in the HPA axis with the depressive response associated with separation or loss.

14. Temperature, blood pressure, hormonal secretions, blood sugar, and dozens of other aspects of bodily activity wax and wane according to varying schedules. These schedules occur approximately every 24 hours and are called circadian rhythms. Many of these rhythms are molded by the daily changes of the light–dark cycle. It may be that mood disorders are temporal disorders in which the timing of biological rhythms is temporarily—but pathologically—altered.

15. People who are depressed go into their first period of REM sleep sooner than people who are not depressed. The sleep architecture of depressed patients is different than that of nondepressed people.

16. The human circadian system is controlled by at least two coupled clocks or pacemakers: a strong one controlling body temperature, REM sleep, and cortisol secretion; and a weak one controlling the sleep–wake cycle and sleep-related hormone secretion. It is the relationship of one to the other and to outside time cues such as light or temperature that serve to establish a pattern of temporal order within the body. It is possible that these two pacemakers are dissociating—beating out of phase with each other—and result in the symptoms we know as mania or depression.

17. A number of studies that have examined circadian rhythms such as rest-activity cycles have noted that the circadian rhythms of patients with affective disorders tend to drift even though they are not isolated from light and time cues. These patients might lack the capacity to process time and light cues.

18. The suprachiasmatic nucleus (SCN) is localized in an area of the hypothalamus. It is one of the "pacemakers" and it stimulates the pineal gland to transform serotonin into the hormone melatonin. Patients with affective disorders have a disturbance in the melatonin-circadian secretion pattern. Dr. Julien Mendlewicz found that the normal nighttime increase of melatonin was absent in three of four depressed patients studied, and that in patients with bipolar disorder, the melatonin rhythm was desynchronized. That this altered pattern persisted beyond the episode of illness has led to the speculation that the pattern of melatonin secretion may be a stable biological "trait" marker for bipolar disorder.

19. An additional model, the kindling-sensitization hypothesis, which derives from the fact that repetitive exposure to a stimulus can activate or arouse the central nervous system, attempts to account for the pattern of cyclicity typical of affective illness. According to this concept, once a particular stressor has initiated an episode in a genetically predisposed individual, the susceptibility of the individual to further episodes increases such that successive episodes can be set off by less significant stressors.

It is still a mystery as to how these different aspects of the illness combine with a genetic vulnerability to produce the common symptoms of mania and depression. It is, however, encouraging to think that much of the information presented in this chapter was unknown even fifteen years ago. Judging from this perspective, there is every reason to hope that the next decade will see an exponential increase in our understanding of the causes of the major mood disorders—and perhaps similar leaps in their treatment.

TWO

ABOUT THE TREATMENT

5

THE SOMATIC THERAPIES: MEDICATIONS AND ECT

In ancient Phoenicia, the mentally ill were boarded on ships—the "ships of fools"—and set adrift to roam the seas in search of more hospitable harbors. In the Middle Ages, exorcists coaxed the "demons" from the bodies of those who acted strangely. Shock treatments were administered to eighteenth-century patients by twirling them on stools until their ears bled, and by dropping them through trap doors into icy lakes.

More humane treatments were developed in the nineteenth century, but effective medical treatments still did not exist. In 1937 Sigmund Freud wrote: "The future may teach us how to exercise a direct influence, by means of particular chemical substances, upon the amount of energy and its distribution in the apparatus of the mind. It may be that there are other undreamed of possibilities of therapy."

Freud would have been fascinated with what happened. When he died in 1939, only electroconvulsive shock treatments were effective for serious depression. Ten years later, John Cade discovered the true value of the salt lithium. In 1952 the French psychiatrists Jean Delay and Pierre Deniker tested chlorpromazine for calming psychotic agitation. Not long afterward, the antidepressant drugs were added to the new-found psychiatric armamentarium.

The effectiveness of these new drugs is now firmly established through research studies. Mood swings are prevented or ᵇᵉᶜome less severe; lives are returned to more normal paces. In 14 studies of bipolar disorder, the percentage of patients having a recurrent episode of either mania or depression during 1 year after the start of treatment was significantly reduced by lithium maintenance in contrast to placebo. In most of these studies, the number of recurrences was reduced by 50 percent compared with that of the placebo, and the recurrences were less severe.

Other controlled studies have shown that treatment with lithium or antidepressants can substantially prevent the recurrence of unipolar depression. In most patients, lithium and tricyclic antidepressants decrease the frequency and/or intensity of recurrences. Dr. Jan Fawcett wrote that when he started his practice, families of patients who required hospitalization anxiously asked him whether they would ever come out of the hospital. In the 1970s families of patients began asking him why they were not out and well in two weeks!

A new deal? Yes. A cure-all? Not quite. While some people respond to the medications completely and do not suffer side effects, a smaller population responds only partially or finds the side effects uncomfortable or intolerable. The drugs do not cure the illnesses; they *control* them. For now they're the best we have, and the effect they have on the quality of life is impressive.

LITHIUM THERAPY

Forty years ago, when I was ten, my mother was taken away to an asylum because she was "mad." Eventually and because nothing could calm the turbulence in her mind, she was given a lobotomy. She never came home from the hospital, and all these years of custodial care depleted the huge trust fund that her father had provided. Last year we had to transfer her to a less expensive hospital.

When my brother began to act strangely, everyone

thought he had a bit of the family taint. He continued to have periods of illness and became intrusive and even frightening at times. One day he took a flight to England, next we heard from him in Switzerland, and then the family got a call from the Australian Consulate in Sydney reporting that he was found on the beach, alone, and screaming bizarrely at the sky.

We managed to get him home and, like my mother before him, he was hospitalized. Only, this time it was different. The doctor who saw him took a careful look at the symptoms, enquired about the family history, and treated him with lithium. Four weeks later, he left the hospital and began to put his life back together.

Because we now know my brother's diagnosis, I finally realize—after so many years—that my mother was not "mad" or schizophrenic, or that it wasn't just something peculiar to our family. She had manic-depression, and it is now very treatable. If she had become ill today, she would have come home to her family. My beautiful, elegant mother was born too soon.

Lithium has been the long-standing drug of choice in the acute treatment of mania and for the maintenance treatment of bipolar disorder. It protects a person by reducing the possibility of future episodes of mania and depression. This medication, most of it mined in the state of North Carolina, literally makes the difference between lives of chaos and disruption and lives of stability and productivity.

Trace amounts of lithium exist in the human body, in plants, and in mineral rocks. It was inserted into the chemists' periodic table as the lightest of the alkali metals when it was described in 1817 by a young Swedish chemist, August Arfwedson. He christened his new element lithium, from the Greek word "lithos," stone.

Interesting intuitions about lithium go way back. About 1,800 years ago, the Greek physician Galen formulated a treatment for mania by bathing patients in alkaline springs and by having them "take" (drink) the waters. There was probably lithium in those springs. The medicinal connection began in earnest in the 1840s when it was thought that lithium, combined with carbonate or citrate—it then forms a salt—was a good treatment for gout. It wasn't, but for some reason known only to history lithium was touted as a cure for epilepsy, diabetes, cancer, even sleeplessness. This cure-all was never proven all that effective, but something about this drug led it to turn up constantly in new incarnations.

In the late 1940s, lithium chloride was tried as a salt substitute for patients with kidney or heart disease who required low-sodium diets. Later it was learned that lithium is particularly dangerous for people on low-sodium diets, and for those with congestive heart failure or kidney failure, because lithium exchanges for sodium. If a person is salt-depleted, lithium enters the brain cells, occupies the sites normally taken up by sodium, and soon rises to toxic levels. Some people suffered poisoning; a few people died.

Meanwhile, in 1949, in a primitive laboratory in Australia, an unknown psychiatrist named John Cade discovered the true value of lithium. What a quirk in timing. After a century of misapplication, Cade got on the right track just as alarming stories about lithium poisonings spread throughout America.

Dr. Cade began with a hunch that uric acid caused manic behavior. He intended to inject guinea pigs with uric acid, but he needed to control its potency by keeping it in soluble form. And what solution did he use? Lithium salts.

The guinea pigs became calm and unexcitable. Cade could put them on their backs and they would lie there, unresponsive to any poking or prodding. Dr. Cade reasoned that the lithium might have the same calming effect on people with mania, and he switched the drug to human test subjects: ten manic patients, six schizophrenics, and three "melancholics." In the *Medical Journal of Australia* for September 3, 1949, Cade reported:

W. B., a male, aged 50-one years, had been in a state of chronic manic excitement for 5 years, restless, dirty, destructive, mischievous, and interfering, had long been regarded as the most troublesome patient in the ward. His response was highly gratifying. From the start of treatment on March 29, 1948, with lithium citrate he steadily settled down and was enjoying the unaccustomed surroundings of the convalescent ward. . . . He remained perfectly well and left hospital on July 9, 1948, on indefinite leave with instructions to take a maintenance dose of lithium carbonate, five grains twice a day. . . . He was soon back working happily at his job. However, he became lackadaisical about his medicine and finally ceased taking it. His relatives reported that he had not had any for at least six weeks prior to readmission on January 30, 1949, and was becoming steadily more irritable and erratic. He ceased work just before Christmas. On readmission to hospital he was at once started on lithium carbonate, ten grains three times a day, and in a fortnight had again settled down to normal. . . . He is now (February 28, 1949) ready to return to home and work.

Ten case histories of lithium's profound effects on manic patients were reported in this landmark article, but its argument failed to galvanize the medical community. The lithium poisonings in America closed people's minds to the subject.

Danish psychiatrist Mogens Schou, the world expert on the use of lithium in psychiatry, was determined to bring lithium to world attention. He began his campaign in 1957. By the 1960s, lithium was being used in several other countries, but the U.S. Food and Drug Administration (FDA) restricted its use to small experiments.

Many scientific papers later, the FDA partially lifted the nonapproved status of lithium and allowed physicians to prescribe it for the treatment of acute mania illness, but it wasn't until 1974 that the FDA permitted doctors to prescribe lithium in order to prevent future episodes in bipolar disorder. Today hundreds of thousands of people are living normal lives because of it.

Determining Dosages

Before a patient can be started on lithium therapy, he or she needs a medical evaluation including a medical history, physical examination, and simple laboratory tests of blood and urine. Because lithium is almost entirely eliminated from the body by the kidneys, laboratory tests of kidney functions are done before starting the lithium, and at regular intervals thereafter. Tests of thyroid function also are advised since lithium can occasionally cause goiter (a treatable and reversible enlargement of the thyroid gland) or a mild decrease in thyroid function (hypothyroidism). Blood tests of the level of thyroid and thyroid stimulating hormones usually are done at regular intervals.

In order for lithium to be effective, its concentration in the blood must be held at a proper level. Although too little is ineffective, too much can be toxic—and there is not much leeway between what is necessary and what is a dangerous excess. Therefore, the person who takes lithium must have regular blood tests in order to determine the lithium concentration in the blood. At the start of treatment, blood levels usually are monitored every few days. The blood sample is drawn about 12 hours after the last evening dose and before the patient takes the morning dose. Since the result of a blood test taken more than 60 minutes before or after the 12 hours has elapsed may be misleading, the timing of blood tests should be planned carefully.

A lab report is sent to the physician and he or she will look to see that the level remains in the area of 0.6–1.0 for outpatients and 0.75–1.2 units for someone experiencing an acute manic episode. (These measurements are in units of milliequivalents of lithium per liter of blood.) Once the level of the drug has stabilized in the bloodstream, monitoring is needed only at one- to three-month intervals. Lithium treatment takes ten days to two weeks to become effective.

Several preparations of lithium are now available. Most are 300-milligram, immediate-release lithium carbonate tablets or capsules. The least expensive preparation is lithium carbonate tablets, which have the added advantage of being scored so that they can be broken in half and the dosage adjusted by 150-milligram increments. Capsules are sometimes preferred because they may be easier to swallow and because tablets may have an unpleasant taste. A liquid form of lithium citrate is also available.

When a person takes any of these forms of lithium, the drug is immediately absorbed and, as a result, produces relatively high peak blood levels. For this reason, a divided dosage regimen is prescribed—often three or four times a day. A conventional release formulation produces a peak blood level from one-half to three hours after the patient takes the medication. Several pharmaceutical companies now produce different forms of release designed to minimize the swings in drug levels. One of these is a slow-release form (Lithobid). This preparation releases the lithium slowly so that the peak blood levels are flattened—the blood level peak is approximately four hours. There are reports that the slow-release form reduces side effects. Another of these release designs is called sustained-release (Eskalith CR). The lithium is embedded in a nondigestible carrier that delays absorption even longer, as much as 12 hours after administration. This allows the drug to be given less frequently, perhaps only twice a day. (It should be noted that some patients complain of lower abdominal cramps or diarrhea with these preparations, perhaps because of their delayed absorption in the gut.)

Slow-release and sustained-release preparations are more expensive. Individual preference, cost, and side-effect considerations will influence a choice or change in lithium preparations.

A patient might find it useful to purchase a clear plastic box with divided compartments for lithium storage. (Most health food and vitamin stores and pharmacies sell them.) Each compartment can be labeled with a day of the week and filled with the daily dosage, and a glance will tell a patient whether or not it has been taken. A routine, such as taking the dose at a mealtime or at the hour of sleep, can be established so that forgetfulness is not a problem.

Should a person forget a dose of lithium, he or she should *not* double the next. It is relatively safe to skip a dose, but very risky to double one.

Lithium is taken by mouth, rapidly and fully absorbed into the bloodstream, and carried to all body and brain tissues. It is excreted almost entirely by the kidneys. Sodium is also excreted by the kidneys in competition with lithium, so a normal sodium balance is important to ensure a reliable lithium balance. The less sodium in the body, the less lithium is excreted, and the greater chance of lithium buildup and possible toxicity. Diuretics that cause the kidneys to excrete sodium and low-salt diets top the list of things to avoid. But patients should also be aware that a severe loss of fluids and salts (such as those caused by fevers, vomiting, and diarrhea) can cause the lithium level to rise in the bloodstream to potentially toxic levels (greater than 1.5 mEq/L). If any of these conditions exists, the patient will most likely be instructed to get a lithium level assay and to lower the daily dose of lithium.

TYPICAL COSTS OF LITHIUM PREPARATIONS

**A patient taking the equivalent of 1200 mg of
lithium carbonate a day would spend the following
for a one-month supply of these available formulations:**

Generic name	Trade name	Formulations	Cost of one-month supply*
lithium carbonate	Eskalith	300 mg tablets or capsules	$21.00
	Lithane	300 mg tablets	23.00
	Lithotabs	300 mg tablets	19.00
	Eskalith CR (sustained-release)	450 mg tablets	42.00
	Lithobid (slow-release)	300 mg tablets	39.00
lithium citrate	Cibalith-S	8 mEq/5 ml (500 ml bottles)	29.00/bottle

*Based on 1996 prices for 120 tables or capsules.

How Does Lithium Work?

Researchers and physicians have unequivocal data that proves the effectiveness of lithium therapy, but no one is sure how it works, especially why it works in both mania and depression. Some researchers have found that lithium affects a complex biological system called the phosphatidyl inositol cycle inside many types of cells. This cycle is a "second messenger" system that relays and amplifies signals from neurotransmitters, hormones, and other molecules. Lithium apparently inhibits or throttles down the activity of this pathway, which may be overactive in mania and depression (see Chapter 4 for a more complete discussion of lithium's effects on this complex pathway).

Side Effects

Lithium is nonsedating and nonaddictive. It is safe at appropriate dosages, although when taken in excess it can produce intoxication and potentially dangerous side effects.

Most of the common side effects are both harmless and easily dealt with. Stopping treatment is rarely necessary.

Early Side Effects   The following early side effects occur in perhaps 40 percent of those taking lithium and usually subside in several days:

- Gastrointestinal symptoms: nausea, vomiting, diarrhea, stomachache. These side effects can usually be alleviated through adjustments of dosage and timing of administration. Simple changes, such as taking a few tablets or capsules at a time, taking them on a full stomach, or taking them with a glass of milk, are often effective.
- Fine tremor of the hands at rest, which may cause a change in handwriting.
- Thirst and frequent urination.
- Fatigue, a dazed feeling, muscle weakness.

Persistent or Later-Beginning Side Effects   The side effects that are most likely to persist or begin later in lithium treatment are:

- Hand tremor. An individual inconvenienced by continued tremors beyond the first weeks of treatment should speak with his or her doctor. After ensuring that the hand tremor is not an indication of early toxicity, the doctor may choose to vary the dosage schedule, change to a slow-release preparation, or lower the dose. If all of these options fail and this side effect interferes with the patient's livelihood (for example, if the patient is a jeweler or a teacher who must write on a blackboard), then the doctor may prescribe small doses of propranolol (Inderal) to steady the hand tremor.

- Severe thirst and frequent urination, which may be reversed by lowering the dose of lithium, or by careful use of a thiazide diuretic (water pill) such as hydrochlorothiazide.

Other Side Effects

- Increase in weight. It is not clear why some patients tend to gain weight on lithium, but a few theories have been proposed, including an altered fat and carbohydrate metabolism, improved appetite after the resolution of an affective episode, increased fluid intake and retention, and diminished thyroid function. It seems that people who are overweight before starting lithium therapy are more likely to gain weight. At any rate, a recent study showed that weight gain was one of the major factors in lithium noncompliance. Therefore, in order to avoid the distress of weight gain, patients should drink noncaloric beverages to quench their thirst and watch their calorie consumption. Many people in support groups reported that they increased their weekly exercise routines in order to combat the problem and found this to be effective.

- Hypothyroidism. A small percentage of patients (mostly women) on lithium develop hypothyroidism—the thyroid gland becomes underactive and enlarges in size. The following symptoms may appear: tiredness, slow reactions, or slow thinking, feeling cold, dry puffy skin, unusual weight gain, hair loss, muscle aches, or menstrual changes. These symptoms should be reported to the doctor, who will evaluate the thyroid gland by ordering thyroid function studies. If there is a problem, it can be easily and effectively treated with (v)Levothyroxine Sodium (Synthroid or Levothroid), a synthetic thyroid hormone replacement.

Less Common Side Effects

- Metallic or bad taste in the mouth, a worsening of acne or psoriasis, skin rashes, hair loss, and short-term memory loss. Hair loss (alopecia) has been occasionally reported by patients taking lithium. One summary of seven cases of hair loss revealed that six of the seven were women, two had abnormal thyroid function (hair loss can be a symptom of this), and three had hair regrowth even though they continued taking lithium. There appears to be no explanation for the hair loss, which is really more of an increased shedding or thinning. It can appear as early as 5 months into treatment and as late as 54 months. Should this side effect occur, thyroid functioning should be checked before any decisions about reducing or discontinuing lithium are made.

    There are mixed reports concerning short-term memory loss. Patients have occasionally complained of it, but several memory tests have failed to reveal lithium-induced memory dysfunction. Dr. Mogens Schou and his research team made an attempt to address the issue some years ago. They took lithium experimentally for periods of one to six weeks and noted that though they felt no mental side effects at normal preventative doses, they did experience some difficulty concentrating and memorizing at higher doses. Patients who experience this side effect should be assured that lithium's effects on mental functioning are reversible and disappear when lithium is discontinued.

Signs of Trouble

High levels of lithium in the blood can be severely intoxicating, brain damaging, or even fatal. Therefore, patients and their families should take careful note of the following signs of an impending problem:

SIGNS OF IMPENDING LITHIUM TOXICITY

Fatigue	Coarse or worsening hand tremor
Sleepiness	Unsteady gait
Confusion	Tremor of the lower jaw
Muscle weakness	Muscle twitches
Heaviness of the limbs	Nausea, stomachache, diarrhea
Slurred speech	Tinnitus (ringing in the ears)

Some of these symptoms could be caused by other illnesses. No matter what the underlying cause, the patient should not take any more lithium, but should call the doctor and report the symptoms. An immediate blood test to check the lithium blood level will give firm evidence of the problem, and if necessary, the dosage can be adjusted.

Can You Drink Alcohol or Take Other Medications While on Lithium?

Patients often ask whether they can drink while taking lithium. While one or two drinks will probably do no harm, alcohol can interact with lithium and cause excessive sedation and confusion contributing to intoxication. Moderation is the key here.

Several antibiotics, most notably tetracycline, erythromycin, and the medication known as Flagyl, as well as antiinflammatory agents such as ibuprofen (Motrin, Rufen, Advil, and Nuprin) and mefanamic acid (Ponstel), can lead to an increase in the plasma lithium level. Should a patient need to take these drugs while on lithium, serum blood levels should be checked every four or five days until the extent of the drug interaction is clear. Other medications can interact unfavorably with lithium and are listed in the chart below. (Some of these medications may still be prescribed in conjunction with lithium, but the patient should be monitored closely throughout the period of joint prescription.)

Is It Safe to Suddenly Stop Lithium Treatment?

Dr. Gianni Faedda and colleagues from McLeans Hospital in Massachusetts surveyed 14 previous studies seeking to clarify the risk over time of recurrence for a manic or depressive episode following discontinuation of apparently effective long-term lithium maintenance treatment. They defined a relapse as any new episode of mood disorder that required rehospitalization or that was sufficiently severe as to require pharmacological or electroconvulsive therapy. Their survey revealed a 28-times higher monthly risk for recurrence in the patients who discontinued lithium.

INTERACTIONS OF LITHIUM WITH OTHER DRUGS

Lithium May Interact With	Resulting In
NONSTEROIDAL ANTI-INFLAMMATORY DRUGS	
Ketorolac (Toradol)	Increased lithium
Ibuprofen (Advil)	level
Indomethacin	
Naproxen (Aleve, Naprosyn)	
Phenylbutazine	
ANTIBIOTICS	
Erythromycin	Increased lithium
Metronidazole	level
Spectinomycin	
Tetracycline	Reports conflict as to tetracycline's increasing or decreasing lithium levels

INTERACTIONS OF LITHIUM WITH OTHER DRUGS (cont.)

Lithium May Interact With	Resulting In
BRONCHODILATORS	
Aminophylline	Significantly increased lithium excretion
Theophylline	
ANTIHYPERTENSIVES	
Clonidine	Decreased antihypertensive effect
Methyldopa	Increased lithium level
CARDIAC MEDICATIONS	
Ace Inhibitors	Increased lithium level, increased potassium
Calcium channel blockers (verapamil, etc.)	Possible increased rate of lithium excretion
Digoxin	Serious dysrhythmias if lithium levels are elevated
Quinidine	Decreased lithium effect, possible cardiac conduction effects may be potentiated by lithium
DIURETICS	
Thiazides	Increased lithium concentration, decreased potassium
Indapamide	Increased lithium level
Potassium-sparing agents (amiloride, etc.)	Increased lithium concentration
INSULIN AND ORAL HYPOGLYCEMICS	Increased glucose tolerance (careful monitoring of glucose levels is necessary)

INTERACTIONS OF LITHIUM WITH OTHER DRUGS (cont.)

Lithium May Interact With	Resulting In
ANTICONVULSANTS	
Carbamazepine	Increased carba-mazepine toxicity unless doses of both drugs are modified
Divalproex	Possible decreased lithium level
NEUROLEPTICS	Increased risk of neuro-toxicity, tardive dyskinesia
SODIUM BICARBONATE	Decreased lithium effect

There was a relatively high risk of recurrence of mania following more-or-less abrupt discontinuation of a previously successful lithium maintenance regimen in bipolar-I patients, with over half of the instances of mania arising within the first three months. In addition, these researchers found that the rate of recurrence of new episodes of illness in bipolar-I patients was greater after being taken off lithium treatment than would have been predicted by a patient's earlier course before treatment was initiated, or by a general knowledge of the natural history of the illness. These findings support the widely accepted conclusion that long-term lithium treatment can exert a powerful protective action in many responsive bipolar patients.

In a separate study, these investigators and their collaborators at Centro Lucio Bini in Cagliari, Italy, found that both the risk and speed of recurrence were much higher when lithium treatment was discontinued rapidly—in less than two weeks. Rapid withdrawal of lithium was associated with early recurrence of mania in bipolar-I patients and of depression in both bipolar-I and bipolar-II patients. Slowing the withdrawal of lithium may delay, but not reduce the risk of mania in bipolar-I patients, while it could delay and reduce the risk of recurrences of depression in both bipolar-I and bipolar-II patients.

These studies point to the advantages of gradual discontinuation of lithium—over a period of at least a month—and/or the use of alternative treatments to prevent recurrences, particularly when rapid discontinuation is medically necessary.

How Long Should One Remain on Lithium?

Whether a person should remain on long-term lithium therapy after a bipolar episode has ended depends on many individual factors, and it is a decision requiring close cooperation and discussion by the patient, and doctor, and usually the family as well. Treating someone for a mild illness or one that is not likely to recur for many years, if ever, unnecessarily exposes the patient to all the potential risks and expenses that come with prolonged use of any drug. Unfortunately, it is rarely possible to predict what the course of illness will be. The pattern of recurrence and the severity and the duration of each episode help govern the decision. If episodes are minor and are widely separated in time, long-term medication may not be necessary, although it is usually best to continue treatment for at least four to six months after recovery from an acute episode. Other patients, who experience more severe and frequent episodes, may need to take lithium indefinitely. Dr. Robert Prien of the National Institute of Mental Health reviewed the research on the issue of who should receive long-term lithium therapy and concluded that in either of the following situations, the doctor, patient, and family members should seriously consider long-term lithium therapy:

1. If a patient has two or more severe episodes within a five-year period
2. If one of the episodes was life-threatening or profoundly disruptive to the patient's and family members' lives

But is it safe to take lithium indefinitely? Well, one of John Cade's patients (one of the ten who were first treated with lithium) died of an unrelated illness after 32 years of lithium therapy. He holds the world record for length of recorded lithium treatment.

According to the report on this patient, "B. D.," he had no known episodes of lithium intoxication, and the severity of his mood swings remained attenuated. His kidneys were normal for his age. The 1984 Consensus Development Conference at the National Institute of Mental Health concluded that, with the exception of possible thyroid problems, there are few significant permanent risks from long-term lithium therapy. Earlier fears of functionally significant kidney damage now seem greatly exaggerated. Physicians remain cautious as to the length of time someone should take maintenance lithium; still, these reports are encouraging.

But when all is said and done, how do patients themselves feel about lithium? We asked this on the questionnaire we used in preparing this book and received responses such as these:

- "To finally be off that roller coaster is great."

- "A necessary evil and yet a blessing."

- "Lithium has literally saved my life. Without it, I know I would have committed suicide."

- "I think it's great, except for the weight gain. However, I decided it's better to be fat and sane than skinny and crazy."

- "It is necessary and it works, but I hope for better medications with less side effects in the future."

- "Fine stuff!"

OTHER ANTIMANIC MEDICATIONS

Lithium has gained worldwide acceptance for the treatment of mood disorders, and approximately 70 to 80 percent of bipolar patients respond to it and are not troubled by serious side effects. But where does that leave the 20 to 30 percent who either don't respond or respond only partially, who can't tolerate the side effects or who, for medical reasons, can't take lithium at all? Especially difficult to stabilize are the group of patients known as "rapid cyclers." These are people who have four or more episodes of illness in a one-year period, and their response to lithium is often partial—they still have breakthroughs of mania or depression. If these patients become depressed, the doctor can treat them with an antidepressant, but at a risk of reinducing mania. And so the cycles begin again.

Fortunately things are looking up. There are alternative treatments for these groups of patients. Studies completed within the last few years in Japan and the United States show that two drugs introduced for temporal lobe epilepsy, carbamazepine (Tegretol) and valproic acid or divalproex sodium (Depakene, Depakote), can be effective treatments for acute mania, have uncertain effects in acute depression, and work to prevent future episodes of bipolar illness.

Carbamazepine

Not only has carbamazepine proved effective in the treatment of patients with rapid-cycling bipolar disorder (alone or in combination with lithium), but patients with mixed bipolar states (see pages 47–49) may respond better with carbamazepine than to lithium in both the acute phase of the illness and in the long-term treatment phase. Also, patients who first experience a depressive episode, and then go on to suffer a manic one, with a well interval following, may be better treated with carbamazepine alone or in conjunction with lithium, as opposed to lithium alone.

Determining Dosages Before a patient is started on carbamazepine, he or she needs a medical evaluation, including blood tests to evaluate liver function, blood cell and platelet counts, and iron concentration. These blood tests contribute to the safe use of this agent, and, when repeated, provide a baseline assessment of the functioning of body systems affected by the medication.

The usual starting dose of carbamazepine is 200 to 400 milligrams, which is usually taken in two equal doses in the morning and evening. The dose is gradually increased, based on the individual's capacity to tolerate increasing levels, with the target of reaching a blood level of 6 to 12 mg/ml.

Because carbamazepine strongly induces the activity of oxidative enzymes in the liver, and this causes the drug to be metabolized faster, the carbamazepine level may drop somewhat after the first month of treatment. It is not uncommon for the dosage to be increased at this time. Blood tests are needed more frequently in the beginning of treatment, and every three months or so afterwards. The blood should be drawn 10 to 14 hours after the patient's last dose, usually in the morning before the first dose of the day.

Conversely, several of the newer antidepressants (Prozac, Zoloft, Luvox, and Serzone) inhibit liver enzymes (see chart on pages 141–142) and thereby increase levels of carbamazepine. Combined therapy of carbamazepine and one of these antidepressants should be carefully monitored and will likely require a reduction in the dosage of carbamazepine.

If a dose of carbamazepine is forgotten, the patient should call his or her doctor. Most likely, if less than three hours has elapsed since the dosage time, the patient might be told to take it. If more than three hours has elapsed, he or she may be told to skip that dose and resume taking the allotted medication at the next regularly scheduled time.

The most common side effects of carbamazepine are dizziness, drowsiness, unsteadiness of gait, confusion, headaches, double vision, nausea, diarrhea, and rash. Many of these side effects don't last beyond the first week or so of treatment.

There have been some reports of bone marrow suppression (aplastic anemia) with carbamazepine. While very rare— one in 50,000 cases—this is a life-threatening condition. Therefore, it is good practice for the patient to have a red blood cell count weekly at first, and every three months thereafter. Photosensitivity (the skin's extreme sensitivity to sunlight), easy bruising, fever, sore throat, and purple spots on the skin may be early symptoms of this potentially lethal development, and the carbamazepine should be stopped immediately. After the first few months on carbamazepine, the risk of aplastic anemia becomes smaller.

Carbamazepine should always be stored away from sources of heat and out of contact with direct sunlight. The medication should not be kept in the bathroom medicine cabinet or in any humid place because humidity may cause it to lose one-third or more of its effectiveness. The tablets can absorb the moisture, harden, and so become less soluble and less well-absorbed when taken. The FDA recommends that carbamazepine be dispensed in limited amounts during humid weather, using moisture-proof containers.

Women on birth control pills should understand that carbamazepine interferes with the contraceptive ability of the pills (it accelerates their normal breakdown and makes them less reliable). There are other drugs that interact adversely with carbamazepine, and they are listed in the following chart.

INTERACTIONS OF CARBAMAZEPINE WITH OTHER DRUGS

**Increased Carbamazepine Levels and
  Toxicity Produced By:**
Erythromycin (and similar agents)
Triacetyloleandomycin
Viloxazine
Isoniazid

INTERACTIONS OF CARBAMAZEPINE WITH
OTHER DRUGS (cont.)

Verapamil
Diltiazem
Fluoxetine (Prozac)
Sertraline (Zoloft)
Fluvoxamine (Luvox)
Nefazodone (Serzone)
Propoxyphene (Darvon and others)

Decreased Carbamazepine Levels Produced By:
Phenobarbital
Phenytoin (Dilantin and others)
Primidone

Carbamazepine Diminishes Effects Of:
Neuroleptics (decreases blood level)
Phenytoin (decreases levels of both drugs)
Valproate
Ethosuximide
Theophylline
Dexamethasone
Dicumarol
Warfarin
Pregnancy tests
Oral contraceptives
Thyroid hormone (decreases thyroid levels)
Corticosteroids (decreases levels and therapeutic
   response to steroids)
Barbiturates
Tricyclic antidepressants
Benzodiazepines

Divalproex Sodium (Depakote)

Reports of the antimanic effects of the anticonvulsant drug valproic acid were published over 25 years ago. Since then, well-
controlled studies and the growing clinical experience of
psychiatrists indicate that valproic acid (Depakene) and its
sodium salt, divalproex (Depakote), are similar to lithium in
efficacy, may benefit patients who do not respond to lithium or

carbamazepine, and are often better tolerated than either. Divalproex sodium is not only effective during a manic phase, but acts to prevent or reduce the severity of further mood swings.

As with carbamazepine, before a patient is started on divalproex, he or she needs a medical evaluation to gauge liver function, blood cell and platelet counts, and iron concentration. These tests contribute to the safe use of divalproex sodium and, when repeated, provide a baseline assessment of the body systems affected by the medication.

Divalproex sodium (Depakote) is supplied in 125, 250, and 500 milligram tablets or capsules. A patient is usually started on 250 to 500 milligrams a day and the dose is increased by 1 or 2 tablets or capsules a week to obtain plasma concentration of 50 to 100 mg/ml (usually at 1000–1500 milligrams a day). Some patients, however, may require up to 5,000 milligrams a day of the drug. Most people improve gradually after starting divalproex sodium and it may take up to several weeks for the drug to take effect. It is not uncommon for a physician to prescribe additional medications on a short-term basis until the divalproex sodium takes hold.

Blood tests to ensure a therapeutic level are needed more frequently when divalproex sodium therapy is started and less frequently as blood levels are stabilized. The blood should be drawn 10 to 14 hours after the patient's last dose, usually in the morning before the first dose of the day.

The side effects of divalproex sodium are generally mild. Drowsiness, indigestion, nausea, and vomiting sometimes occur, but these side effects usually subside a week or two after the target dose is achieved and the body adjusts to the medication. Taking divalproex sodium with meals may diminish any nausea. A thinning or loss of hair has been reported, but is usually resolved over time, even with the continued use of the medication. The use of a multivitamin with zinc and selenium is often used to protect against this unwanted side effect.

A rare side effect of divalproex sodium is liver toxicity (hepatotoxicity). Most cases of this potentially catastrophic side effect have been reported in children under the age of ten who had been taking the drug for the treatment of a seizure disorder. In almost all of the cases that involved an adult, the patient was taking divalproex sodium with another anticonvulsant, including carbamazepine, phenobarbital, phenytoin (Dilantin), or barbiturates. Therefore, it is contraindicated to combine any of these drugs with divalproex sodium for the treatment of bipolar disorder.

As mentioned above, liver function studies via a simple blood test are measured before a patient is started on divalproex sodium; every week at the beginning of the treatment, and less frequently after the first few months. Nausea, vomiting, fatigue, weakness, swelling of the ankles, jaundice (yellowing of the eyes or skin), or easy bruising may be signs of liver toxicity and must be reported to the physician immediately.

The chart below lists the drugs mentioned above as well as some others which should not be taken in combination with divalproex sodium.

Always store divalproex away from sources of heat and out of contact with direct sunlight and *always* out of reach of children. Do not store the medication in the bathroom medicine cabinet or in any humid place because heat and moisture may cause it to break down.

Unlike carbamazepine, divalproex sodium does not interfere with the contraceptive ability of oral contraceptives.

DRUGS TO BE AVOIDED WHEN TAKING DIVALPROEX SODIUM

Barbiturates
Benzodiazepines (clonazepam [Klonopin*], diazepam [Valium], lorazepam [Ativan*])
Phenytoin (Dilantin)
Phenobarbital

DRUGS TO BE AVOIDED WHEN TAKING
DIVALPROEX SODIUM (cont.)

Carbamazepine (Tegretol)[†]
Alcohol (valproate and alcohol may produce central
nervous system depression)

Note: Caution is suggested with aspirin because the interaction of aspirin
and valproate may cause higher valproate blood levels. There also may be
an adverse interaction with the blood thinner warfarin (Coumadin) and the
risk of bleeding may be increased.

---

[*]Although the additive effect of Klonopin or Ativan in combination
with divalproex may produce sedation, some clinicians use this combination
to enhance sleep, decrease anxiety, and diminish hypomanic symptoms.

[†]Severe bipolar disorder unresponsive to a single mood stabilizer may
rarely lead to combination treatment of carbamazepine with divalproex.
Blood levels of both drugs should be monitored carefully.

Clonazepam and Lorazepam

Another anticonvulsant drug, clonazepam (Klonopin), as well
as the anti-anxiety agent and sedative lorazepam (Ativan), can
provide clinically useful sedation in acute mania. These members of the benzodiazepine family produce no movement disorder or anticholinergic side effects (see pages 149–151). Like
neuroleptics, they act more rapidly than lithium in acute mania
and commonly are used while waiting for lithium to work.

While clonazepam and lorazepam control manic features
such as pressured speech, racing thoughts and hyperactivity, they
have not been demonstrated to be effective for psychotic symptoms such as delusions and hallucinations and have not been
shown to have sustained mood-stabilizing effects like lithium and
the anticonvulsant divalproex sodium and carbamazepine.

Lamotrigine and Gabapentin

Although there have been no controlled clinical trials to prove
its efficacy as a mood stabilizer, the anticonvulsant lamotrigine

(Lamictal) has been found to be effective in some cases of refractory bipolar disorder and treatment-resistant depression. It's possible that lamotrigine has more of an antidepressant effect than other anticonvulsants, but this also remains to be studied.

When lamotrigine is used as an antidepressant or as a mood stabilizing agent, the final dose of the drug is usually between 100 and 200 milligrams daily, although some individuals require dosages as high as 400 milligrams.

Most people tolerate the drug well, but side effects such as gait disturbances, dizziness, and headaches have been reported, as well as dosage-related allergic skin rashes. Because divalproex sodium (Depakote) can double the blood levels of lamotrigine, patients already on Depakote require a halving of the lamotrigine dosage.

Gabapentin (Neurontin), a new anti-epileptic drug that was designed to mimc the action of the inhibitory neurotransmitter GABA, is also increasingly being prescribed for patients with refractory mood disorders. Because the drug is quickly metabolized, it needs to be taken three times daily.

The drug seems to have few adverse effects; however, there have been reports that some children with attention deficit disorder with hyperactivity (ADDH) and developmental delays can develop an intensification of behavioral problems, such as tantrums and aggressive behavior. In adults the most common reason for discontinuing treatment with gabapentin is sedation.

ANTIPSYCHOTIC MEDICATIONS

Patients who suffer from severe mania, psychotic depression, and schizoaffective illness may also suffer delusions and hallucinations and may also hear "voices." The antipsychotic (or neuroleptic) drugs such as Thorazine and Haldol—the same class of drugs that calm and reduce the symptoms plaguing a schizophrenic patient—calm and stabilize the patient experiencing acute mania and psychotic depression. While lithium or an anticonvulsant would prevent states like this from occurring in the future, they can take days to weeks to become effective. Meanwhile, in order to make the patient more comfortable and ensure his or her safety during a particularly vulnerable period, an antipsychotic drug might be used during the first week or two. As the lithium or anticonvulsant takes hold, the antipsychotic is discontinued slowly.

Antipsychotic medications have another use in treating some patients. There are a certain number of people for whom lithium by itself does not work. In such cases, a supplementary drug such as an antipsychotic or an anticonvulsant (discussed on pages 139–146) is sometimes added to the medication regimen.

Antipsychotic drugs were originally used for their antihistaminic quality in surgery. French physician Henri Laborit quickly noticed that patients who were given an antihistaminic became remarkably calm. In one of the great understatements in history, Dr. Laborit commented to his colleagues, "It must have an application in psychiatry."

He began to talk to the French psychiatric establishment about his findings, but he failed to arouse much enthusiasm. "Psychiatrists didn't believe that chemical molecules could have an effect on the human brain, especially when it came to human pathology," he recalled in an interview with Richard Restak for *The Brain.* One surgeon who attended a conference given by Laborit went home and told his psychiatrist brother-in-law, Pierre Deniker, about the Laborit findings with the antihistaminic chlorpromazine. By 1952 Pierre Deniker and another psychiatrist, Jean Delay, completed their first clinical trials with chlorpromazine and reported its enormous potential. The drug diminished delusional thought and hallucinations. Before long, this new psychiatric drug was being used all over the world.

The chart on the next page lists the eight different chemical classes of antipsychotic drugs, their generic names, and their trade names. (Generic refers to the official name for the chemical compound; trade names are the brand names used by drug companies for marketing purposes. For example, Thorazine is the trade name of the generic chemical chlorpromazine.)

Because there is up to a 50-fold difference in the milligram potency (the antipsychotic effect per milligram) of each drug, there is a correspondingly large variance in the prescribed doses. For instance, because haloperidol (Haldol) is approximately 45 times as potent as chlorpromazine (Thorazine), a patient given 450 milligrams of chlorpromazine would be receiving approximately the same amount of antipsychotic benefit as a patient given 10 milligrams of haloperidol.

Generally the antipsychotic medications are prescribed in tablet or liquid form, and usually are taken once or twice a day. Many of these drugs can be given as a short-acting intramuscular injection. Fluphenazine decanoate (Prolixin) and haloperidol decanoate (Haldol) can be given as a long-acting "depot" injection in oil that lasts from two to four weeks.

COMMON TYPES OF ANTIPSYCHOTIC MEDICATIONS

Type	Generic name	Trade name
aliphatic phenothiazines	chlorpromazine	Thorazine Chlorprom Largactil
	promazine	Sparine
piperidine phenothiazines	thioridazine	Mellaril
	mesoridazine	Serentil
piperazine phenothiazines	fluphenazine	Prolixin Permitil
	trifluoperazine	Stelazine Pentazine
	perphenazine	Trilafon Phenazine

COMMON TYPES OF ANTIPSYCHOTIC MEDICATIONS (cont.)

Type	Generic name	Trade name
thioxanthines	thiothixene	Navane
	chlorprothixene	Taractan
butyrophenones and cipheryl butyl piperidine	haloperidol	Haldol
	pimozide	Orap
	droperidol	Inapsine
	loxipine	Loxitane
dibenzoxazepines	clozapine	Clozaril
dihydroindolone	molidone	Moban
		Lindone
benzisoxazole derivative	risperidone	Risperdal
pirenzepine	olanzapine	Zyprexa

Side Effects

Among the most common side effects of an antipsychotic drug are constipation, blurring of vision, drowsiness, and dry mouth, but these often diminish or disappear as a person becomes accustomed to the medication.

Also common (but extremely frightening to a patient who has not been warned of them) are the side effects that involve movement and posture: dystonic reactions, akinesia, and akathisia. These are transient, treatable, and reversible and are defined as follows:

- Dystonic reactions. These are involuntary muscle contractions that cause bizarre and uncontrolled movements of the face, neck, tongue, and back and an uncontrolled rolling of the eyes (counteracted in minutes by the antiparkinson agents such as Artane or Cogentin).
- Akinesia. This is characterized by stiffness and diminished spontaneity of gestures, physical movement, and speech (counteracted by Artane or Cogentin).

- Akathisia. This is a feeling of internal restlessness—inability to sit still, as well as a subjective sensation of discomfort often described as anxiety, and often mistaken for agitation rather than a side effect of the antipsychotic drug (counteracted by propranolol [Inderal]).

These movement disorders can be dealt with by lowering the dose of the antipsychotic medication, adding an antiparkinson drug, or switching to another class of neuroleptic. Generally, the more sedating the neuroleptic, the less likely it is to cause movement disorders. A physician might want to select a low-potency, more sedating drug such as a thioridazine (Mellaril) or chlorpromazine (Thorazine) to minimize the likelihood of movement abnormalities for the patient.

Antipsychotic drugs can cause menstrual changes in women, breast discharge in both sexes, and a diminished sex drive. They can also cause sexual dysfunction in men, for example, retrograde ejaculation (ejaculation occurs but the seminal fluid passes backward into the bladder), anorgasmia (the inability to have an orgasm), or impotence.

There may be a tendency to gain a great deal of weight on an antipsychotic medication. The reasons why this occurs have not been conclusively determined, but it could become a serious problem and should be watched carefully.

Another side effect (especially common with low-potency neuroleptics) is the development of a sensitivity to the sun, or photosensitivity. Patients who have it may burn very easily. Exposure to the sun should be very limited, and sun-screen lotions with a high sun-protection factor should be used.

Tardive Dyskinesia

Perhaps the most publicized side effect of antipsychotic drugs is tardive dyskinesia, "late appearing movement disorder." It is

THE SOMATIC THERAPIES | 151

characterized by involuntary facial grimacing, lip smacking, chewing and sucking movements, cheek puffing, and wormlike movements of the tongue. Writhing movements of the body, or jerky, purposeless movements of the arms and legs, complete this disfiguring but unpainful picture. Tardive dyskinesia may not reverse itself, and the peak risk for the patient occurs when he or she has been on a neuroleptic for one to two years.

There are ways to minimize the risk. A person should be put on the lowest dose necessary to control the psychotic symptoms, and the doctor should regularly attempt to reduce the dose. Frequent monitoring by the physician will reveal early symptoms of tardive dyskinesia and the medication can be discontinued.

Before the FDA approved the use of lithium for manic-depressive illness, neuroleptics were the only drugs that could control some of the psychotic symptoms of a manic phase. Today the use of lithium and anticonvulsants prevents manic or psychotic depressive episodes to a degree that alleviates the need for long-term use of neuroleptics at high doses. As stated earlier, if an antipsychotic drug is needed, it is usually for only a short period of time, or if it is part of a drug regimen, it can usually be prescribed at low doses. The specter of tardive dyskinesia, while still a possibility, is not now the threat it once was for people with manic-depressive disorders.

Atypical Antipsychotics

Newer atypical antipsychotic medications like Clozaril and Risperidone have far fewer movement side effects and are increasingly used in place of older antipsychotic drugs. Indeed, several uncontrolled studies indicate that Clozaril may be quite effective in the treatment of schizoaffective disorder. Many anecdotal reports point to a mood elevating effect that may make it particularly useful for patients with schizoaffective disorder in depressed states.

MEDICATIONS FOR DEPRESSION

A psychiatrist or physician can treat a person suffering from depression in a number of ways: with tricyclic antidepressants; with monoamine oxidase inhibitors (MAOIs); with new types of antidepressants like Prozac, Zoloft, Wellbutrin, or Effexor; and with electroconvulsive therapy (ECT). If there is a history of recurrent depression, the patient may be treated with lithium or an anticonvulsant and an antidepressant during the acute depressive episode, and remain on the lithium or anticonvulsant alone thereafter in order to prevent future episodes.

Tricyclics and Related Antidepressants

Tricyclic antidepressants were discovered in the 1950s when the Swiss pharmaceutical firm Geigy tested a compound that resembled chlorpromazine's chemical structure. The animal data looked good, so they gave the new compound, imipramine, to psychiatrist Roland Kuhn. Dr. Kuhn began trials with schizophrenic patients, but imipramine did little to help their delusions and hallucinations. It did, however, have remarkable effects on depressed patients, as it elevated mood and activated behavior.

Dr. Kuhn reported his results with the drug in a paper given at the Second International Congress of Psychiatry at Zurich in 1957, but only about 12 people attended the session. Fortunately the news spread rapidly thereafter. A new class of drug was added to the psychiatric armamentarium, and many, many patients were helped. The other pharmaceutical houses in Europe and America rushed to produce their slightly altered versions (the "me too's") of tricyclic antidepressants.

The tricyclics (named with a nod to their three-ring chemical structure) were just the beginning. Today there are antidepressants with a four-ring structure (Ludiomil), and an atypical antidepressant called trazodone (Desyrel) that doesn't resemble the tricyclics or the tetracyclics. Newer antidepressants such as fluoxetine (Prozac), sertraline (Zoloft), and paroxetine

(Paxil) act directly on the serotonergic system and have relatively few side effects.

Typically, a psychiatrist may start a patient on 25 to 50 milligrams of a tricyclic antidepressant and increase the dosage each day until the effective daily dosage is reached. Patients should not expect to feel better immediately. For reasons the researchers are still puzzling out, it often takes three to four weeks for a person to experience relief from depression (see pages 83–84 for a possible explanation). Some patients, after a few weeks of the treatment, feel their depression lift almost overnight. They simply wake up feeling good. Others report that their symptoms improve slowly over a period of days to weeks.

Although all patients have individual response patterns, the usual sequence of events that occurs when a person is treated with a tricyclic antidepressant is as follows:

1. The patient notices an improvement in sleep disturbance within the first few days of therapy.
2. Other people note the changes, although the patient may not feel greatly improved.
3. Within two to three weeks the patient finds himself or herself more interested in people, in surroundings, and in activities.
4. The patient feels better as the symptoms recede or disappear.

Side Effects

Each of the antidepressants can cause varying degrees of side effects, which fall into the following three categories:

- sedation (drowsiness or sleepiness)
- anticholinergic effects (dry mouth, blurred vision, constipation, difficulty urinating, increased heart rate)

- orthostatic hypotension (light-headedness or dizziness
  when rising quickly from a sitting or lying position)

The more infrequently reported side effects of tricyclic antidepressants are:

- skin rash
- sweating
- tremor
- altered orgasmic function
- weight gain

In the best of all possible worlds, the drugs that doctors
prescribe would affect only target symptoms—those for which
relief is sought. This, unfortunately, is not the case, especially
with the tricyclic antidepressants. In addition to interacting
with the chemical substances norepinephrine or serotonin, the
tricyclic antidepressants block the acetylcholine receptors at
the junctions between nerve fibers and internal organs or the
brain. The blockade at the salivary glands is responsible for dry
mouth; the blockade at the iris of the eye causes blurred vision.
Constipation and urinary retention can occur because these
drugs affect the system that regulates the contractions of the
intestines and bladder. These side effects are called *anticholinergic,* and they are usually more annoying than worrisome.

If a drug has weak anticholinergic activity, the blockade is
less complete and the side effects are less noticeable. High or
strong anticholinergic activity means a patient can usually expect
more of the dry mouth, blurred vision, constipation, and so on.
However, it is important to keep in mind that many patients
respond well to antidepressants with higher anticholinergic
activity, and that side effects may decrease with continued use as
the body adjusts.

There are several ways to minimize the categories of side
effects caused by antidepressants. The symptoms of dry mouth

can be alleviated partially by stimulating the saliva by sucking on *sugarless* candies or chewing *sugarless* gum. When a patient is particularly troubled by the symptom, a doctor may prescribe a saliva-stimulating medication like pilocarpine. Because a lack of sufficient saliva may indirectly lead to tooth decay and gum problems, it is very important that the patient pay attention to oral hygiene.

While constipation is indeed a possible side effect of a tricyclic antidepressant, it is associated frequently with the depressive syndrome itself and may actually stop being a problem as the antidepressant begins to have an effect. If constipation does occur as a side effect of the antidepressant treatment, the patient should increase intake of fruits, vegetables, and other sources of fiber and ensure adequate fluid intake. If these measures fail, the psychiatrist may prescribe a stool softener or a laxative or switch the patient to an antidepressant with less risk of anticholinergic side effects.

The light-headedness caused by orthostatic hypotension can be minimized by rising to a sitting position slowly, and sitting for a few seconds before standing.

Some people are helped by the sedating side effects of some antidepressants: they begin to sleep better, and they are less troubled by anxiety and agitation. But there are those who find the sedation troubling and would like to get up in the morning feeling less groggy. Then, too, some people have to drive or operate machinery and cannot afford to feel sedated or drowsy. There is always the possibility of switching to another, less sedating antidepressant, or lowering the dosage or taking the medication at the hour of sleep.

The chart on pages 156–157 outlines the range of dosages and the side effects of the commonly prescribed antidepressants.

Some patients require a higher dose of an antidepressant than others. One of the reasons for an incomplete response is the failure of some doctors to prescribe adequate doses of antidepressants. (Many patients who are referred to affective disorders clinics because they do not respond to treatment are found to have been treated with inadequate doses of the medications. They often recover when the dosage is raised.) A depression not treated aggressively is demoralizing and potentially dangerous to a patient. Therapeutic blood levels can be recommended for several of the tricyclic antidepressants, most notably nortriptyline and imipramine. To ensure that the dosage of medication is adequate, the physician may order blood tests to determine the antidepressant level.

Caveats

It's ironic that the very drugs that treat depression and stave off suicidal impulses can be used to express them. An acute overdose of 10 to 15 times the usual adult therapeutic doses can cause convulsions, a coma, or even death in adults, and even smaller amounts may prove fatal to children. For this reason, a doctor faced with a potentially suicidal patient may choose to administer the treatment in a hospital setting, or to limit each prescription to a one-week supply and to monitor the blood levels to ensure that the patient is not saving up a supply, or to prescribe fluoxetine (Prozac), which has little capacity to cause death if a patient takes an overdose.

COMMON ANTIDEPRESSANT MEDICINES

Generic name	Trade name	Usual daily starting* dose (mg)	Usual effective daily dose* (mg)	Relative sedative effects	Relative anticholinergic effects	Relative hypotensive effects
"Tricyclic" and related antidepressants						
amitriptyline	Endep Elavil	50–75	150–300	high	very high	more

*Lower doses (often ⅓ to ½ of the usual dose) are used with older patients.

COMMON ANTIDEPRESSANT MEDICINES (cont.)

Generic name	Trade name	Usual daily starting* dose (mg)	Usual effective daily dose* (mg)	Relative sedative effects	Relative anticho- linergic effects	Relative hypo- tensive effects
amoxapine	Asendin	50 three times daily	150–400	medium	low	less
clomipromine	Anafranil	25	100–150	more	high	more
desipramine	Norpramin Pertofrane	50	100–300	low	moderate	more
doxepin	Adapin Sinequan	75	75–300	high	high	more
imipramine	SK-Pramine Tofranil	50–75	150–300	medium	high	more
nortriptyline	Aventyl Pamelor	50	50–150	low	medium	less

Atypical antidepressants

Generic name	Trade name	Usual daily starting* dose (mg)	Usual effective daily dose* (mg)	Relative sedative effects	Relative anticho- linergic effects	Relative hypo- tensive effects
bupropion	Wellbutrin	100 two times daily	300–450	very low	low	low
fluoxetine	Prozac	20 before 3 p.m.†	20–80	very low	low	low
nefazadone	Serzone	50 twice a day	200–400	medium	low	low
paroxetine	Paxil	20	20–50	low	low	very low
sertraline	Zoloft	50	150–200	low	low	low
venlafaxine	Effexor	75 two– three times daily	150–250	low	low	medium

†Insomnia may result if taken too close to the hour of sleep.

Adapted and reprinted with permission from *Depression and Its Treatment* by John H. Greist, M.D., and James W. Jefferson, M.D. (Washington, DC: American Psychiatric Press, Inc., 1984).

A psychiatrist would rarely give a tricyclic antidepressant to a person with cardiovascular disease, cardiac arrhythmia, thrombophlebitis, hyperthyroidism, or a history of narrow-angle glaucoma or increased intraocular pressure. Therefore, it is good medical practice for the patient to have a physical examination, electrocardiogram, and routine blood tests before an antidepressant is prescribed.

Bipolar patients should be aware that treatment of depressive episodes with antidepressants may induce a rapid switch into hypomania or mania, or increase the frequency of cycles of illness. For these reasons, antidepressants administered without a mood-stabilizing medication (lithium, Depakote, or Tegretol) are contraindicated for long-term use in bipolar patients. The newer antidepressant, bupropion (Wellbutrin), discussed on pages 167–168, may be less likely to induce cycling in bipolar patients.

Patients who wear soft contact lenses and take antidepressants may have some special problems. The anticholinergic side effect of decreased tearing may lead to excessive deposits of thick mucoid secretions on the contact lenses, and this may cause an itching, gritty sensation under the lenses. A patient should be sure to mention the use of contact lenses to his or her physician. Should a problem occur, the doctor can prescribe a different antidepressant, reduce the dosage, or prescribe the use of artificial tears.

Older patients often can tolerate a lower dosage of antidepressants and are most likely to tolerate agents with a low risk of anticholinergic side effects (see chart, page 238).

The Matter of MAOIs

At about the time that tricyclic antidepressants made their debut, doctors noticed that an antibiotic, iproniazid—a monoamine oxidase inhibitor used for the treatment of tuberculosis—was producing a euphoric effect in the patients taking it. Because the patients felt too good to take proper precautions with their illness, the physicians switched them to another medication, and the antibiotic retreated to the drug company's shelf inventory.

Two American psychiatrists, George Crane and Nathan Kline, reported favorably on its mood improvement characteristics and helped resurrect the drug. Within one year, approximately 400 thousand people were given iproniazid.

Many were helped, but unfortunately the rose hid thorns: several people who took the drug developed problems ranging in seriousness from headaches, jaundice, or cerebral hemorrhage. The FDA recommended iproniazid's removal from the market, and the drug company complied.

Today, there are three classes of monoamine oxidase inhibitors (MAOIs as they are called) used in this country. Although doctors are concerned that they can cause dangerously high blood pressure if patients are not careful about what they eat and that there can be adverse reactions when they are taken with certain other drugs, the MAOIs are increasingly recognized as a useful treatment in depression. The drugs lack the severe anticholinergic side effects of the tricyclic antidepressants, and they can be used by patients with heart disease. Moreover, these drugs often work when all others fail, and seem to be increasingly useful for patients with so-called atypical depression (those who eat excessively, sleep for irregularly long periods of time, are lethargic, feel worse later in the day, experience extreme anxiety or fear, or are hypochondriacal). For certain patients who do not respond to tricyclic antidepressants, or who will not opt for electroconvulsive therapy, the MAOIs just might make the difference and return the patient to health.

The three MAOIs available in the United States are phenelzine (Nardil), tranylcypromine (Parnate), and selegiline (Eldepryl).

MONOAMINE OXIDASE INHIBITORS

Generic name	Trade name	Usual daily therapeutic dose*
phenelzine sulfate	Nardil	60–90 mg
tranylcypromine sulfate	Parnate	30–50 mg
selegiline	Eldepryl	50–60 mg

*All the dosages noted above are approximate. Some patients respond to lower dosages than those listed; others may require higher dosages.

The common side effect profile of the MAO inhibitor drugs include: low blood pressure or dizziness after standing up, but also mild, sustained increases in blood pressure; weight gain; sleep disturbance (which may be insomnia for some patients and sleepiness for others); delayed orgasm or the inability to have an orgasm (anorgasmia); and fluid retention in the ankles and fingers. Less common side effects resemble those characteristically caused by tricyclic antidepressants (dry mouth, constipation, blurry vision, and difficulty urinating), and, in some patients, a hypomania.

The two most commonly prescribed MAO inhibitors in this country are phenelzine sulfate (Nardil) and tranylcypromine sulfate (Parnate). Nardil seems to cause more weight gain than Parnate, but Parnate is more activating and tends to cause more sleep disturbance for patients.

Restrictions When Using MAOIs

The dietary prohibitions for patients taking MAOIs need some explaining. The body has within it a marvelous mechanism for halting neurotransmitter activity. The monoamines norepinephrine, dopamine, and serotonin are "retired from service" by an enzyme located within nerve endings and in other tissues called monoamine oxidase (MAO). It breaks down the monoamines to alcohols or acids. But since depression is thought to be caused by a deficiency of norepinephrine or serotonin, the inhibition or blockade of the monoamine oxidase increases the amount available for transmission.

Certain foods contain the amine tyramine or other blood-pressure-elevating monoamines. Normally tyramine is metabolized by monoamine oxidase in the gut and liver, but a person taking an MAOI cannot metabolize it efficiently, and the tyramine enters the general circulation in abnormally high concentrations. Once there, it can stimulate the release of norepinephrine, whose levels are increased also by the MAOI treatment, and so cause a sudden, sometimes dangerous increase in blood pressure. Such a hypertensive reaction can cause symptoms ranging from throbbing headaches, nausea and vomiting to a potentially catastrophic rupture of blood vessels in the brain—leading to stroke or death. Therefore, although an MAOI definitely combats the problems of depression, its use is safe only in the absence of the foods, drinks, and medications that in combination with an MAOI would be dangerous for the patient. (They are listed on the next pages.)

The signs of elevated blood pressure are: a headache at the back of the neck, a stiff neck, a pounding heart, nausea and vomiting, or sudden collapse. If a patient feels any of these symptoms, he or she should stop taking the MAOI and go immediately to a doctor's office or a hospital emergency room. The patient should explain the type of medication he or she is taking and have his or her blood pressure taken. If it is dangerously elevated, the medical personnel will probably prescribe a blood-pressure-lowering agent such as phentolamine (Regitine). Some doctors instruct their patients to carry a medication called nifedipine (Procardia, Adalat) with them at all times. If the symptoms of elevated blood pressure develop, the patient should place a capsule under his tongue, and proceed to the nearest emergency room. The nifedipine will bring the blood pressure down quickly, but the staff at the emergency room should be informed immediately that the patient is on an MAOI and may be experiencing a hypertensive crisis. Patients taking MAO inhibitor medications should also investigate the possibility of wearing a medical alert bracelet or carrying a medical alert card in their wallet.

In addition, a person taking an MAOI must not use nose drops or cold remedies such as Contac or Nyquil—anything that shrinks the mucous membranes. These cold medications are pharmacologically similar to tyramine and norepinephrine and thus can't be metabolized when an MAOI is in the picture.

They'll concentrate in the blood and also provoke increases in blood pressure by releasing norepinephrine or by their own direct actions.

FOODS AND BEVERAGES TO BE AVOIDED WHILE TAKING MONOAMINE OXIDASE INHIBITORS

The following foods should be avoided completely:
Aged cheeses of any kind and foods prepared with them, such as pizza and fondue (cottage cheese, cream cheese, and farmer's cheese are allowed)
Yogurt
Liver (including pâté)
Fermented sausages (bologna, pepperoni, salami, summer sausage)
Pastrami, corned beef
Bean curd, miso soup; soy sauce, teriyaki
Salted or smoked fish (lox, nova, etc.)
Caviar, snails (preserved)
Pickles
Pickled fish (herring, etc.)
Fava beans, lima beans, Italian beans, or Chinese pea pods
Yeast products (Bovril, Oxo, Marmite, dietary supplements containing brewer's yeast). *Note:* Baked goods made with yeast are allowed.
Avocado (especially overripe; guacamole)
Figs (overripe, canned, or spoiled), bananas (overripe)
Soups (canned and "instant soup" powders)
Chianti, champagne, imported beers, nonalcoholic beer, whiskey, Chartreuse, and Drambuie

The following foods and beverages may cause problems in large amounts, but are less troublesome in small quantities:

Alcohol	Caffeinated beverages
Sour cream	(coffee, tea, cola, cocoa)
Chocolate	Sauerkraut

Warning: One can "cheat" on this diet with impunity at one time and go on to suffer a hypertensive crisis at the next ingestion of that same food or liquid.

Only fresh foods—no overripe, fermented, or spoiled foods—should be eaten.

DRUGS TO AVOID WHILE TAKING MAO INHIBITORS

Cold remedies (Contac, Nyquil, TheraFlu, Alka-Seltzer Plus, CoTylenol, Dimetine Decongestant, etc.)

Nasal decongestants, nose drops

Most sinus, allergy, hay fever, and asthma medications

Local anesthetics that contain epinephrine (dentists have Novocain without epinephrine)

Demerol

Barbiturates and surgical anesthetics

Stimulants such as cocaine, amphetamines (for example, some diet pills)

Opiates and some nonopiate analgesics such as meperidine

Tricyclic antidepressants

Fluoxetine (Prozac)

Bupropion (Wellbutrin)

Certain amino acids, especially 5-hydroxy-tryptophan (5HTP)

Other MAO inhibitors, especially Parnate

A patient on an MAOI should take *no other medications* unless they've been cleared by the physician prescribing the MAOI—especially no barbiturates or opiates. Demerol, in particular, is potentially lethal because of a central nervous system reaction of unknown basis. Patients who need surgery and require a surgical anesthetic should be taken off the MAOI several days prior to the operation.

So who is a candidate for the value MAOIs have to offer? Obviously someone with a good memory, someone with the ability to look at a piece of pizza and think, "cheese," and someone with the desire to sacrifice and stick to the dietary prohibitions in order to recover health. They're tricky, without a doubt. They also work—sometimes when nothing else does.

Prozac

The late 1980s saw the introduction of two novel antidepressants that have very quickly established themselves as useful tools in the psychiatric armamentarium: fluoxetine (Prozac) and bupropion (Wellbutrin). Prozac has garnered more patient testimonials and media publicity than almost any drug in history, and it made more money in its first two years on the market than any other psychotropic drug.

Newsweek magazine placed a giant Prozac capsule on its March 1990 cover and subtitled its report "A Breakthrough Drug for Depression." *New York* magazine also devoted a cover to the drug emblazoned with the words "A New Wonder Drug for Depression." The propaganda aside, it is obvious why patients and doctors like Prozac. For most people, the drug has fewer side effects than the tricyclic antidepressants or the MAO inhibitors. Prozac doesn't cause the distressing weight gain of those medications; in fact, it can promote a small weight loss in some people. Of greater significance, Prozac has little capacity to cause death if a patient takes a substantial overdose. Early reports indicate that the medication may prove to have an important place in the treatment of chronic depression and dysthymia (see pages 51-52) and other psychiatric disorders such as obsessive–compulsive disorder, panic-agoraphobic syndrome, and bulimia nervosa.

Prozac is a selective serotonin-uptake inhibitor; initially, it acts principally to increase the levels of serotonin at synaptic junctions. Because the drug is highly selective for the serotonergic system, it produces fewer of the side effects associated with the traditional antidepressants, such as dry mouth, constipation, dizziness, and blurred vision (the anticholinergic side effects discussed on pages 149-151). Many patients on Prozac report that they don't even feel they are taking a medication, but the common side effect profile includes insomnia, nervousness or agitation, nausea, diarrhea, and headaches. For many patients, these side effects subside after the initial adjustment period of two or three weeks. The sleep problem can sometimes be dealt with by taking the drug in the morning. Sometimes a sleep medication is prescribed along with the Prozac.

Less common side effects include drowsiness, yawning, increased sweating, and rashes. Many men and women have complained of a delay of orgasm or of difficulty having an orgasm or of a loss of libido while on the medication. These sexual side effects may be countered or reversed with the adjunctive use of bupropion (Wellbutrin) or yohimbine (Yocon).

It should be noted that all classes of antidepressants, including the new SSRIs (Prozac, Zoloft, Paxil, etc.), can cause an acceleration in the frequency of cycling in bipolar depressed patients. Should hypomania develop, the treating psychiatrist should be notified immediately and the drug should be stopped. A different antidepressant might be tried later, often in conjunction with lithium or Depakote (see pages 172–175).

Prozac now comes in 10 and 20 milligram capsules and in a liquid formulation. Most people get the antidepressant effect with 20 milligrams a day, but some people seem to need and can tolerate higher doses. There are also some patients who receive the antidepressant benefit by taking one pill every other day. The capsules are not cheap; they cost over $2.00 apiece. Like the other drugs used to combat depression, Prozac may take three to five weeks to deliver a full antidepressant effect.

Perhaps the greatest area of concern about Prozac has centered around a handful of accounts that imply the drug might be associated with suicidal or other aggressive thoughts or actions for some patients. This came to national attention when Dr. Martin Teicher and his colleagues, researchers at Harvard, reported the cases of six patients who became obsessed with violent suicidal thoughts two to seven weeks after starting treatment with Prozac. Four of the six attempted to hurt or kill themselves.

In their report in the *American Journal of Psychiatry,* Dr. Teicher and his team carefully explained all the possibly confounding factors (rarely did Dr. Teicher explain them on all the televised interviews that followed): four of the patients were on other medications as well as Prozac, and five of the patients had contemplated suicide or attempted it in the past, although none seemed actively suicidal at the time they began treatment with Prozac. There is some speculation that because Prozac is specific to the serotinergic system—the system that may contribute to mediating aggression—it may, for a few people, "tip the balance in the wrong direction, toward violence and aggression," according to Dr. Teicher.

However, a study conducted by Drs. Maurizio Fava and Jerrold Rosenbaum from Harvard Medical School failed to confirm the Teicher group's findings about Prozac. Knowing of the imminent Teicher report, Drs. Fava and Rosenbaum surveyed 27 psychiatrists who had treated some 1017 depressed outpatients with antidepressants during 1989. The surveyed psychiatrists knew nothing of the Teicher findings and were relatively unbiased.

Patients included in the study had been treated with Prozac alone, Prozac and tricyclics, tricyclics alone, or with lithium. None of the patients reported intense suicidal thoughts to the degree described in Dr. Teicher's six cases. Dr. Fava and Dr. Rosenbaum point out in their report that the Teicher patients had been unresponsive to earlier treatments and had severe side effects to Prozac, which included marked agitation or anxiety. The Prozac doses were raised rather than reduced despite the agitation, and other drugs were prescribed with Prozac—drugs that can also cause agitation (antipsychotics, stimulants, etc.). Drs. Fava and Rosenbaum concluded that though their study was not vast, the difference in suicidal ideation occurring only after initiation of treatment was not significant between patients treated with Prozac alone and those receiving other antidepressant treatments (a worsening of symptoms and suicidal preoccupation have been very rarely reported with other antidepressants). In the evaluation of these reports, one must take into account that suicidal thinking and behavior are commonly experienced during depressive mood states, whether or not the patient is taking an antidepressant.

Unfortunately, the Teicher report drew the attention of the Church of Scientology, which has used it to wage a propaganda campaign against psychiatry in general and the Eli Lilly Company, the developer and manufacturer of Prozac. Following the cult's long-held belief that "Psychiatry Kills," it has targeted Prozac and issued highly negative press releases (which have been picked up and published by newspapers around the country), appeared actively on the talk-show circuit, and even lobbied Congress and the FDA to ban Prozac. (In the past, this group has gone after the makers of Ritalin for hyperactivity in children.)

Dr. Teicher has stated publicly that the Scientologists's use of his paper is "absolutely irresponsible." He feels they are distorting his research to "advance their purpose, which is to destroy psychiatry."

Eli Lilly countered the charges by publishing the results from the clinical trials conducted before Prozac entered the American market. The data on over 3000 depressed patients actually revealed a lower tendency toward suicidal thinking with Prozac than with other antidepressants, or with the placebos given to a control group.

Today, some 21 million people world-wide have used Prozac safely and effectively. Prozac's entry into the marketplace was glitzy and dramatic, yet it was accompanied not only by hype, but hope. Long-term data has yet to reveal anything untoward, and for many, many people it has proved to be a miraculous ally against the shadow of depression.

Bupropion

Bupropion (Wellbutrin) is an antidepressant of the aminoketone class that is pharmacologically distinct from tricyclics, MAOIs, and SSRIs. It acts primarily on the noradrenergic system and has some weak dopaminergic properties, with no effect on serotonin.

Following its first introduction in the United States, it was quickly withdrawn from the market because of its tendency to induce seizures. This association with seizure risk, however, may have been overstated. In dosages less than 450 mg, the seizure incidence is comparable to that of most tricyclic antidepressants.

Like that of the SSRIs, the side effect profile of bupropion is different from that of the traditional antidepressants. Dr. Dennis Charney of Yale reported that in the placebo-controlled studies that he and his colleagues conducted, side effects only rarely allowed the clinicians to guess who was on bupropion and who was on placebo, but excitement and agitation, high blood pressure, insomnia, nausea, and tremor have been reported. Other adverse reactions include headaches and rashes. Weight gain and sexual dysfunction rarely occur with bupropion. In fact, it is commonly used in lower dosages (75–100 mg) adjunctively to reverse the sexual side effects of the SSRIs.

Bupropion may offer a particular advantage for bipolar patients because of the reported diminished likelihood to induce hypomanic episodes and cycle acceleration. While no controlled studies exist to confirm this belief, it has become the antidepressant of choice for many clinicians who treat bipolar patients.

Bupropion is supplied in 75 milligram and 100 milligram tablets. A patient is usually started at 75 milligrams two or three times a day, with doses taken at least six hours apart, but not after 6:00 P.M. The usual effective daily dose is between 200 and 300 milligrams, with some patients requiring up to 450 milligrams. Because of the increased risk of seizures at higher doses, a patient should not take more than 150 milligrams in any one dose, unless directed to do so by a physician.

A new sustained-release-dosage form is currently under evaluation. Wellbutrin SR reduces the drug peak serum levels that can provoke a seizure, and in trials of 4000 patients who received the investigational dosage form, only 3 patients experienced a seizure. This 0.08 percent incidence is comparable to that observed with the SSRIs.

Newer SSRIs

Sertraline (Zoloft), paroxetine (Paxil), and fluvoxamine (Luvox) were marketed in the United States after Prozac and are equally effective antidepressants that share a similar side effect profile. The most common side effects are sleepiness, insomnia, agitation, nausea, diarrhea, dry mouth, and abnormal ejaculation. Many of these side effects may dissipate over time as the body adjusts to the medication.

All of the SSRIs can produce withdrawal symptoms— including withdrawal hypomania—and therefore need to be tapered slowly during the discontinuation period. This is even more important with Paxil and Luvox because of their shorter half-lives.

Like all other antidepressants, the SSRIs may induce hypomania or mania in bipolar patients, although some clinicians have observed that they may be less offensive than the tricyclic antidepressants. If one of the SSRIs is used in combination with a mood stabilizer for the treatment of a depressed bipolar patient, it would be wise to choose one with a shorter half-life for quick clearance of the drug should a hypomania develop.

Nefazadone (Serzone) Serzone was introduced in 1995 and shares many of the properties of the SSRIs. Indeed, it is a serotonin reuptake blocker but also acts as an antagonist of the $5HT_2$ receptor. The initial treatment dose recommended by the manufacturer was 100 mg twice daily, but for many patients this dose was found to produce sedation, mental confusion, and low blood pressure. Therefore, many clinicians initiate treatment with a lower dosage strength—usually 50 mg for the first few nights— and then increase the dose to 50 mg twice daily to prevent these unpleasant side effects.

After the initial adjustment period, many patients require a dosage higher than 50 or 100 mg a day. In fact, some clinicians have found it necessary to prescribe in excess of the maximum recommended dose of 600 mg daily, in order to receive a full response.

As with all SSRIs, Serzone can produce nausea in the early treatment phase, but it appears to promote sleep and to be less offensive in causing sexual dysfunction—in particular delayed orgasm. It causes neither weight gain nor weight loss.

Venlafaxine (Effexor)   Effexor has a unique pharmacological profile suggesting that it may have clinically meaningful effects on both the noradrenergic and serotonergic systems. It combines the properties of an SSRI and a tricyclic antidepressant without the anticholinergic side effects such as dry mouth, blurriness of vision, constipation, and orthostatic hypotension. Effexor was introduced with the promise that it would produce a faster antidepressant effect, and several inpatient studies have suggested that this in fact may be the case.

The usual starting dose is 75 mg administered two or three times daily. Depending on tolerability and clinical effect, the dose is increased at no less than four-day intervals.

Effexor has been found to have a potent dose-dependent antidepressant effect with the rate of response increasing as the dosage is increased. For this reason it may prove particularly useful for more severely depressed patients.

One of the disadvantages of Effexor is that it must be administered twice or three times daily, depending on the dosage prescribed. It also has a tendency to elevate blood pressure, and therefore it is recommended that blood pressure be monitored regularly when dosages of greater than 100 mg are prescribed.

NEWER ANTIDEPRESSANTS AND THEIR EFFECTS ON LIVER ENZYMES

Prozac, Zoloft, Paxil, Luvox, Serzone, and Effexor, to varying degrees, inhibit one or another of the liver enzymes that metabolize certain other medications. These enzymes are known as P-450 isoenzymes, and their inhibition can result in increased levels of the medications listed in the following chart.

ANTIDEPRESSANT INHIBITION OF CYTOCHROME P-450 ISOENZYMES

Prozac	Zoloft	Paxil	Luvox	Serzone	Effexor
phenytoin (Dilantin)	phenytoin		theophylline, caffeine, TCAs, tacrine		
diazepam (Valium)	diazepam				
hexobarbital	hexobarbital				
methobarbital	methobarbital				
tolbutamide	tolbutamide				
propranolol (Inderal)	propranolol				
TCAs, antipsychotics, type IC antiarrhythmics, codeine, beta blockers	TCAs (weak), antipsychotics, type IC antiarrhythmics, codeine, beta blockers	TCAs, antipsychotics, type IC antiarrhythmics, codeine, beta blockers			TCAs, antipsychotics, type IC antiarrhythmics, codeine, beta blockers
carbamazepine (Tegretol)	carbamazepine	alprazolam (weak)	carbamazepine	carbamazepine	
alprazolam (weak) (Xanex)	alprazolam		alprazolam	alprazolam	
triazolam (Halcion)	triazolam		triazolam	triazolam	
terfenadine (Seldane)	terfenadine		terfenadine	terfenadine	
astemizole (Hismanal)	astemizole		astemizole	astemizole	
				cigapride (Propulsid)	

Therefore, if a patient is taking any of the medications listed, careful consideration should be given to the choice of SSRI. If there is no alternative but to take a medication that interacts with one of the SSRIs, then blood levels must be monitored if possible (not all drugs have such tests) and/or the dosages of both interacting medications should be reduced and any and all side effects noted.

How Long Should One Remain on an Antidepressant?

Studies show that about 70 percent of depressed patients who stopped taking an antidepressant 5 weeks or less after they became symptom-free relapsed; 42 percent of those who discontinued treatment 11 to 20 weeks after becoming symptom-free relapsed; but the relapse rate fell to 14 percent among those who had been symptom-free for over five months before discontinuing treatment. In other studies, the risk of relapse after coming off medication at 6 and 12 months following initial recovery from an acute episode of unipolar major depression was approximately 65 percent and 50 percent, respectively. In other words, a longer period of time on the medication lessens the chances of the patient falling ill again, even after the clinical recovery from an acute depressive episode.

Therefore, many psychiatrists prescribe an antidepressant for at least six months to a year after an episode of major depression. Afterward, there is a carefully supervised process during which the dosage is reduced gradually over a period of several weeks. Abruptly discontinuing the medication may precipitate withdrawal symptoms such as restlessness and anxiety, as well as various bodily discomforts.

Combined Antidepressant and Lithium Treatment for Depression

Studies from the NIMH Collaborative Project on the Psychobiology of Depression indicate that approximately 25 percent of patients with severe depressions show little or no improvement despite antidepressant trials that appear to be adequate with respect to dose (at least 150–200 milligrams per day of imipramine or its equivalent) and duration (4 to 6 weeks). Another group of patients whose depressive illness remits for only brief periods of time may relapse even with intensive treatment. Such patients are referred to as "treatment resistant," and, lately, much attention has been focused on their improved treatment.

Several prominent research groups have reported that many patients with true treatment-resistant depressions have improved considerably when they were given a combination of a standard antidepressant *and* lithium. In one study, 31 percent of previously unresponsive patients had a complete remission of symptoms while 25 percent improved significantly. Dr. Dennis Charney of Yale has reported that about 10 percent of patients whose tricyclic antidepressant was augmented by lithium had a "miracle response" in a matter of days. Fifty to seventy percent responded within one to three weeks.

Something else is also becoming apparent as more clinicians institute combined lithium and antidepressant treatment. Not only does lithium enhance the response to the antidepressant drug, but this combined treatment appears to accelerate the response rate by as much as 50 percent: Some patients seemed to recover from acute depression in 7 to 10 days rather than the several weeks it usually takes for recovery on an antidepressant alone.

Drs. Linda Austin, George Arana, and James Ballenger called attention to this early-response phenomenon of lithium augmentation in an article in the *Journal of Clinical Psychiatry.* We've extracted one of their case reports here to illustrate their findings.

Ms. C, a 49-year-old woman with a DSM-IIIR diagnosis of major depression with psychotic features, recurrent, had a 3-week history of depressed mood, extreme anhedonia, severe psychomotor retardation, loss of energy, decreased ability to think and speak, fearfulness, poor hygiene, and mild paranoid ideation. Ms. C. had been hospitalized for severe depression three times previously; her hospitalizations ranged from four to nine months in duration. On one occasion she had responded to ECT and fluoxetine. However, she failed to comply with the prescribed regimen of medication as an outpatient and quickly relapsed.

At admission, Ms. C lay all day in bed, refusing to speak. On day four after admission, she was treated with nortriptyline (a tricyclic antidepressant) and gradually increasing doses of lithium. By day eight, her blood levels of the medications were where the doctor wanted them to be. (Ms. C was also treated with 10 milligrams of the antipsychotic medication Haldol for 15 days because of the paranoid ideation.)

Ms. C remained in bed except for brief periods until day 11 (after 7 days of nortriptyline therapy); on that day she was found out of bed, dressed, and wearing jewelry and makeup. Her affect remained flat and constricted, but by the next day she was able to attend occupational therapy and became social with the staff and patients. On day 13, after 9 days of lithium and nortriptyline medication, Ms. C smiled, joked and socialized normally. She was discharged on day 25. Ms. C was eventually maintained on her regimen of discharge medications and remained normal at follow-up nine months later.

The authors of the report felt that the side effects of the combined treatment may be minimized by using the combination of lithium and the antidepressant for the initial month of treatment only and subsequently maintaining the patient on tricyclic treatment alone.

These findings have particular implications for inpatient care. Not only would the terrible suffering of a patient be curtailed by using a lithium-augmentation therapy, but the length of stay within a hospital would be shortened significantly. Today, this treatment strategy is becoming more and more common.

A New Treatment Strategy For Recurrent Unipolar Depression

As we mentioned in the first pages of this book, not all people who suffer a major depression suffer a recurrence, but there are a significant number of patients who go on to develop repeated episodes. Psychiatrists typically have combattled recurrence in a number of ways: Each episode was treated separately with an antidepressant that was withdrawn several months after clinical recovery, or the dose of medication was slightly lowered and continued for an extended period. Alternately, lithium carbonate therapy can be instituted or added. But even with these maintenance strategies, recurrences can and do occur.

Now the results of a sizable, well-controlled study by Dr. Ellen Frank and her colleagues at the University of Pittsburgh reveal that an established antidepressant (imipramine) combined with interpersonal psychotherapy kept the majority of patients from relapsing into depression for the five-year duration of the study.

Actually, the investigators found that if they continued the patients on the same dosage of antidepressant given to pull them out of the depression rather than lowering the dosage to a hypothetical "maintenance" level, they could prevent another episode from developing 80 percent of the time. In other words: "The dose that gets you better, keeps you better," said Dr. David Kupfer, co-principal investigator of the study when interviewed by *The Psychiatric News.*

This study was unique in that only patients with a history of two or more previous episodes of depression were enrolled and each patient's previous episode had to have occurred no longer than two and a half years prior to the present episode. (It should be noted that, before entering the study, this group of patients had been experiencing a recurrence of depression at approximately six-month intervals.) The 128 patients selected were assigned to one of the following five treatment plans:

1. Twenty-eight of the patients received the antidepressant imipramine at an average daily dose of 200 milligrams.
2. Twenty-three of the patients were given placebos.
3. Twenty-six patients received no medication but were in talking therapy once a week for the first twelve weeks of treatment, then every other week for eight weeks, and then monthly for the rest of the three-year period. (The talking therapy was one specifically designed for depression and known as Interpersonal Psychotherapy (IPT). This type of therapy is discussed on pages 205–206.)
4. Twenty-six of the patients received a placebo and the talking therapy described.
5. Twenty-five patients received the full dose of imipramine as well as the talking therapy.

At the end of the 3–5 year study period, those who received only a placebo had a 20 percent chance of remaining relapse-free; the group who received full doses of imipramine and psychotherapy had an 80 percent chance of remaining episode-free for the entire period. These excellent results of the combined medication and psychotherapy treatment suggest the possible added value of a talking therapy in the comprehensive treatment of recurrent unipolar depression. (Psychotherapy will be discussed in more detail in Chapter 6.)

Which patients will likely benefit from long-term antidepressant treatment? Those who have experienced a rapid recurrence of illness (two episodes within a two- to three-year period), patients who experience residual symptoms between episodes, and those with multiple episodes (several over a five-year period) or a history of early onset.

While this farsighted view of treatment—focusing on preventive strategies—will likely benefit many, a note of caution needs to be sounded. Frequent recurrent episodes of depression, particularly those that don't respond to antidepressants, should raise the suspicion that the patient may actually have an undiagnosed bipolar disorder. The increased use of antidepressants for longer durations of time, then, may provide a more fertile setting for the induction of hypomanias and manias, as well as cycle acceleration in these patients.

As psychiatrists begin to address the issue of recurrence in unipolar depression, no doubt other effective treatment strategies will evolve. However, the findings from this long-term study offer hope to those whose lives are paralyzed by the dreadful anticipation of future depressive episodes.

ARE GENERICS JUST AS GOOD?

Once a medication regimen is decided upon, the psychiatrist will write the prescription for the drug or drugs. At this point, the patient may have a choice between using a generally more expensive brand name drug or a generic version. The question then arises: Is the generic version just as good as the brand name drug?

Maybe. With a few exceptions, most generic companies have good reputations, but in order to make an informed decision, all patients should understand what a generic drug is and what kind of standards the generic manufacturers are held to by the Food and Drug Administration (FDA).

Most people assume that a generic drug is precisely the same as a brand name one. They reason that once a drug is off patent, a generic company—unburdened by the astronomical costs of research and development laboratories, sales forces, and advertising—can hand a patient the same drug for less. While there's a bit of truth to this (the generic companies usually spend far less to conduct business), generic drugs are not identical to their brand name counterparts—nor are they required to be identical.

The active chemical ingredients of a brand name or a generic drug must be the same, and the strength, the route of administration, and the dosage form (tablet versus capsule) must also be identical. But the FDA allows other variables: The inert ingredients such as binders, fillers, color, and flavoring can differ, as well as the manufacturing process itself. And these variables can affect the "bioavailability" of the drug: the amount of the drug that enters the bloodstream and thus can reach the central nervous system.

Because it is rare for two products to be perfectly super-imposable, the FDA has chosen to pick what appears to be a reasonable percentage deviation—the so-called "20/20" rule (alternately referred to as the 80/80 or 20/80 rule). This means that 80 percent of the 18 to 24 healthy volunteers taking a single dose of the generic product should achieve a blood level that is within the range of 20 percent above or 20 percent below the level achieved when these healthy volunteers take a single dose of the brand name medication. Many generics are on the average no more than 10 to 15 percent different than the brand name product, and some brand name manufacturers produce their own generics so as to ward off other generic manufacturers and retain market share.

Because a brand name company has its name before the public eye and wishes to maintain and extend the confidence of physicians, pharmacists, and patients, the brand name manufacturer constantly monitors its products, undertakes postmarketing surveillance studies in the population of people who are sick and being treated with the medication and whose ages vary widely (generic companies are not required to do this), and usually has more quality control of its product. This is not to say that there are not highly ethical and reliable generic manufacturers. The problem is that a patient on a long-term prescription can be doing well on a generic medication, but there is no guarantee that month after month the pharmacy will fill the prescription with that same product by that same manufacturer. Availability and price and profit-margin factors influence the pharmacist's or the supplying distributor's buying patterns. At the very least, patients who find that their symptoms are controlled on a particular generic prescription should get the manufacturer's name from the pharmacist and request the same manufacturer's drug the next time the prescription is filled. Patients who understand the vagaries of non-brand-name prescription filling can alert the treating psychiatrist if the side effect profile changes or if the drug seems less effective. If a patient switches to or from a generic, the psychiatrist should monitor blood levels after the switch.

SAMPLE MONTHLY COST COMPARISON OF THREE BRAND NAME DRUGS AND THEIR GENERIC COUNTERPARTS*

	Agent	mg/day	Dollars/month
Brand name	Tofranil	150	$93.57
Generic	imipramine	150	25.77
Brand name	Elavil	150	$64.09
Generic	amitriptyline	150	12.89
Brand name	Norpramin	150	$104.21
Generic	desipramine	150	84.99

*Based on 1996 data.

It behooves all patients to comparison shop for their medications. There is a wide variance in price, as the chart indicates. Also, buy the largest-size tablet or capsule available, consistent with the dose needed. A patient taking 150 milligrams of imipramine a day would pay less for three 50 milligram tablets than if he or she takes the daily dose in six 25 milligram tablets.

ELECTROCONVULSIVE THERAPY (ECT)

During the writing of this book, we reviewed a videotape that had been made to teach medical students at the Albert Einstein College of Medicine in New York how to administer electroconvulsive therapy or ECT. The tape began with an interview of a woman suffering from severe depression. She had been unresponsive to medications, had been depressed for eight months, and sat hunched in a chair. She refused to look at the doctor conducting the interview, and she gave short, irritable, and hopeless-sounding answers to the questions asked of her. When the ECT treatment was described to her, she didn't seem to feel it (or anything else) could help.

Toward the end of the tape, and after three treatments of ECT, the viewer sees this woman sitting in the same chair, in the same room, but now dressed up and not only looking directly at the doctor, but also laughing and teasing him about something he's said. The woman, at the end of the video, actually tells the doctor that she would recommend the treatment to other people in her situation. The before–after differences in the woman are so marked that it occurred to us that a person viewing this tape and unfamiliar with ECT would strongly suspect that the talents of an actress had been employed to convince people that ECT wasn't really so bad.

ECT has been an option in the treatment of depression (and intractable mania) for over 50 years. There's been a resurgence of interest in it because it has evolved into a safe option, and one that works. But for a public influenced by Ken Kesey's *One Flew Over the Cuckoo's Nest,* whose associations with electric shock start with the electric chair and move on to lightning bolts, electric eels, and third rails, it makes for queasy conversation, for all of us. Let's replace a few of the myths with facts.

The idea that electrical stimulus can be a therapeutic agent goes back to before A.D. 43, when the torpedo fish was used to shock people to treat headaches. Physicians in the twentieth century (erroneously) thought that schizophrenia was rare among epileptics and decided that seizures might prevent the schizophrenia. Somewhere in the 1930s, Dr. Ladislas Meduna injected patients with the stimulating drug metrazol, induced a seizure, and found that 70 percent of his depressed patients got well. At about the same time, Dr. Manfred Sakel used injections of insulin to produce coma in depressed patients and noted that there was improved functioning after the treatment. Two physicians in Italy, Drs. Ugo Cerletti and Luigi Bini, began to look at the data on this chemical convulsive treatment and thought that they could achieve a desired neural discharge by applying an electric current to the temples of a human being. They gave the treatment the distressing label *l'elettroshock.*

Before we describe the procedure, let us state that ECT has a higher success rate for severe depression than any other form of treatment. It can be life saving and produce dramatic results. It is particularly useful for people who suffer from psychotic depressions or intractable mania, people who cannot take antidepressants because of problems of health or lack of response, and pregnant women who suffer from depression or mania. A patient who is very intent on suicide, and who would not wait three weeks for an antidepressant to work, would be a good candidate for ECT because it works more rapidly. In fact, suicide attempts are relatively rare after a course of treatment has started.

ECT is usually given three times a week. A patient may require as few as 3 or 4 treatments or as many as 12 to 15. Once the family and patient consider that the patient is more or less back to a normal level of functioning, it is usual for the patient to have one or two additional treatments in order to prevent relapse. Today the method is painless, and with modifications in technique it bears little resemblance to the treatments of the 1940s.

The patient is put to sleep with a very short-acting barbiturate, and then the drug succinylcholine is administered. This medicine temporarily paralyzes the muscles so that they do not contract during the treatment and cause fractures. Then an electrode is placed above the temple of the nondominant (usually right) side of the head, and a second is placed in the middle of the forehead (this is called unilateral ECT); or one electrode is placed above each temple (this is called bilateral ECT). A very small current of electricity is passed through the brain, activating it and producing a seizure. Because the patient is anesthetized and the body is totally relaxed by the succinylcholine, he or she sleeps peacefully while an electroencephalogram (EEG) can be used to monitor the seizure activity and an electrocardiogram (EKG) monitors the heart rhythm. The current typically is applied for a fraction of a second, and the patient breathes pure oxygen through a mask. The duration of a clinically effective seizure ranges from 25 seconds to sometimes longer than a minute, and the patient wakes up 10 to 15 minutes later.

Upon awakening, a patient may experience a brief period of confusion, headache, or muscle stiffness, but these symptoms typically ease in a matter of 30 to 60 minutes.

The setting and composition of the treatment team are important factors in reducing the risks associated with ECT. During the few seconds following the ECT stimulus there may be a temporary drop in blood pressure. This may be followed by a marked increase in heart rate and a rise in blood pressure. Heart rhythm disturbances occasionally occur during this period of time, but generally subside without complications. For this reason, however, and because there is always risk (although very small) associated with even very short-acting anesthetics, a hospital setting with a treatment team composed of a psychiatrist, an anesthesiologist, and nursing personnel trained in ECT procedures and recovery can decrease the risk of complications. A patient with a history of high blood pressure or other cardiovascular problems should have a cardiology consultation prior to treatment.

Because as many as 50 percent of the people who respond well to a course of ECT relapse within 6 months of the treatment, a maintenance treatment of antidepressants or lithium is advisable. Patients who have responded to a course of ECT and who may not be able to tolerate, or have been unresponsive to trials of antidepressant medication, may be advised to continue single ECT treatments at monthly or six-week intervals. While there is no research support for this maintenance ECT practice, it may be of use in the preventive treatment of recurrent depression.

Short-term memory loss has always been a concern to patients who receive ECT and the doctors who administer it, but several studies conclude that patients who received unilateral ECT performed better on attention/memory tests than those who received bilateral ECT. However, there is a question as to whether the unilateral method is as effective. Experts agree that changes in memory function do occur and persist for a few days following treatment, but that patients return to normal within a month. A 1985 Consensus Conference convened at the National Institute of Mental Health concluded that while some memory loss is frequent after ECT, it is estimated that less than one-half of 1 percent of ECT patients suffer severe memory loss. Memory problems resulting from ECT usually clear up within seven months of the treatment, although there may be a persistent memory deficit for the period immediately surrounding the ECT treatment.

How Does ECT Work?

Animal research shows that ECT enhances dopamine sensitivity, reduces the reuptake of serotonin, and activates the systems in the brain that use norepinephrine. It also increases the amount of the major inhibitory neurotransmitter, GABA, yet much remains unclear about its mechanism of action.

How Distressing Is ECT to Patients?

While there are certainly patients who perceive the treatment as terrifying and shameful, and some who report distress about persistent memory loss, many—like the woman in the video— speak positively of the benefits. An article entitled "Are Patients Shocked by ECT?" reported on interviews with 72 consecutive patients treated with electroconvulsive therapy. The patients were asked whether they were frightened or angered by the experience, how they looked back at the treatment, and whether they would do it again. Of the patients interviewed, 54 percent considered a trip to the dentist more distressing, many praised the treatment, and 81 percent said they would agree to have ECT again. Those are comforting statistics about a treatment that has an ugly name and ugly connotations but sometimes beautiful and even lifesaving results.

6

WORKING THROUGH: DENIAL, ACCEPTANCE, AND THE PSYCHOTHERAPIES

Prior to the availability and widespread use of lithium and antidepressants, individuals in this country who had mood disorders were treated with psychotherapy. This process involved the therapist and the patient in a dialogue intended to reveal unconscious causes or determinants of the symptoms. Today, thanks to ever-expanding knowledge about the nervous system and the medicines that affect it, and a more refined system of diagnosis, treatment practice has moved in a different direction—these disorders are viewed primarily as medical disorders. In the rush to spread the good word about the new drug treatments, psychotherapy was dismissed by some or viewed as unnecessary.

This view was short-sighted. Simply relegating these disorders to the realm of physiological disturbances that require only medical treatment is a serious clinical oversight and a gross scientific presumption, similar to those of the earlier psychological oversimplifications and prejudices. Complex psychological and biological factors combine before, during, and after an episode of depression and mania, and it is often difficult to know which of these elements are primary and which are secondary to the development of a mood disorder. Psychological conflicts can produce attitudes and behaviors that are maladaptive and that can encumber an individual, while also serving to precipitate episodes of illness or to retard recovery. These disorders affect mood, thinking and behavior, and vitally influence a person's view of himself and his relationships with others. The problem—as well as its solution—now rests firmly in the realms of medicine *and* psychology.

AN INTEGRATED TREATMENT APPROACH

A widely accepted strategy in a commonsense treatment plan is to relieve painful symptoms by the appropriate medication while educating the patient and his family members about the nature and course of the disorder, as well as the expected effects and course of treatment. Medications can indeed relieve the symptoms of depression and mania for most people, but the alleviation of symptoms is not the whole story, especially for those who suffer recurrent episodes. The advent of a recurring or chronic illness such as an affective disorder represents a significant loss for an individual. There is a loss of function and a loss of confidence and security. Questions—Why me? What did I do to deserve this? Will I be able to accomplish my life goals? What will happen to my relationships? Can I have a family?—will loom large for an individual. Each person will deal with the questions and the answers in his or her own way, but make no mistake: there will be an emotional response to the illness. All will have to come to terms with feelings of anger, sadness, and shame. (These issues become even more complicated if parents, siblings, or other relatives have the illness—not an uncommon occurrence with a disorder that is heavily familial.) These feelings and questions need to be addressed, but that can happen only in the context of an integrated treatment plan where the therapist and patient talk about more than symptoms and prescriptions. An adjunctive psychotherapy is recommended.

In the most fundamental sense of the word, psychotherapy is a dialogue between two people in which the patient has the respectful attention of a professional trained to elicit information. The professional, through clarification and interpretation, helps the person see things about himself or herself in a realistic light—one not clouded by a lingering sense of worthlessness or victimization. In the treatment of a recurrent affective disorder this can mean many things. Psychotherapy can strengthen the capacity to cope, help the person to understand and come to terms with the vulnerability, and develop an adaptive way of coping with interpersonal problems that emerge or are magnified as a result of the illness.

This respectful dialogue between patient and therapist may at first focus on the acceptance of the need to take medication. The taking of any medicine, and especially a psychotropic drug, can raise highly charged psychological issues. The medicine may become a concrete symbol of a chronic illness, a nagging reminder that something within is not working as it should. For anyone, a deficit—something that makes one more vulnerable in relation to others—has the potential for decreasing one's sense of self-worth. This deficit may be experienced as a slight that is reinforced daily by the taking of medications. There may be a wish to deny the illness, and this may lead to a person's discontinuing the prescribed drugs.

Many people feel: "I've been well for a while; I've beaten this. I don't need the drugs anymore." It is not uncommon for patients to go off the medications a number of times, testing their limitations. This often (but not always) results in further episodes. Unless there is an early recognition of the symptoms of an impending swing and a treatment intervention, there will again be disruptions in family life, work, and social relationships. This returns the patient to square one and further disturbs his or her sense of self-worth.

Some patients are very upset by the idea that it is not their own will but a medication that is responsible for preserving control over their behavior, mood, or judgment. They may view the lack of psychological control as a weakness. These feelings can lead to a rather negative attitude about the taking of medication and may complicate or prevent accepting the disorder and its medical treatment and entering into a collaborative relationship with the doctor.

An illness that changes mood and affects thought processes makes it extremely difficult for the person experiencing the changes to sort out which feelings are valid and should be acted upon and which are symptoms of an impending swing. Often, a person with recurrent mania or depression will need to learn to distinguish between normal human mood changes and episodes of illness. One young man in California complained that he felt disenfranchised from his feelings. If he was elated, he worried that it was the beginning of a hypomanic period, and if he was blue, that it was the beginning of a descent into a hellish depression. He spoke about his worries and doubts with his psychiatrist, and after noticing on repeated occasions that the mood change did not progress to extremes, he was better able to accept his normal expression of emotion.

This sort of discussion and learning about oneself is a critical element in the treatment of affective disorders. If an individual can learn to recognize the symptoms of an impending mood swing, it can be short-circuited by talking to the doctor. The physician, alerted early, is then in a position to adjust the medication and hopefully prevent relapse.

Furthermore, if a person can recognize changes in behavior, alterations in thinking, and changes in the pattern of relationship with others early during periods of mood swing, he or she may be able to temper this behavior and thus prevent potential embarrassment. One 24-year-old man said that when he becomes slightly hypomanic, he presents his employer with all kinds of ideas. Sometimes he is given the go-ahead to implement a project, and then finds himself out of the hypomanic period and out of steam—thus risking his credibility. He has learned to wait and consider things carefully before racing ahead. A woman who begins manic cycles with buying sprees has decided to divest herself of credit cards in order to protect against financial ruin. Self-awareness and the capacity for control can be enhanced. On the other hand, a person mustn't stifle and inhibit ambition and creative drive; a balance must be achieved. These complicated issues are fruitful areas for discussion and clarification with an informed therapist.

How else can psychotherapy be useful? An ongoing dialogue that examines fears and behavior can help one relinquish the defenses and coping strategies that were marshalled during episodes of illness, but which may no longer be adaptive or necessary once maintenance medication has stabilized the mood swings. Some people have become overly dependent on family members; others have withdrawn from all social situations. When asked to name the most enduring and painful aspect of having this disorder, one woman said, "I personally hesitate to be in any kind of a group for fear that I'll do something embarrassing that I'll later regret." This fear and inhibition about being with other people is a persisting problem for many who suffer mood disorders, even years after they have been stabilized on a medication. Others never lose the painful sense of humiliation about what they did during a manic episode and how people reacted toward them afterward. The shame of one's behavior during a manic episode can linger long after the symptoms of the episode have disappeared.

Bipolar patients suffer another kind of humiliation during the recovery period. During the manic episode they may have felt more creative and intelligent, more able to accomplish things they never thought possible. These feelings of great exaltation, self-importance, and power are difficult to give up. Once out of the manic phase, however, the patient needs to face himself and assess his natural limitations and the realities of his life. The insult to the patient's self-respect can be enormous when he realizes that he not only had a false sense of his abilities, but must also now deal with the fact that he has a psychiatric disorder.

A woman with a bipolar disorder elegantly summed up her need for an integrated treatment combining medications and psychotherapy when she wrote:

> I cannot imagine leading a normal life without lithium. From startings and stoppings of it, I now know it is an essential part of my sanity. Lithium prevents my seductive but disastrous highs, diminishes my depressions, clears out the webbing of my disordered thinking, slows me, gentles me out, keeps me in relationships, in my career, out of a hospital, and in psychotherapy. But psychotherapy heals, it makes some sense of the confusion, it reins in the terrifying thoughts and feelings, it brings back hope, and the possibility of learning from it all. Pills cannot, do not, ease one back into reality. They bring you back headlong, careening, and faster than can be endured at times. Psychotherapy is a sanctuary, it is a battleground, it is where I have come to believe that I someday may be able to contend with all this. No pill can help me deal with the problem of not wanting to take pills, but no amount of therapy can prevent my manias and depressions. I need both.

But psychotherapy does more than pick up the pieces in the aftermath of an episode. There are often personality traits, issues of early loss, unconscious conflicts, and stressors that can contribute to the development and course of a mood disorder: these can be identified, explored, and worked through in psychotherapy. A person with low self-esteem, or negative expectations of life and people, or one who is unduly dependent on others may be predisposed to depression. (Conversely, these personality traits may be engendered or amplified by repeated bouts of illness.) An introverted person who cannot reach out to people and who is socially withdrawn may also be susceptible. While these personality traits may not cause depression, they could serve to reduce the threshold for mood disorder or foster the onset of an affective illness.

Early or unmourned loss may significantly reduce the threshold for a mood disorder. A person may have a "psychological fault line," so to speak, which can amplify or trigger a genetic vulnerability. This geological metaphor proposes that some people have a profound vulnerability in the psyche—a childhood trauma, real or perceived, or a loss of attachment that is buried and denied and never set right. Individuals with this vulnerability may have developed constraining and stressful thought and behavioral patterns in order to avoid dealing with the emotional pain that resulted from the trauma or conflict. As the years go by, the pressure builds, and, if other acute or chronic stresses are experienced, an emotional earthquake can be triggered.

The early loss of a parent or a significant loved one can produce such a fault line. A young child's experience of stable, consistent, and supportive parents gives him or her a sense of self-worth, a belief in the predictability and trustworthiness of others, and a favorable model on which to build future relationships. Within such a nurturing atmosphere, personality becomes structured adaptively, a child develops resiliency and becomes increasingly capable and independent. If all goes moderately well, a person may be able to respond with some equanimity to life changes, separations, and losses. An untimely loss of a parent by death or divorce or illness, however, may result in a lasting vulnerability or worsen a preexisting genetic vulnerability, thus predisposing an individual to depression in adulthood.

Caroline, an unusually competent professional woman who had managed to steer clear of the residue of feelings and inner conflict surrounding the death of her father at an early age, turned as an adult to the task of helping others in her professional life as a pediatric nurse. Then, at the age of 40, she discovered that her husband was having an affair. At first, she reacted to this infidelity with hurt and anger, threatening to leave her husband if he continued seeing the other woman. Yet within days Caroline sank into the depths of a severe depression, overwhelmed by intense feelings of worthlessness and by her fear of being alone and uncared for. Her sleep became interrupted and fitful, her appetite greatly diminished, and anxiety overwhelmed her ability to concentrate on the details of everyday life. She berated herself for making a poor choice of a marital partner and began to view her whole life as meaningless. These symptoms persisted for several months.

By our current definitions, Caroline had lapsed into a major depression. Her husband's infidelity and the potential loss of a 14-year relationship naturally unleashed a torrent of feelings, but these feelings about her present situation were suffused with and complicated by the long-withheld, unmourned loss of her father.

Entering into therapy with a psychiatrist, Caroline began to unburden herself by expressing the intense feelings of loneliness she felt. Slowly, the buried memories of deep yearning for her father became conscious. While the antidepressant the psychiatrist prescribed provided relief from the acute and paralyzing symptoms of agitation, guilt, loss of appetite, and sleeplessness, only the psychotherapeutic dialogue was able to bring her into touch with her own feelings and submerged needs. Caroline and her therapist were able to understand that some of the anger and disappointment she felt about her father were indirectly displaced onto her husband, thus contributing to his estrangement. Over time, Caroline and her husband were able to work out their problems, improve their communication, and thus the quality of their relationship. Psychotherapy sealed the fault line and Caroline began to better understand herself, her husband, and the problems that had come between them.

All of the above helps build the case for a treatment approach that combines psychopharmacological and psychotherapeutic treatment. The following list illustrates the principal elements of a combined treatment approach that integrates medical, psychological, and educational aspects.

Principal Elements of an Integrated Treatment Approach

Medical

- The physician establishes an appropriate medication regimen for the treatment of the acute episode.
- The physician and patient develop a retrospective and prospective record of cycle frequency (see Chapter 7 about charting the illness).
- The physician and the patient determine the need for intermediate or long-term maintenance medications.
- The physician reviews periodically the effectiveness of the medications.
- If the patient is taking lithium, the physician monitors levels on a monthly basis and assesses thyroid and kidney functioning every six to twelve months.

Psychological

- The patient engages in a collaborative and trusting relationship with the therapist.
- The patient and therapist explore the psychological meaning of taking the medications for the treatment of the disorder.
- The patient and the therapist review past episodes and examine their effect on self-esteem, life goals, and relationships.
- The patient and therapist assess defenses and coping strategies—adaptive and maladaptive.
- The patient and therapist determine whether there have been psychological contributions to the onset of the illness, such as unresolved issues of early loss of attachment or personality traits that may reduce the threshold for mood disorder.

- The patient begins to get in touch with unconscious stressors, negative patterns of thinking, and behavior limited by conflicts and defenses. (Admittedly, it is difficult to know what negative elements are primary versus secondary to a mood disorder.)
- The patient confronts the stigmas associated with the diagnosis, symptoms, and treatment and learns how to deal with any limitations imposed by the illness.
- The patient accepts the disorder.

Educational

- The patient and family learn about the disorder: course, symptoms, medications and their side effects.
- The patient and family learn about the symptom patterns of the illness in the affected individual (early signs and symptoms of an episode, seasonality, yearly patterns).
- The patient learns to differentiate normal mood variations from episodes of illness.

EDUCATING THE FAMILY

Ironically, because of the efficacy of lithium and antidepressant treatment, and because individuals with mood disorders usually experience periods of well-being, there has been a tendency to underestimate the disruptive fallout these illnesses can cause the patient and his or her family. In many cases a profound rupture in familial ties persists long after the episodes of illness end. Children of a mother who was severely depressed who no longer trust her love and nurturing capacity need help in understanding what she was experiencing in order to reestablish the bond; a father who perceives his daughter as a tramp following a hypomanic episode needs the opportunity, through education, to see that her excessive sexuality was yet another manifestation of the illness.

Families could be a tremendous support to the patient if they were given information and an active role in the treatment. Every person we interviewed felt that family involvement and education made a critical difference in the posthospitalization period and beyond.

A model program to educate patients and family members was developed at the Albert Einstein College of Medicine. It is based on the psychoeducational work of Drs. Carol Anderson, Gerald Hogarty, and Douglas Reiss with schizophrenic patients and their families in Baltimore and Pittsburgh. The approach is a practical one that goes far, in a short amount of time, toward clearing up the myths surrounding the illness. It seeks to increase the stability of the family environment by decreasing the family members' anxiety about the patient and increasing their self-confidence and knowledge about the disorder. It improves the family's capacity to react constructively to the patient during episodes of illness. The approach typically requires 5 to 10 patient and family meetings.

If the first of these sessions takes place following an initial episode, or if the family has not been involved in previous episodes, it is often the case that each member has a theory about the disorder. The goal of the first meeting, then, is to understand the family members' theories. Family members are then asked to entertain the new standard medical hypotheses about the possible causes of the disorders and are given a copy of the pamphlet *Mood Disorders: Major Depression and Manic-Depression* (written by Demitri F. Papolos, M.D., and published by the National Alliance for the Mentally Ill), which describes in a question-and-answer format the nature, symptoms, and course of major mood disorders.

The provision of information usually sparks a lively discussion between the family members and the therapist at the second session. There are often emotional responses to the idea that the illness has a biological basis and is familial. Questions about medication efficacy, side effects, and criteria for long-term maintenance are also discussed. In the meetings that follow, the patient is encouraged to describe his or her subjective experience of the symptoms and the limitations they impose, and the family members begin to pinpoint how they each responded to the loss of the ill member during episodes of depression or mania. How did each person try to rouse the patient from his illness during episodes of depression? How did each family member attempt to set limits for the patient during episodes of mania? What feelings were aroused when these attempts failed?

During the final sessions, the therapist and the family review what has been learned: the nature, course, and treatment of the disorder, the effects on the relationship system, and the strategies developed to avoid the conflicts that arose as a consequence of the patient's change in behavior during an acute episode of illness.

In summary, the goals of the psychoeducational approach are to:

- enable the patient and family to accept the idea that the patient has a medical disorder that may be recurrent and produces symptoms that affect mood, self-esteem, thinking, speech, activity, sleep, appetite, and social and sexual behavior
- identify and label the specific symptoms that occur at the onset of an episode
- allow family members to acknowledge that the most recent and/or past episodes have had an impact on the way they view the patient, and to identify and describe any change in their attitudes toward the patient and in the pattern of their relationship with the patient during and after an episode of either mania or depression
- examine the changes that occur in the usual caretaking roles during an acute episode
- teach that major affective disorders are familial disorders and may therefore affect others in the family

- aid in an understanding of the potential advantages and risks of preventive treatment, as well as of no treatment, from the time the acute episode is under control
- teach the importance of long-term monitoring, including laboratory tests, and of the family's sharing in the decision to initiate maintenance treatment
- distinguish medication side effects from the symptoms of illness (for example, fatigue as a side effect of lithium or sedation due to an antidepressant or other agent that may be misconstrued as a depressive symptom)

If all goes well, the conflict between family members is decreased, healthy coping skills are attained, and the family becomes more supportive of the patient.

The following cases demonstrate how a psychoeducational approach worked for two patients and for their family members:

> Joanne Summers is a young single woman. As a teenager she had her first episode of hypomania, in which she became uncharacteristically and excessively sexual, propositioning family friends and strangers. She also had symptoms of insomnia and pressured speech and felt euphoric. This first episode ushered in a period of promiscuity and drug abuse.
>
> Thinking that she was a "bad girl" who had disgraced the family, Joanne's father reacted violently, beating her for her sexual indiscretions. She became more and more agitated and eventually required hospitalization. At the hospital she was diagnosed as having schizophrenia, treated with haloperidol, an antipsychotic drug, and discharged several weeks after admission when her agitation subsided.
>
> Joanne continued to suffer periodic exacerbations of her illness over the next several years. During the hypomanic episodes her behavior bewildered her family, since

they assumed she had received appropriate treatment and they did not attribute her excessive sexuality and argumentativeness to a disorder. Her father continued to lose his temper, to confine her to the home, and to beat her severely.

Following a second hospitalization, the diagnosis of bipolar affective disorder was established, and she responded well to a trial of lithium. Relations with her parents eased somewhat, but they never fully understood the periodic nature of her disorder. The threat of physical violence loomed over the household, yet Mr. and Mrs. Summers feared that any confrontation or stress might trigger another episode.

A few months later Joanne's lithium level fell below the therapeutic range. She felt herself becoming ill and her boyfriend drove her to the hospital, where she requested voluntary admission. She told the resident in the emergency room that she hadn't slept for a week, had racing thoughts, and noticed increased sexual feelings. Her speech was pressured and she was hypertalkative on admission. The dosage of lithium was increased and within a week she was free of symptoms.

Joanne's psychiatrist felt that the Summers family could benefit from the psychoeducational approach, and the social worker invited the family to participate in the five-session family therapy.

In the first family meeting it became apparent that Joanne had a profound fear of her father as a consequence of the beatings she had suffered. Mr. Summers expressed a desire to learn more about his daughter's illness, although initially he did not read the pamphlet *Mood Disorders* that was given to him. When asked about his response to Joanne's illness, he reported that he would typically stop talking to her when she appeared agitated, lest he set her off again. He felt that the only solution to the problem was for his daughter to move out of the house.

During the family sessions, Mr. Summers reported how very guilty he felt over the way he had treated his daughter. He admitted that the guilt and the outrage at his daughter's behavior left him feeling helpless.

During the sessions, the nature of Joanne's periodic disorder was explained to the family. The social worker clarified that Joanne's hypersexual behavior was a symptom of the illness and not the volitional act of a "bad child." This led the family to the realization that she had been punished and shunned for behavior that was out of her control. Mr. Summers apologized for the years of physical abuse, and the family elected to continue in family treatment to further work through their responses to Joanne's illness.

Elliot Anderson was a young man who began to suffer periods of hypomania and depression during his college years. Despite these interruptions, he persevered, graduated from college, and found meaningful work. While Elliot's episodes had been muted by the medications he took, he continued to have mood swings. These periods of hypomania and mild depression flew in the face of his attempts to establish himself independent of his parents, so he continued to live at home. Elliot was encouraged by his parents after each setback, but he felt a growing sense of isolation and a loss of credibility in the aftermath of each episode. He was having a great deal of difficulty understanding and coping with his family's reaction to his illness. Elliot's mother appeared nervous around him and was overly sensitive to any changes in his mood. His father denied that Elliot's problems were very serious (he kept making light of Elliot's concerns) and his younger brother, once his closest confidant, refused to be seen with him or to invite friends to his home.

The Anderson family sought help and agreed to participate in a family therapy that used a psychoeducational approach. Initially, the conversation centered around

Elliot's medication regimen and the fact that he continued to have brief periods of depression and hypomania. This was unacceptable to the family and meant to them that Elliot was being treated incorrectly. Moreover, he was having trouble with lithium-induced tremor and this was a source of embarrassment to the family. Elliot expressed his anger that his mood and behavior were a focus of concern in the household and he felt under increasing pressure to explain even minor changes in his mood. He was troubled both by his mother's anxiety and his father's seemingly cavalier attitude.

A number of things began to change as a result of the family sessions: Elliot's mother learned that her desire to protect her son from any further episodes by scrutinizing his every change in mood was creating an unbearable tension in the household, sapping her energy, and needlessly alienating her son. She lessened the demands on Elliot as well as her own unrealistic expectations that treatment could fix things so that it would be as if the illness had never struck their family.

Elliot's father, an officer at a bank, had a great deal of difficulty acknowledging the emotional impact of his son's condition. He had chosen to minimize and downplay Elliot's symptoms and explained that he thought it best to reassure Elliot rather than offer him sympathy. He initially spoke about the cost of psychiatric treatment and focused his anger on the discriminatory policies of his firm's insurance coverage.

Not long into the family sessions, however, Mr. Anderson acknowledged that he too had experienced numerous episodes of depression without ever seeking treatment. He had chosen to tough it out. As he spoke in more depth about his own experience with depression, he confided a secret that had been kept from his family for years. His own father had suffered from manic-depression and committed suicide.

Mr. Anderson had been unable to face the idea that

there was some association between his own depressions, the suicide of his father, and his son's condition. As a result of the family treatment, he came to realize that the denial of his own illness had been dangerous for him and had contributed to his minimization of Elliot's symptoms. Denial, fear, and shame had cast long shadows, from grandfather to father to son. (These powerful forces can handcuff and immobilize even the most caring of families. With an illness that is heritable like manic-depression, far more than the genetic vulnerability can span the generations.)

After learning about and accepting the biological basis of the condition and its heritability within his own family, Elliot's father was, for the first time, able to seek treatment for himself and to empathize with his son's struggle. He reported that he felt moved by Elliot's courage and determination in the face of this illness and felt an immense pride in his eldest child. Unshackled by shame and denial, Mr. Anderson was now free to find ways to help himself and his family work together rather than at cross-purposes. As a result of the psychoeducational and family treatment, they were able to redirect their energies toward developing a more comprehensive and meaningful understanding of the emotional impact of an illness that had played havoc with three generations of their family, and then to go on to resolve some of the conflicts and apprehensions that threatened to derail the next.

Recently Drs. David Kupfer and Ellen Frank of the Western Psychiatric Institute and Clinic in Pittsburgh underscored the value of the psychoeducational approach when treating patients with recurrent unipolar depression. They found a significantly reduced relapse rate following the acute episode and a markedly increased compliance to treatment in those patients exposed to the combination of imipramine, psychotherapy, and family psychoeducation. They stated that the overall clinic approach that offers this psychoeducational workshop fosters a climate of clinician–patient–family member alliance that leads to a collaborative participation in the treatment.

MARITAL THERAPY

The person most intimately involved with the individual suffering a depression—the spouse—often responds to a partner's loss of interest, withdrawal, diminished sexual arousal, and hopelessness in a very personal way. One woman described the year prior to her husband's receiving treatment for depression as one in which she felt inadequate, guilty, and angry. She began to feel detached from him and to think of separation and divorce.

During her husband's depressive episode, he experienced an extreme loss of interest in her and in their children. He felt worthless and guilty, and, in the worst moments, told her over and over again how anguished he was that he no longer loved them. His wife, not understanding this outpouring of feelings in the context of his major depression, felt confused and shaken. She knew that there was something terribly wrong but continued, as he did, to find cause for their problems within their immediate situation. Later she learned that these expressions of guilt were largely an outgrowth of his general loss of interest in the world around him.

The effects of an illness that alters mood, thinking, and behavior will clearly have an impact on the way one sees oneself and, in turn, the way one relates to and feels about others. Interpersonal problems, especially in the marital arena, can lead to serious and painful repercussions when not understood as part of a medical condition. This is no less true for episodes of mania or hypomania.

Individuals experiencing hypomania or mania are often driven to impulsive acts. Sexual indiscretions, perhaps uncharacteristic during well periods, are common. The experience of infidelity can scar a marriage and easily abrogate basic trust. It is a tragic fact that, while time-limited, episodes of affective illness can persist for months to years if undiagnosed and untreated. Since individuals experiencing hypomania frequently do not come to psychiatric attention, the episodes—and their impact on a marriage—may continue indefinitely until either a severe depression intervenes or the hypomania escalates to mania.

The relationship between marital problems and depression has been examined in a number of clinical studies, most notably those involving women with depression. Drs. Myrna Weissman and E. S. Paykel found that marital relationships were the most impaired areas of social functioning in acutely depressed women and that the impairments were slow to resolve and persisted long after the symptoms of the illness resolved.

In a study of 76 depressed women treated for 8 months with individual psychotherapy and/or antidepressant drugs, Drs. Bruce Rounsaville, Brigitte Prusoff, and Myrna Weissman found that, by comparison, those women who came into treatment complaining of marital disputes experienced less improvement in their symptoms and had a greater tendency to relapse than those women who had no marital disputes at the onset of treatment.

These studies stress the need for couple's therapy in conjunction with the pharmacological treatment of the acute episode. Clearly, educating both patient and spouse about the course and nature of an affective disorder can go a long way toward reducing the interpersonal conflicts that commonly develop between partners in a relationship where one member has the disorder. Once treatment has stabilized the acute symptoms, a retrospective review of the relationship and the course of illness is helpful for both parties, as the origin and intensity of current marital disputes often can be traced back to the onset and evolution of the depressive or manic symptoms.

SHORT-TERM THERAPIES SPECIFICALLY
FORMULATED FOR DEPRESSION

We can't close this chapter without mentioning two short-term therapies designed specifically for depression. These therapies are especially worth discussing because in May 1986 a 6-year $10 million study funded by the National Institute of Mental Health concluded that *cognitive therapy* and *interpersonal psychotherapy* were as effective as imipramine in reducing the symptoms of depression and improving the functioning of patients.

The study was conducted at three sites—the University of Pittsburgh, George Washington University, and the University of Oklahoma—and involved 240 moderately or severely depressed patients and 28 therapists. The patients were divided randomly into three groups: the first and second groups received 16 weeks of either cognitive or interpersonal psychotherapy, and the third group received the tricyclic antidepressant imipramine. A control group was given a placebo plus some verbal support and encouragement by psychiatrists.

Initially there was a faster response to imipramine, but after 3 months the talking therapies caught up. At the conclusion of 16 weeks, all 3 treatments had eliminated serious depressive symptoms in more than half the patients.

What follows is a brief description of cognitive and interpersonal psychotherapy (IPT) as well as an indication of their availability in this country at present.

Cognitive therapy, developed by Dr. Aaron Beck, is a time-limited, structured approach based on the proposition that an individual's affect—moods and emotions—is determined by his or her thoughts and ideas. Therefore, by modifying the ideas, one modifies the moods and emotions.

According to the theory, depressed patients consistently distort their interpretation of events so as to maintain negative views of themselves, their environment, and their future. This predisposition stems from the development of early negative assumptions or "schemas." For example, a child may develop the schema that nothing he or she will ever do will be good enough. This assumption may be unconscious until a life event, such as being fired from a job, activates it. Once the schema springs to life again, the patient processes the experience so as to maintain the failure schema. The distortions in thinking magnify until depression and hopelessness set in and take over.

Cognitive therapy seeks to change this type of depressive thinking and thus alter the depressed mood. The therapist and patient achieve this by examining and modifying the depressive ideas that the patient maintains. The patient is asked to do "homework" assignments between sessions and is instructed to keep a journal. The sessions are aimed at overcoming hopelessness, identifying problems, setting priorities, demonstrating the relationship between cognition and emotion, and labeling errors in thinking. The patient learns to question negative assumptions and put them "to the test" by examining evidence and trying graded tasks. By the end of the therapy, patients begin to view themselves and their problems more realistically, change their maladaptive behavioral patterns, and feel better.

Should you wish to find out if cognitive therapy is available in your area, call or write the Center for Cognitive Therapy at Science Center, 7th Floor, 3600 Market St., Philadelphia, PA 19104 (215) 898-4100. They have an extensive referral list throughout the country and abroad. Normally the therapy is conducted over a 12-week period including 15 to 20 sessions. There is an evaluation fee, and each session costs approximately $140.

Interpersonal psychotherapy was developed by Drs. Gerald Klerman and Myrna Weissman and the New Haven–Boston Collaborative Depression project. It is similar to cognitive therapy in that it is structured and time-limited, but it emphasizes social bonds and relationships and works to improve a person's self-concept and communication skills. Issues such as grief and social and family role transitions are the focus, as is the patient's ability to form and sustain adequate and nurturing relationships. The interpersonal psychotherapist recognizes the role of genetic, biochemical, developmental, and personality factors in causation of and vulnerability to depression.

There are approximately 12 sessions to the treatment, and fees also average about $140 per session. There is, however, a great problem in locating a practitioner to administer the treatment outside of research centers. This should change as efforts are being made to train practitioners across the country.

7

CHARTING MOOD DISORDERS: THE COURSE OF ILLNESS

The first manifestation of a mood disorder may not always be obvious. Some people have brief, mild episodes that are self-limiting and subside on their own. A person experiencing a first episode of hypomania may not recognize it as an illness that needs treatment, and may even look back on it as a special, invigorating time when much was accomplished and many creative ideas were expressed. Unless the hypomania accelerates into mania or until a depression follows, it is difficult for a person to have a perspective and begin to glimpse the larger picture—one that includes the possibility of a recurrent psychiatric illness that insidiously waxes and wanes.

Mood disorders have biological and genetic components, but they are disorders that express themselves through the psychology, perception, and behavior of a human being, and they are illnesses that sometimes can be triggered by stress or environmental change. Early in its course, even a psychiatrist might be perplexed trying to tease apart the tell-tale symptoms and episodic nature of an illness from the emotional history of a person who is involved in both the everyday and the dramatic struggles of life. Yet patterns do emerge if one is alert to them, and research is proving that the more specific a pattern that can be recognized, the more skillfully the illness can be treated.

That is why a picture really *is* worth a thousand words. Charting the illness is an important part of a long-term treatment strategy.

A cycle chart is a chronological account of changes in mood, energy, activity, and sleep. The chart specifically details the patient's course of illness, including the circumstances preceding the initial onset, the cycle length, the nature and duration of subsequent episodes, the treatments received, and the responses to that treatment. This recording of the changes over time brings a view of the course of illness into focus. The chart also helps guide diagnosis and treatment in the acute period of illness, guides decisions concerning maintenance treatment, and identifies periods of heightened vulnerability when a breakthrough episode might occur and where the doctor should be on the alert to modify or augment the medication regimen or the frequency of therapeutic sessions.

The first chart we will review is a retrospective account of a young woman's five-year struggle with depressive and hypomanic cycles. Had an earlier, more complete understanding of the nature of her illness been provided (and charting would have helped ensure this), more timely interventions could have been made and her suffering greatly curtailed.

In the fall and winter of 1984 and 1985, Sarah suffered episodes of depression. She did not seek a psychiatric consultation, but rather tried to dissipate the depressive symptoms with alcohol. It made her feel less edgy and irritable and it helped her sleep. (Self-medication with alcohol is not at all unusual, and greater than one-third of patients diagnosed with alcoholism have an underlying, untreated mood disorder.)

Sarah continued to drink even as she began to switch into a more active energized state in the spring and summer months of 1986. In the fall, however, depression began to take hold again. The insomnia became so severe that a family doctor prescribed Librium so she could get to sleep. While Sarah's sleep improved somewhat, the depressive symptoms increased in

Sarah's Cycle Chart

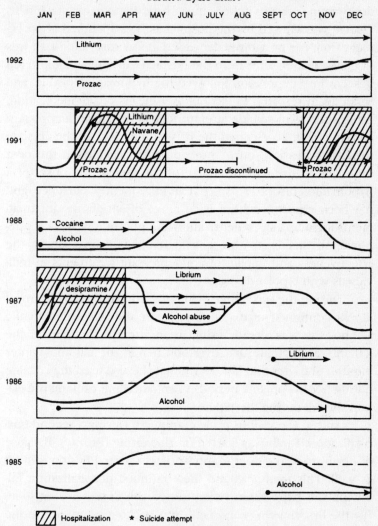

severity and she became agitated, suicidal, and then psychotic. At this point, she was hospitalized and treated as having a psychotic depression complicated by alcohol abuse. There was no attempt to explore the possibility that Sarah might have "high" periods, and within days of starting on the antidepressant desipramine, she switched into a brief hypomanic state. This change was viewed by the hospital staff as a marked improvement from her previously depressed mood state, and Sarah was discharged soon after from the hospital. An often-encountered descent into depression followed the hypomanic episode, and Sarah again resorted to alcohol as a means of self-medication. An unsuccessful suicide attempt followed. The antidepressant had, in effect, accelerated the natural tendency of the episode towards remission, but it probably also accelerated the next sequence in the natural course of the illness: the onset of a hypomanic episode. This is not an infrequent occurrence, and has been reported with a wide range of antidepressant treatments including sleep deprivation and phototherapy. This phenomenon needs to be considered when evaluating the effectiveness and impact of antidepressant treatments in individuals with bipolar disorder.

During the next three years, the annual cyclic pattern of illness continued unabated, and Sarah added cocaine to the alcohol she was already using in an attempt to stave off the lethargy and fatigue that overtook her in the fall and winter months. She later told her doctor that she also used the cocaine during her hypomanic periods to enhance and prolong the elation she felt during these times.

And so the vicious cycle continued. During a second hospitalization, Sarah was started on fluoxetine (Prozac). Because of her history, the doctor appropriately started her on lithium as well. This treatment and the continued hospitalization following the hypomanic swing muted the depressive episode. For the first time in years, Sarah was without symptoms in the springtime. Noting that Sarah was doing well, with no symptoms of depression, and that she was not drinking or taking cocaine, her psychiatrist no longer saw the need to maintain her on an antidepressant. The Prozac was discontinued in August of that year.

If the psychiatrist treating Sarah at this point in the course of her illness had the benefit of a visual chart, he would have been alerted to the fact that Sarah was particularly vulnerable to develop depressions in the fall and would likely have continued her on the Prozac in combination with lithium. Within weeks of discontinuing the antidepressant, Sarah suffered a very severe depression and made another suicide attempt. As of this writing, she has been stabilized on a combination of medications, is in psychotherapy to address personality problems as well as her anger and anguish over the hellish five years she endured, and is in a support group with people who have abused alcohol and drugs.

As mentioned earlier, a great value of maintaining a chart is that it uncovers discrete intervals when the patient may be vulnerable for breakthrough episodes despite treatment with mood stabilizers such as lithium, Depakote, or Tegretol. This classification of the timing of risk allows for a fine-tuning of the treatment regimen. In Sarah's case, a psychiatrist who observed her long-standing pattern of illness of regular depressive episodes occurring in the fall and hypomania in the springtime, would consider the need for adjunctive medications or treatments prior to and during the periods of established vulnerability. For Sarah that might include raising the level of lithium above the usual maintenance dosage prior to the change of seasons in the fall and again in the spring, or alternatively, starting a course of phototherapy prior to the annual depressions. A drug such as clonazepam (Klonopin) or lorazepam (Ativan) might be added to put a "brake" on the increased energy and activity level and to promote sleep during the warmer months. (Conversely, charting would reveal periods of low risk when patients might take a drug holiday, make changes in medication regimens, or attempt to conceive a child.)

There is growing clinical evidence to indicate that sleep loss may induce or intensify episodes of mania or hypomania in predisposed individuals. Dr. Thomas Wehr and colleagues at the National Institute of Mental Health have reported that the majority of a group of depressed, rapid-cycling bipolar patients switched into mania or hypomania the day after they were deprived of sleep for one night. The results of sleep-deprivation experiments strongly suggest that the insomnia caused by mania in turn exacerbates or sustains the mania. In this way, sleep loss arising from a variety of causes (including that caused by jet travel through time zones) could set in motion a hypomanic or manic episode that becomes self-reinforcing or self-perpetuating. This possibility underscores the importance of monitoring the sleep–wake cycle, and of intervening with the appropriate sedative medication to preserve a regular cycle.

In addition to the more planned and deliberate decision making about medication interventions, the psychiatrist and patient should explore which life events seem to precipitate and complicate breakthrough episodes. Significant losses have long been viewed by clinicians as precipitating causes of depression. Sarah made serious suicide attempts following the breakups of important relationships with men and following the death of her father (which coincided with her fall depression). The loss of these important relationships rekindled powerful feelings of rejection, isolation, and vulnerability and were major precipitants leading Sarah to express suicidal impulses during her periods of fall depression. More frequent contact with her doctor or therapist may have allowed Sarah to vent her feelings of disappointment, loss, and anger and would have helped her feel supported and less isolated during such critical times in her life. A confiding relationship and the healing that takes place in psychotherapy should not be underestimated. In combination with appropriately administered pharmacological treatment, psychotherapy is a potent ally.

Recently, psychiatrists have begun to pay closer attention to the pattern and form of the various cycles of depression and mania. Research has begun to focus on the following questions: Which type of episode begins the cycle—a manic episode or a depressive one? How often are the episodes of mania and depression linked with no "well interval" separating them? Does the person experience a period of mania after a depression, or are recurrent depressive episodes the predominant pattern before the later appearance of a cycle of hypomania or mania? To what extent is the pattern of episodes linked to seasonal change? Do these factors serve to define more specific subtypes of the illness?

The casual observer might ask, "Why bother to make these kinds of distinctions? Will they really make a difference in terms of treatment?" In fact, it's turning out that the answers to some of these questions may be very significant when psychiatrists decide which maintenance medications to choose for patients. The pattern of cycling may help predict whether an individual will respond to lithium, or whether carbamazapine or sodium valproate might better be the first line of treatment.

In 1980, Drs. Athanasio Koukopoulos and Daniela Reginaldi reported that a bipolar patient's response to long-term preventive treatment with lithium may vary according to the previous pattern of course of the illness. They distinguished four distinct patterns in a group of patients:

1. Mania, depression, free-interval (MDI). The cycle starts with mania, a depression follows, and then a normal period of mood ensues.
2. Depression, mania, free-interval (DMI). The cycle starts with depression, a manic episode follows, and a symptom-free interval ensues.
3. Continuous circular course (CC). A continuous circular course with no free interval between cycles of depression and mania, in which the cycles may be long or rapid.
4. Irregular course (IRR). No pattern to the cycles of depression, mania, and normal periods of mood.

In the Koukopoulos and Reginaldi study, the patients in the MDI, CC (with long cycles), and IR groups had the best

The Patterns of the Illness

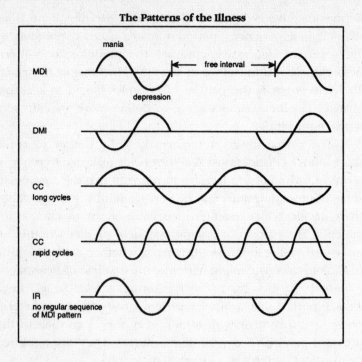

response to maintenance lithium therapy. The DMI group's response to lithium was not as good. In this case, the lithium actually appeared to increase the frequency of recurrence even though the episodes were shorter and milder. The pattern of illness defined as DMI was the one that was most prone to rapid cycling. Rapid cyclers and patients with the DMI course responded well to lithium when antidepressant drugs were not administered during depression. This finding in many ways was a further confirmation of Dr. Mogens Schou's findings. In 1979, Schou reviewed the results of the controlled studies of bipolar and recurrent unipolar patients maintained on lithium and tricyclic antidepressants or placebo treatment. He found that on lithium therapy alone, relapse rates for patients of either polarity decreased dramatically. However, bipolar patients who were administered tricyclic maintenance medication had a relapse rate as high as those patients receiving placebo. The striking difference was the direction of the relapse: bipolar patients taking placebo relapsed primarily to depressive episodes, while those taking tricyclics relapsed to manic episodes. All of the above alerts a psychiatrist to the potential problems inherent in the use of antidepressant medications; for example, the likelihood of inducing manic, hypomanic, mixed states, or more frequent cycles and thereby altering the course of the illness.

CREATING A CYCLE CHART

While charting the course of illness is by no means commonplace in clinical practice, it is apparent that this effort on the part of the patient and his or her psychiatrist could be of significant benefit. This section describes how a person might log and use a cycle chart. A sample chart that may be photocopied from this book for personal use is included in Appendix I on page 363.

A cycle chart is divided into 12 monthly intervals, January through December. This allows one to plot the course of mood, activity, sleep, and significant life events, as well as the dosage and levels of medications, on separate chronological scales. This type of chart converts a great deal of information into a visual form that is easily reviewed, and that over time presents a clear and detailed picture of the episode frequency, the pattern and form of episodes, the relationship of episodes to seasons and to life events, as well as the effectiveness of a particular medication or psychotherapeutic regimen.

Quantifying gradations in mood and behavior is not an easy task even for someone who is a trained observer, and certainly it is far more difficult for someone buffeted about by rapidly changing moods, but the following definitions provide some guidelines for measuring changes in mood, activity, and sleep along a continuum from mild to severe. These definitions are based on what is called a mood scale. The mood scale reflects three levels of elated or irritable mood and three levels of depressed mood: mild, moderate, and severe. (Naturally, a mood rating approaching the severe level will need to be assessed either retrospectively or by a family member or friend.) Use the mood scale to determine the course of mood for the cycle chart.

- Severe = 10. Euphoric/irritable. Mood swings quickly from elation or irritability to tearful outbursts. The person is easily angered or argumentative, and often preoccupied with sexual or religious concerns. Very distractable and unable to concentrate. Agitated, suspicious of others, and unable to participate in a group without trying to monopolize the conversation or becoming the center of attention. Delusions and hallucinations, particularly those of a grandiose or paranoid nature, are common.
- Moderate = 5. Elated, with some mood lability. Increased social gregariousness. Sexual thoughts, racing thoughts, somewhat distractible, less difficult when participating in groups but still intrusive with poor judgment and impulsive decisions such as buying sprees.
- Mild = 2. A pervasively optimistic or irritable mood is common during the hypomanic episode. Often the "life of the party." Productive but distractible and often impulsive.
- Mild = –2. Periodic sadness or irritability, some tearfulness, decreased energy, listlessness, some interest in daily activities. One can force oneself to socialize, but there is little motivation to engage with others.
- Moderate = –5. More pervasive sadness or irritable mood. Increasing social withdrawal, decreased energy, appetite changes, sleep disturbance may be quite pronounced.
- Severe = –10. Overwhelming depression. One is unable to experience pleasure in any activities of daily life.

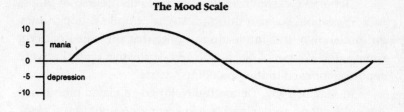

The Mood Scale

Thinking is slowed, there is an absence of emotion. Loss of appetite and libido. Patient can be paranoid or delusional.

Because changes in sleep patterns and levels of activity often preceed a full-blown hypomanic, manic, or depressive episode, separate time-lines are used to chart these changes as they occur. Carefully documenting changes in these behaviors can be helpful in the early recognition of cycle onsets and offer the opportunity for early intervention by the treating physician. A time-line that denotes stressful life events provides the opportunity to identify specific precipitants of an episode. These precipitants may reflect childhood traumas or psychological conflicts that need to be explored in a psychotherapeutic treatment. Resolving these traumas may serve to diminish the intensity of their effect as precipitants for future episodes.

It is not uncommon for a patient with a recurrent mood disorder to have tried a variety of medications. Careful and consistent documentation of the dosages and duration of medication trials, as well as the side effects sustained, provides the treating psychiatrist with vital information. The medication time-line, then, offers a rapid review of what has and hasn't worked. It also indicates whether the levels were adequate or the trials of long enough duration. In addition, the medication time-line reveals whether a particular class of drug has altered the cycling pattern over time.

Deborah's cycle chart demonstrates the course of illness in a 35-year-old woman during a 1-year period. Although they are not shown, it is interesting to note that this same pattern, timing, and course of her manic and depressive episodes were reported for each of the preceding 3 years.

In May of 1987, Deborah developed an elated mood, had difficulty falling asleep, and began staying up until two o'clock in the morning. Her activity level gradually became increased until she required hospitalization in a state of acute mania. Looking back, we can see that her sleep pattern began to change days to weeks prior to the onset of the full manic episode. She had trouble getting to sleep, went to sleep later, her sleep was fitful with frequent awakenings, and she experienced early-morning awakening. For the next year, Deborah plotted her sleep cycle and activity level. Once again, in the spring, her sleep became irregular and her activity increased rather dramatically. She notified her psychiatrist after a few days of this pattern and he prescribed clonazepam (Klonopin), two milligrams. This intervention helped to reduce the severity of the impending manic episode. When Deborah nevertheless experienced a subsequent depression, she was treated early with buproprion (Wellbutrin), a medication which has been reported to be less likely to cause an increase in the frequency of cycling in bipolar patients than other antidepressants. Before the introduction of the Wellbutrin, however, her lithium was raised to a dosage that corresponded with a blood level of 1.4. While she was taking the antidepressant, the lithium level was maintained at this high level with the aim of preventing an antidepressant-induced mania and an increase in the frequency of cycling.

She came out of the depression, but remained on the Wellbutrin for nine months. The Wellbutrin was then discontinued and she has been maintained on lithium alone. She continues to do well and has suffered only minor mood swings since that period of time.

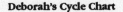

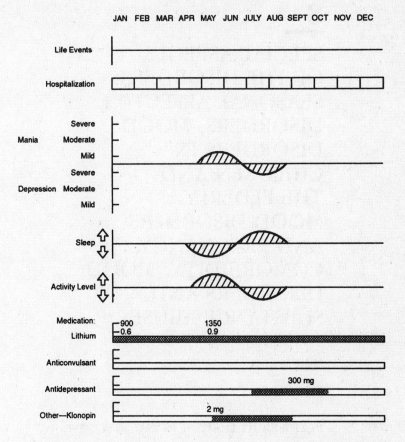

Systematic collection of this type of information from patients and families is a necessary part of the routine clinical evaluation of bipolar disorder. Such information yields a more accurate view of the course of illness and allows the psychiatrist to more fully understand the relationship between the person and the illness. Retrospective and prospective measures of cycles, treatments, and life events, particularly in bipolar patients, are critical to an understanding of the variable but often predictable course of mood disorders.

8

SPECIAL ASPECTS OF THE DISORDERS: SEASONAL AFFECTIVE DISORDERS, MOOD DISORDERS IN CHILDREN AND THE ELDERLY, MOOD DISORDERS AND PREGNANCY, COMORBIDITY: MOOD DISORDERS AND SUBSTANCE ABUSE

IN THE RIGHT LIGHT: SEASONAL AFFECTIVE DISORDER

Seasonal affective disorder (SAD) is a syndrome characterized by recurrent depressions that occur nearly every year at the same time. When the days grow shorter in the fall, these patients experience depression, extreme sluggishness, irritability, and anxiety. They begin to sleep for longer and longer periods of time, and to withdraw from social activities. In effect, they "hibernate" for the winter. But in marked contrast to depressed patients who stop eating and lose weight, they binge on carbohydrates and often gain between ten to twenty pounds during the winter months. Once spring comes and the photoperiod lengthens, people with SAD experience new energy, shed the gained pounds, and find their mood returning to normal or slightly elevated levels.

This depressive syndrome, defined by Dr. Norman Rosenthal and his colleagues at the National Institute of Mental Health, received much media attention because of an unusual treatment devised for it: patients who met the criteria for SAD were seated in front of a bank of high-intensity, full-spectrum lights for three hours before dawn and three hours after dusk. Through the re-creation of the photoperiod of a summer day, almost all the patients experienced partial or complete remission of their depressive symptoms. When the light treatments were stopped, a number of the patients relapsed.

In order to understand the causes of seasonal depressions and why this form of light treatment was effective, researchers are focusing attention on the pineal gland—a small reddish gray structure that sits near the center of the brain. Its name is derived from the Latin word for "pine cone" because early viewers glimpsed a resemblance.

All vertebrates possess a pineal gland, and in certain reptiles and birds the gland is situated close enough to the top of the skull to monitor the intensity of sunlight. This "third eye" appears to help the animal adjust to changes in the day–night cycles of the yearly seasons. Although the seventeenth-century philosopher René Descartes thought the human pineal to be the seat of the rational soul and the second-century physician Galen believed it to be the valve that regulated the flow of thoughts out of storage in the brain, modern scientists until recently felt that the buried-down-under human pineal had been abandoned by the roadside of human evolution. No longer a third eye, they believed it had no present function.

Not so. In the midsixties, researchers discovered that the pineal gland secretes an important hormone called melatonin.

It is now clear that information about light is brought by special nerve pathways to the pineal gland, where it affects the secretion of melatonin (see the illustration on page 108). It is the secretion of melatonin that may provide a link to depression. There are several reasons for this. First, the neurotransmitter serotonin (believed to be associated with depression) is a precursor of melatonin. Also, melatonin is a sleep-inducing hormone, produced in the dark, which appears to depress both mood and mental agility; its secretion is at its highest levels in winter. To build the case further, studies by Dr. Alfred Lewy found that, compared to others, bipolar patients had a supersensitivity to light as evidenced by a markedly increased suppression of melatonin on exposure to bright light. Melatonin is also thought to have a part in the synchronization of circadian (daily) rhythms.

Today scientists accept that a kind of biological clock in the human organism establishes a fundamental daily rhythm for bodily functions such as body temperature, the release of cortisol, rest/activity levels, and the secretion of melatonin. But nature has built some flexibility into the organism so that the body can adjust and synchronize to the ever-changing environmental rhythms—such as longer and shorter photoperiods in summer and winter.

Apparently some people do not adjust so easily. Dr. Lewy hypothesized that certain depressed people have a desynchronization in their 24-hour internal clock rhythms. For instance, their sleep, temperature, and cortisol cycles may be in synchrony with each other, but be out of step with other 24-hour rhythms, thus causing their internal clocks to run a few hours behind or ahead of schedule. They either start and stop releasing melatonin earlier than usual (leading to evening sleepiness and early morning awakening), or start and stop releasing melatonin later than usual (leading to difficulty sleeping at night as well as difficulty getting up in the morning). In 1980, Dr. Lewy was able to determine that bright light inhibited the level of melatonin secreted. By exposing the first group of patients—those who experienced evening sleepiness and early morning awakening—to bright light for three hours in the evening, he delayed the release of melatonin, and the symptoms of depression improved; by exposing the second group—those who had trouble sleeping at night and couldn't get up in the morning—to bright light in the early morning, he phase-advanced the patients by shutting off the melatonin levels at a more normal time. Again the symptoms of depression improved. The 24-hour rhythms seemed to resynchronize.

Dr. Daniel Kripke and his research group in San Diego are exploring the impact of light and the secretion of melatonin from the perspective of the hibernation response. Melatonin triggers hibernation and mating cycles in animals. Perhaps the depression of seasonal affective disorders in humans is a vestigial hibernation response. Dr. Kripke's group looked at the hibernation cycle in hamsters and discovered that it was triggered by a lack of light during a specific period in the early morning. Conversely, if there was exposure to light during that critical period, the hibernation response was inhibited. Kripke and his colleagues wondered whether there is such a point in the human circadian cycle, possibly occurring right after awakening. Perhaps depressed patients are reaching this critical point earlier than normal people—while they are still sleeping and cannot be exposed to the light. Researchers have indeed found that circadian cycles occur earlier in some depressed patients.

Hoping to reset or phase-advance the cycle, Kripke awakened the depressed patients two hours before their normal waking time and exposed them to bright light for one hour. The results were mixed. It should be noted, however, that Dr. Kripke's patients had depression but not SAD. Dr. Rosenthal's patients met the criteria for seasonal affective disorder and had a more robust response to the light therapy.

Without doubt, this noninvasive treatment for depression

has great appeal. Following the publicity, quite a few psychiatrists reported a flurry of phone calls from depressed people inquiring where they might buy the light banks. Self-treatment is not advised as the phototherapy must be precisely timed and the brightness calibrated for effect and safety. Moreover, this form of treatment might be applicable to only a small subgroup of patients. The mechanism of the effect of bright light treatment is unknown, and the studies still require further validation.

Still, these new looks at the relationship between circadian and seasonal cycles and sunlight and depressive disorders are important. Future reports could help to further define and document the physiology of depression.

Recurrent Summer Depression

As researchers increasingly studied patients who suffered recurrent winter depressions, they began to identify a group of patients who had a reverse pattern of SAD: summer depressions that typically began in May and ended in September. Often the periods of summer depression were followed by hypomanic bouts during the winter months.

In addition to their opposite times of occurrence, winter and summer SAD seem to have opposite types of symptoms. While the patients who experienced winter depression had "atypical" depressive symptoms such as oversleeping, overeating, carbohydrate craving, and weight gain, the patients with summer depression had insomnia, loss of appetite and weight, anxiety, and agitation.

Interestingly, many of the patients interviewed reported that a change in latitude and temperature could bring relief of the symptoms. If these patients traveled north, for instance, leaving Washington, D.C., for New England, the symptoms abated. One patient was able to obtain relief of depressive symptoms by swimming in an icy cold lake in New Hampshire. These "climatotherapy" cures suggest a possible association between elevated brain temperature and depression. However, since the depressive symptoms are similar to common forms of major depression, most psychiatrists treat summer depressions with standard antidepressants or lithium.

It is worth noting that the NIMH researchers working with Dr. Thomas Wehr found summer SAD only 20 to 25 percent as prevalent as winter SAD, but Dr. Gianni Faedda and his colleagues at Harvard Medical School studied a group of 175 patients in Caligari, Italy, whose periods of depression followed one of two patterns: either they suffered fall–winter depression with or without spring–summer mania or hypomania, or spring–summer depression with or without fall–winter mania or hypomania. The two patterns occurred with almost equal frequency in this patient population. Dr. Faedda is not sure how to explain this differing epidemiological ratio. The clinical unit in Caligari, Sardinia, is located at the same latitude as Bethesda, Maryland (39°N), where SAD has been intensively studied, and the two sites have almost identical seasonal variations of daylight hours, although the Mediterranean climate of Sardinia is more temperate. He writes: "While there is no obvious geographical explanation for the high prevalence of spring–summer depression and seasonal mania in Sardinia, it is possible that unidentified climatic, cultural, or genetic differences are involved. Further research is necessary to test and extend the present findings, and to further clarify the role of seasonal changes as precipitants of recurrences in mood disorders."

MOOD DISORDERS IN CHILDREN
AND ADOLESCENTS

Until the early 1960s, depression in children was rarely (if ever) diagnosed. It was almost never mentioned in textbooks on child psychiatry. Psychoanalytic theory held that a classical depressive syndrome could not occur in prepubertal children. Others felt that what might be regarded as depressive symptoms are merely transitory developmental phenomena that would disappear over time. The debate continued as different factions argued that children do suffer depression but that they have different symptoms than those seen in adults. In 1980 the DSM-III stated that the criteria for depression in children is the same as that for adults, but that the form of expression may be different and related to the developmental level of the child. Although much still remains unclear, there are researchers who feel that depression is an underdiagnosed condition in childhood.

A wide range of depressive symptoms may be noticed by the parents or teachers of a child. These can include an appearance of sadness or loneliness and decreased energy. The child may have difficulty sleeping at night or want to do nothing but sleep. He or she may fail to make expected weight gains, or there may be an unusual change in appetite. Teachers often notice that the child daydreams or has little ability to concentrate, and it is not uncommon for a depressed child to resist going to school, and even to refuse altogether. Any interest in after school or social activities vanishes.

Sometimes children don't say they feel sad, but express feelings of being ugly, stupid or dumb, and useless. They may feel inordinately guilty about things. Their behavior may change with irritability and temper tantrums becoming more frequent. Children can also begin to act aggressively. If the depression becomes severe, the child may experience delusions and hallucinations as well as entertain suicidal thoughts. It is imperative that the parents intervene and have the child evaluated by professionals.

Who Should Diagnose and Treat Children and Adolescents?

Ideally, a child psychiatrist should diagnose and treat psychiatric disorders in children and adolescents. The doctor needs to elicit the information necessary for a diagnosis and must be trained to speak with a child in a way the child can understand, utilize play therapy, and then treat the child in the context of the family unit.

A child psychiatrist is a medical doctor who has completed one year of internship, two or three years of an adult psychiatric residency, and two additional years of a child psychiatry fellowship program.

The best way to go about locating a good child psychiatrist is to talk to the family pediatrician or family practitioner. Also, a school psychologist or guidance counselor might be able to make a referral. If these avenues fail to locate someone competent, the department of child psychiatry at a major teaching hospital would be a very likely resource.

Locating a child psychiatrist in such states as Alaska, Arkansas, Mississippi, Nevada, West Virginia, or Wyoming presents a real problem. Only a few years ago, these states each had fewer than 10 practicing child psychiatrists. In fact, the shortage of child and adolescent psychiatrists is nationwide: there are no more than 5,000 throughout the United States. In the event that a child psychiatrist is not available, an adult psychiatrist with an interest in and a history of treating children would be the likely alternative. A call to one of the patient or family support groups listed in the Appendices of this book would no doubt shorten the search, as the people you contact there could use their networks to help.

The Treatment of Depression in Children

The doctor evaluates the child's symptoms and behavior and gathers additional information through psychological testing and from the parents and teachers. Very often, therapy, support, and parental counseling that could result in a change in the home life or in communication patterns in the home are enough to counteract the depression. Sometimes, however, when the child manifests symptoms of a major depressive syndrome, the physician considers treating the child with an anti-depressant medication since the child's discomforting feelings may so undermine his or her confidence and out-reaching ability as to seriously impair future undertakings and relationships.

Before any pharmacological treatment begins, the physician orders a complete exam. Blood tests, urinalysis, and an electrocardiogram (ECG) will be done. Today, it is likely that one of the SSRIs will be prescribed—either Prozac, Zoloft, or Paxil—because there is far less concern about cardiac toxicity or overdoses with any one of these medications. The drug selected is started at low doses and increased incrementally every few days until the symptoms begin to clear. The dosage is calibrated according to the height and weight of the child. While the child is on the drug, the blood pressure, pulse rate, and heart rhythm should be monitored.

Daily medications should *always* be dispensed by a parent or responsible adult as overdoses can and do happen. In the event of an overdose, the child must be rushed to the nearest hospital, where the cardiac and respiratory functioning will be monitored.

Side Effects of Antidepressants

Antidepressants are generally well tolerated by children and many suffer no side effects, but others report insomnia, some agitation, nausea, dizziness, and headache. Most common side effects, should they occur, abate within the first weeks of treatment. A change in the time of day in which the medication is taken may help, or the psychiatrist may try one of the other drugs in the SSRI class.

How Long Should a Child Be on an Antidepressant?

Typically, a child takes the medication for six to nine months and is then tapered off slowly, but not always. As child psychiatrist Dr. Rosalie Greenberg says:

Mood disorders can be chronic, recurrent illnesses, and though we don't want to wed a child to medication for life, we must look at the previous course of illness. If a ten-year-old has been depressed since the age of five, it is unlikely that he or she will remain well if the medication is discontinued. Depression can take a terrible toll on the psychosocial interaction with peers, teachers and family members, and therefore one needs to weigh seriously the risks and benefits of a longer-term treatment.

Suicide

It is particularly poignant and distressing to think about children suffering with depression, but it is harrowing to think that children attempt suicide and are frequently successful in their attempts. Clinical reports show that children as young as five and six years old have made attempts to kill themselves. Dr. Cynthia Pfeffer of Cornell University Medical College has reported that her studies of children reveal that approximately 75 percent of the children who are psychiatrically hospitalized are suicidal, while about 33 percent of those treated outside the hospital are suicidal. It is estimated that about half of all suicide victims suffer from depressive illness.

The burgeoning statistics on adolescent suicides are shocking. It is estimated that 5000 adolescents kill themselves in the United States each year, and that at least 400,000 youngsters make unsuccessful attempts annually. Suicide is the third leading cause of death in adolescents. Dr. Pfeffer feels that adolescents are particularly at risk for suicide attempts because they progress through a variety of rapid developmental stages. "Besides those that are physiological," she writes, "the youngster may also be biologically vulnerable to psychiatric illnesses such as depression." She adds:

Although the incidence of major affective disorder in preadolescents is relatively low, it increases greatly in adolescents. These young people are in the process of psychologically "leaving home," and the relationship to their family changes as peer relationships become more important. The development of a firm sense of identity is a critically important issue. When this process is hampered or inhibited, adolescents may be especially prone to suicidal behavior.

There are certain signs and symptoms that may warn of an impending suicide attempt in an adolescent. They are:

- depressed mood
- changes in sleep and/or appetite patterns
- decline in school performance
- increased social withdrawal
- loss of interest and pleasure in previously enjoyable activities
- changes in appearance—for instance, no longer caring about one's clothing or hair
- preoccupation with themes of death—the youngster may begin to read books with themes of death and dying
- increased irritability and behavior problems
- giving away important possessions
- use of drugs and alcohol
- history of a previous attempt
- history of abuse and neglect
- history of learning disabilities and a sense of failure
- frequent somatic complaints
- verbal expression about self-death—for instance, a youngster who actually says, "I wish I were dead"
- no longer concerned about making plans for the future

An adolescent who is potentially suicidal may make an attempt following a variety of events. These may include the breakup of a romantic relationship, disciplinary problems with parents, difficulty with school or work, or an injury to self-esteem such as the failure to win an important award or position. The loss of an important person in the child's life may also serve as a precipitant.

Should a parent, a teacher, or another adult suspect that a child is suicidal, the matter should be discussed immediately. Too often people avoid introducing the subject because they think it will "plant ideas." "To the contrary," says child psychiatrist Dr. Rosalie Greenberg, "asking a young person about self-destructive wishes can help make him or her feel more understood and less trapped. Ignoring suicidal thoughts or behavior is a way of making suicide more likely to happen."

Once it becomes clear that an adolescent is at risk for suicide, it is crucial that he or she be seen immediately by a psychiatrist (ideally by a psychiatrist familiar with the treatment of adolescents). This doctor can then assess the risk of suicide and decide whether protective hospitalization is necessary, what kind of therapy the child needs, and whether or not medications are indicated. The family will need information and support at this time also, and the psychiatrist should work closely with family members and possibly the personnel at the child's school.

Manic-Depression in Children and Adolescents

Manic episodes can begin early in life. A look back at the histories of adults with bipolar symptoms often shows that mood swings began around puberty, but there are many case reports of manic symptoms seen in prepubertal children.

Some of the most common manic symptoms in children are increased psychomotor activity (hyperactivity, distractibility), a push of speech, sleep disturbances, a low frustration tolerance, and outbursts of rage. The early histories of individuals diagnosed with childhood onset bipolar disorder frequently reveal the experience of pronounced separation anxiety associated with excessive clinging to a parent, school phobias, difficulty going to sleep, fear of being alone at night, and night terrors. These symptoms often precede a pattern of cycling that differs from that classically observed in adult patients: the cycles are frequently rapid, of 24–48 hour duration, with brief periods of depression alternating with hypomania or mania, and often characterized by irritable moods, aggressive behavior, and angry outbursts. Older children may have racing thoughts and flights of ideas, as well as grandiose thinking.

Manic-depressive illness is not easy to diagnose in children as many of the symptoms overlap with attention deficit disorder (ADD). Symptoms of ADD include easy distractibility and inattention and impulsive and hyperactive behavior; the picture can resemble aspects of a manic episode. A differential diagnosis must be made between ADD and manic-depressive disorder.

The following is a case history of manic-depressive illness in a young boy:

> Milo, a 13-year-old boy, had a family history of bipolar illness. His paternal grandfather reportedly had been "explosive and temperamental," and two cousins had been hospitalized for manic episodes. Milo's paternal grandmother had had four hospitalizations for manic or depressive episodes and was receiving lithium maintenance.
>
> The father had had two depressive episodes that were treated with tricyclic medication. Milo's 16-year-old brother had dysphoric moods, and a 14-year-old sister had had a learning disability since age 7.
>
> Milo was referred by the school because of poor academic achievement, lack of concentration, and distractibility. He had a history of extreme separation anxiety

in infancy, phobias, tantrums, bed-wetting, hypersensitivity to noise, and "thoughtless behavior" (e.g., destructiveness). His parents reported that he had a low frustration tolerance and that his moods varied from "ecstasy to black despair."

Milo was treated for two years with psychotherapy. The school reported increasing numbers of incidents such as unprovoked school fights, vandalism, and minor theft. A violent attack on a schoolmate led to Milo's expulsion. Lithium carbonate was begun and there were no further reports of uncontrolled explosive aggression.

A follow-up study revealed excellent academic achievement and improved social skills until Milo stopped taking the lithium when he was 16. Impulsive behavior, drug abuse, running away, and brief psychotic episodes were reported before psychotherapy and lithium carbonate were restarted, with good results.

Lithium worked very well in this case, and it appears that young people tolerate lithium very well. In fact, because of the efficiency of the kidneys and the speed with which lithium is excreted by children and adolescents, they often need doses similar to those prescribed for adult patients to maintain adequate blood levels of the drug for maintenance therapy (between 0.75 and 1.00 mEq/liter).

Dr. Gabrielle Carlson, in a chapter of the book *Affective Disorders in Childhood and Adolescence,* explains one point of view urging the use of lithium in young people when appropriate:

Even in the case of mild episodes of depression and mania, if they occur with any frequency (at least two per year), the youngster may have a less stormy adolescence on medication and will be better able to cope with the other age-appropriate demands of making relationships,

finishing school, and identifying himself as other than fla-
grantly psychiatrically ill.

In the past few years, many child psychiatrists have begun
to use divalproex (Depakote) as a first line of treatment at least
in adolescents. It is tolerated well, and there is less danger of
toxicity. (See Chapter 5 for a complete discussion of lithium,
Depakote, and antidepressant drugs.)

MOOD DISORDERS IN THE ELDERLY

As attention has turned to the treatment of affective disorders
in children and adolescents, so it has turned to the large population of the elderly. There are nearly 30 million people 65 years
of age or older in the United States, and it is estimated that 15 to
20 percent of them, or about 5 million people, suffer from
depression.

Some of the precipitants may be social or psychological.
The elderly sustain many losses: their work with its meaningful-
ness, income and structured routine, their friends and loved
ones, and their physical strength. Depression is common after
retirement, and it is easy in this society for an aging person to
feel superfluous, isolated, and alone. The burden of these
adjustments could perhaps be lightened with the help of a psychotherapist or counselor.

Other precipitants of depression may be medical illnesses
or the drugs used to treat them. Elderly patients more commonly have diseases that may appear as depression: hypothyroidism, hyperthyroidism, Cushing's disease, Parkinson's
disease, cardiovascular and pulmonary disorders, vitamin B12
and folic acid deficiencies, carcinoma, and stroke. Many of the
drugs that the elderly consume can induce depression in vulnerable individuals.

The following chart lists the medications that are sometimes associated with depression.

MEDICATIONS SOMETIMES ASSOCIATED WITH DEPRESSION

Antihypertensives (for Controlling Blood Pressure)

clonidine (Catapres)
hydralazine (Apresoline Hydrochloride)
methyldopa (Aldomet)
propranolol (Inderal)
reserpine (Serpasil, Ser-Ap-Es, Sandril)

Antiparkinsonism Agents

levodopa (Dopar, Larodopa)
levodopa and carbidopa (Sinemet)
bromocriptine

Hormones

estrogen
progesterone
cortisone
prednisone

It is vitally important that the diagnosing physician know, and better yet see, the bottles of prescription and nonprescription drugs that the patient is taking. This may provide a clue to one of the contributing factors of the depression.

In order for an accurate diagnosis to be made, the doctor needs to spend time talking with and examining the patient. Depression in an older patient may manifest different symptoms than in a younger adult. The aging person often reports less change in mood and attitude and more of the somatic complaints such as constipation, headaches, and fatigue. Moreover, the elderly depressed patient may appear confused, have memory loss, and be agitated, and the deficits in mental functioning may be ascribed too quickly to dementia. Because doctors expect to see dementia in this age group, there is a tendency to overdiagnose it. In fact, approximately 12 percent of the elderly diagnosed as suffering from a dementia are thought actually to have a false dementia arising from untreated depression. The failure to diagnose depression results tragically in unnecessary suffering, suicide attempts, antisocial behavior, premature retirement, overuse of social and medical services, unnecessary hospital and nursing home admissions, and alienation of family and friends.

It takes a highly trained and sensitive physician to determine whether the problem is dementia, depression mimicking dementia, or depression existing alongside dementia. Tests are needed to help rule out dementia, and the patient will be given a series of radiological and laboratory tests, including an electroencephalogram (EEG), a computerized axial tomogram of the brain (CT scan), thyroid function studies, and blood tests.

If the results of these tests indicate that there is no other underlying cause for the mood changes the patient is experiencing and the state of confusion the patient is in, then the doctor should suspect that the patient is suffering from depression masquerading as dementia. A previous history of depression or a family history of mood disorders would further implicate depression as the problem.

One such case was a 60-year-old man who was admitted to the hospital complaining of fatigue, loss of appetite, difficulty sleeping, and confusion, symptoms he had had for a month. When interviewed by the psychiatrist, the patient was disoriented—he could not remember the date or time of year, nor could he remember events from day to day. His mood shifted rapidly from tearfulness to irritability. The family members were extremely disturbed and afraid that he had Alzheimer's disease.

A close examination of the patient's history revealed that he had suffered two previous depressions: one at age 22, the other at age 40. The first depression lifted after seven treatments of ECT, and the second was successfully treated with the tricyclic antidepressant desipramine. Further neurological and neuropsychological examination revealed no evidence of dementia, and the man was again treated with desipramine. Two and a half weeks later, his mood was normal and the confusion and memory disturbance were gone. He was discharged home to his family.

Treatment

If the treating physician decides that the problem is a depression that could benefit from drug therapy, he or she has a complicated prescription task to confront. The side effects of tricyclic medications can be more serious and pose more problems in this age group. An older patient experiencing the dizziness of orthostatic hypotension (see page 154) is more likely to fracture bones in the event of a fall. Also, because an elderly person's heart is more sensitive to the cardiovascular challenge of these medications, there is increased risk of heart attack and stroke. For these reasons, a doctor would want to prescribe a drug that produces less sedation, and fewer effects on the heart and blood pressure (desipramine and nortriptyline are often prescribed).

There is another consideration when prescribing medications for an older patient. The dosage of medication that would be well tolerated by a young person might be toxic to someone older. Psychiatric drugs remain in the elderly patient's body longer, and exert stronger and more prolonged effects for several reasons.

Chemicals circulating through the body are metabolized by the liver and excreted by the kidneys. Because these organs are less proficient as a person ages, it takes longer for a drug to pass through these "breakdown stations." Also, an increase in body fat relative to lean muscle comes with age. Psychiatric drugs can be stored in fat, and often these drugs are sequestered there and released only slowly. This sustained release can cause a buildup in the body. Toxicity is a considerable problem.

Therefore, elderly patients receive lower doses of medication than are normally prescribed to young adults. But before any medications are dispensed, the doctor requests that the patient have a complete physical exam, including a pretreatment electrocardiogram (EKG). Also, because other prescription and nonprescription drugs can interact poorly with the psychiatric drugs prescribed, the physician asks for a complete list of all medications, including such common household remedies as milk of magnesia, Kaopectate, sodium carbonate, analgesics (Motrin, Advil, or Nuprin), antacids, and Dilantin. A discussion of alcohol and coffee consumption is important also.

The chart demonstrates the doses typically prescribed for the average adult and the elderly patient.

DOSE RANGE OF ANTIDEPRESSANTS

Drug	Dose (mg daily)	
	Average adult	Elderly
imipramine (Tofranil)	75–300	20–150
trazodone (Desyrel)	150–400	25–200
desipramine (Norpramin, Pertofrane)	75–300	20–75
nortriptyline (Aventyl, Pamelor)	50–150	10–100
amoxapine (Asendin)	150–300	50–150
maprotiline (Ludiomil)	75–250	25–150
fluoxetine (Prozac)	10–60	10–20
bupropion (Wellbutrin)	200–300	100–200
paroxetine (Paxil)	20–50	10–40
sertraline (Zoloft)	50–200	*
venlafaxine (Effexor)	75–225	*

*Similar to average adult, but caution must be exercised when increasing dosage.

The common side effects of antidepressants are sedation, dry mouth, constipation, urinary hesitancy or retention, precipitation of narrow-angle glaucoma, weight gain, increase in heart rate, and the orthostatic hypotension mentioned earlier.

The patient should tell the doctor whether he or she has previously responded to a certain antidepressant (chances are that it will work again), or if a relative has had a particularly good response to an antidepressant medication (a possible genetic link may render it effective in the patient also).

During the course of treatment with an antidepressant, the elderly patient should have his or her blood pressure and urine output monitored periodically.

In the case of an agitated depression (the patient is extremely anxious, paces around, and can't sit still) or if there are psychotic symptoms, it is appropriate for a psychiatrist to prescribe an antipsychotic medication along with an antidepressant. Doses in the lower ranges of 5–2 milligrams of Haldol may be effective in ameliorating the agitation or psychotic symptoms.

Clinicians have also reported that methylphenidate hydrochloride (Ritalin), a mild central nervous system stimulant, has been effective in the treatment of elderly depressed patients with medical illnesses.

Patients who have serious cardiovascular problems may be treated more safely with ECT. It has fewer and less dangerous adverse effects than the antidepressant medications, and it usually works well in severe depression (see pages 180–184).

Lithium and the Elderly

The use of lithium by the elderly is quite common, but here again, special precautions are taken. Many older patients are on a salt-restricted diet or take diuretics, leading to increased reabsorption of lithium from the kidneys with higher and more dangerous lithium blood levels. The patient is at greater risk for developing lithium toxicity. Therefore, the blood levels are increased cautiously to usual adult levels, and heart, kidney, and thyroid functioning, as well as lithium blood levels, are checked regularly. It may be best to use a slow-release formula of lithium such as Lithobid in order to flatten peak blood levels (see page 127).

Symptoms of lithium toxicity may include nausea, vomiting, restlessness, tremor, confusion, disorientation, fear, and agitation. Should any of these occur, the patient should take no more medication, and he or the family should call the physician immediately.

THE QUESTION OF PREGNANCY

A 31-year-old woman from Maine who had a bipolar disorder wrote: "I started looking around for material on lithium and pregnancy and found literally nothing! I called my obstetrician and found out that he would allow no lithium the whole term of pregnancy, and not just the first three months. That gave me something to think about seriously."

This young woman faced the dilemma that all women who take medications for mood disorders face when they decide to have children: can one get through the nine-month period of pregnancy without the protection of lithium or other antimanic or antidepressant drugs, and what happens if an episode of mania or depression develops?

Any kind of medication exposes the developing fetus to possible risk, and early evidence suggested that the risk of heart malformation is especially high to fetuses exposed to therapeutic levels of lithium in the first trimester (about 13 times higher than that of the general population). A birth defect called Epstein's anomaly, in which the tricuspid valve of the heart is malformed, occurs approximately once in every 20,000 live births. The Langley-Porter Lithium Registry in San Francisco kept track of babies born to women treated with lithium during pregnancy, and found that out of 166 cases, 18 children had malformations, 12 involving the heart and great vessels, and 4 of the 12 had Epstein's anomaly. Because this syndrome is so rare in the general population, its high incidence among lithium-treated pregnancies was worrisome. Even though a significant percentage of women treated with lithium in the first trimester had normal babies, these reports encouraged a conservative approach and suggested that lithium should not be prescribed during the first months of pregnancy when the fetal organs are being formed. Because one-third to two-thirds of the first trimester passes before the diagnosis of pregnancy is made, a drug-free period of one month was advisable before attempting conception.

But in 1994, Dr. Lee Cohen and his colleagues at the Harvard Medical School published the most extensive literature review to date on in utero exposure to lithium and found that the risk of Epstein's anomaly was much lower than originally feared. The original conclusions of higher risk were based exclusively on a voluntary reporting system that tended to underreport healthy fetal births, thereby inflating estimates of Epstein's anomaly.

While this reduced risk factor is welcome news for patients and their physicians, a slightly higher risk is reported nonetheless. But this should be balanced against the substantial risks of an untreated manic or depressive episode. Dr. Lee Cohen's article in the *Journal of the American Medical Association*, "A Reevaluation of Risk of in Utero Exposure to Lithium," offers helpful treatment recommendations to psychiatrists for lithium use in women with bipolar disorder, and we include them here:

TREATMENT RECOMMENDATIONS FOR LITHIUM USE IN WOMEN WITH BIPOLAR DISORDER

I. Encourage careful contraception practices for women of childbearing age

II. Evaluate the need for lithium prophylaxis

   A. In women with single episodes of affective instability and long intervening periods of well-being

      1. Attempt gradual tapering and discontinuation of lithium prophylaxis prior to pregnancy

      2. Maintain lithium-free well-being for the entire pregnancy if possible; reintroduce lithium during the second and third trimesters if necessary

   B. In women with severe bipolar disorder in whom discontinuation of lithium prophylaxis poses substantial risk of increased morbidity

      1. Temporarily discontinue lithium therapy for a period coinciding as closely as possible with that of embryogenesis (the development of the embryo)

      2. Consider reintroduction of lithium and/or treatment with antipsychotic agents if clinical deterioration occurs

   C. In women with severe bipolar disorder in whom discontinuation of lithium prophylaxis poses an *unacceptable* risk of increased morbidity, maintain lithium therapy throughout pregnancy

III. Other considerations for women who take lithium during all or part of the first trimester of pregnancy

   A. Provide reproductive risk counseling as early in pregnancy as possible

   B. Offer prenatal diagnosis by fetal echocardiography and high-resolution ultrasound examination at 16 to 18 weeks gestation

Lithium used at the end of a pregnancy can be a problem also. Fetal distress can occur: the babies may be born lethargic and listless with decreased suck response and Moro reflex (the startle response of newborns). They may have decreased oxygenation and appear bluish.

The mother has a greater risk of lithium toxicity after the

delivery. Increased kidney function during pregnancy results in more lithium's being excreted, so higher doses may have to be prescribed. However, during and after delivery, kidney function returns to normal, and there are major alterations in fluid and electrolyte metabolism. More lithium may be retained in the body, leading to a too-high blood level. Therefore, the lithium dose should be reduced by 50 percent or more in the last week of the pregnancy and stopped completely with the onset of labor. Once the fluids return to normal (approximately three to four days after birth), lithium therapy can be reinstated. Breast feeding is not a good idea because breast milk lithium concentration is about 30 to 50 percent of the mother's blood level. A newborn does not have well-developed systems of excretion, and there have been reports of insufficient oxygenation of the blood (cyanosis) and poor muscle tone in infants breast fed by mothers on lithium.

There was even less information about the problems of antidepressant drugs used during pregnancy or in nursing mothers. These drugs do pass the placental barrier and can be excreted in low levels in breast milk, and there were rare reports of neonatal distress in infants born to mothers given these medications. Some of the babies suffered muscle spasms, an unusually fast heart rate (tachycardia), congestive heart failure, and respiratory distress.

But data has been accumulating in the last few years about antidepressant treatment during pregnancy, and a multicenter collaborative study was published in 1993. Dr. Anne Pastuszak and her colleagues compared outcomes of pregnancy among 128 mothers who took Prozac during the first trimester with those of two age-matched control groups: women who had taken tricyclic antidepressants during the first trimester and women who had taken medications that are known not to cause birth defects.

It appears that the babies who were born to women on Prozac or on tricyclic antidepressants fared as well as the comparison group born to women who were taking drugs known not to cause birth defects. The rates of major malformations were comparable among the three groups and did not surpass rates expected in the general population. Thus, this study reported findings that suggest that neither Prozac or tricyclic antidepressants appear to cause birth defects.

But there were two other notable differences that the study brought to light: the women treated with Prozac and tricyclic antidepressants appeared to have a slightly higher rate of miscarriage than the women exposed to the known nonteratogenic medications; and the infants born to women in the antidepressant-treated groups tended to have more neonatal complications, although, when looked at individually, none of the recorded complications was significantly more common.

The data sent to us by Prozac's manufacturer, Eli Lilly, supports these findings. In 37 clinical trials, 758 women were identified as having been exposed to Prozac in the first trimester, and there was neither a consistent nor a recurring pattern of abnormalities in the newborns.

The possible link between antidepressant drug therapy and miscarriage will require further study along with questions about the effects of psychotropic medicine on the developing brain. In the meantime, the lack of birth defects (teratogenesis) is encouraging, and the risk of antidepressants during pregnancy has to be weighed against the high risk of depressive episodes that can follow discontinuation of the medication.

Antipsychotic drugs may be a problem, however. There continue to be disturbing reports on neurological and behavioral abnormalities in neonatal rats born to rat mothers exposed to these medications. Therefore, their use should be limited in pregnancy if possible, but if they are necessary, a relatively potent antipsychotic such as haloperidol (Haldol) or fluphenazine (Prolixin) should be prescribed in small, divided doses.

Sedatives, benzodiazepines such as Valium or Klonopin

and anticonvulsants such as Tegretol and Depakote should be avoided.

Undoubtedly the safest and most effective way to treat a pregnant woman experiencing a manic or depressive episode is with electroconvulsive therapy (ECT). This treatment option can be used during any stage of the pregnancy and is thoroughly described on pages 180–184. An obstetrician should be a part of the ECT treatment team, and external fetal monitoring should be done before the treatment and for several hours afterward. In the event that the woman is carrying more than one baby, or has high blood pressure, diabetes, a history of premature labor or heart or kidney disease, ECT may not be the right treatment as there may be some concern about premature labor.

All of the above speaks in favor of cautious deliberation when planning a pregnancy. A close-working team of psychiatrist, obstetrician, and patient is critical. A woman should understand the risks of medications, particularly in the first trimester and right around the period of delivery, and decide which options might be preferable.

It goes without saying that pregnancy produces a host of physical and psychological changes in a woman, and there is some debate as to whether the hormonal shifts of pregnancy stress the woman with a mood disorder or whether they have a protective effect. There is, however, agreement that the period immediately following childbirth is a time of increased vulnerability to depression and (in those who are bipolar) mania. Forearmed with this knowledge, a woman should stay in close contact with her psychiatrist who, if necessary, can prescribe medications to stabilize her mood.

We wanted to convey what's known or suspected in the medical arena regarding pregnancy, but the human experience of what a woman faces is virtually absent in the scientific literature. The young woman who couldn't find information when she planned her pregnancy told her story with informative detail:

After I had been stable for about a year, I decided that I should try getting pregnant. On New Year's eve, I stopped taking all medications. I told my psychiatrist that my obstetrician advised no lithium or carbamazapine or valproic acid. If worse came to worst, I could always have electroshock therapy. I just hoped nothing would happen.

I was very, very lucky to become pregnant in one month. When I found out I was pregnant, I began to worry, of course, that I would lose my mind by the end of the week, that I would have to have shock treatments, etc., etc. I remember getting up in the morning, looking in the mirror and thinking: "Well, will you lose it this morning?" After a few weeks (probably about ten weeks) I began to have more confidence that I would not have my ups and downs. Of course I was very moody from the hormones of pregnancy. This is quite common, and most everyone goes through it, but I thought with each mood that "this was it" and I would really have trouble.

I was very fortunate, because I never did have serious mood swings while I was pregnant. I know now that if I would have had trouble, both my obstetrician and psychiatrist would have worked together to make sure both the baby and I were okay. I also know that in my case, somehow, the hormones of pregnancy "insulate" me from serious mood swings. This is not a medical fact, just something I know.

I am now the proud parent of a three-month-old baby girl named Alice. She and I have survived colic and a very serious postpartum depression for me. I think that it took me almost five weeks to recover from the birth (I had a C-section, as Alice was breech). A difficult part of the postpartum weeks is the depression and moodiness that go along with losing all those hormones. I was sure I was going to have to take medication again. However, one day I started feeling better, and although I have moods just like other people do, I am essentially without serious mood swings.

I am attending college again. I have changed my major from business administration to nursing and I'm trying to survive my first chemistry course.

I would certainly encourage women who are on lithium to at least give pregnancy serious consideration. Talk to your obstetrician and tell him or her that you are a lithium-medicated patient and are considering pregnancy. Your obstetrician should speak at length with your psychiatrist and you can all decide how best to handle the pregnancy and the postpartum period. Once you are pregnant, communicate with your partner at all times as to how you are feeling and keep in touch with your psychiatrist as often as is necessary.

COMORBIDITY: MOOD DISORDERS AND SUBSTANCE ABUSE

Sarah's story in the last chapter underscores what clinicians have long observed: alcohol and drug abuse are frequently associated with mood disorders. It was commonly thought that patients with mood disorders who use substances were self-medicating—they were either prolonging the highs of hypomania with stimulants or calming the anxiety of depression and the irritability of mixed states with alcohol.

In the last few years, however, researchers have begun to look more carefully at this "comorbidity" of substance abuse with mood disorders and are asking the following questions: Is this association really due to attempts at self-medication? Is the tendency to crave substances of abuse a heritable phenomenon that travels in the company of the gene or genes that predispose to mania or depression? Or do abused substances induce mania or depression?

Whatever the answer, the comorbidity of substance abuse and affective illness has been vastly underestimated. In a random sample of 500 members of the National Depressive and

Manic-Depressive Association, 41 percent of the members who have bipolar disorder reported that they had abused alcohol or drugs prior to correct diagnosis and treatment of the mood disorder, compared to 13 percent among patients properly diagnosed and treated.

The Epidemiologic Catchment Area data of 1990 pinpointed an even higher statistic. It showed that 61 percent of bipolar I patients had a history of substance abuse. Of that number, 15 percent used drugs alone; 20 percent used alcohol alone; and 26 percent used both alcohol and drugs.

These findings suggest that individuals with undiagnosed bipolar disorders may comprise a larger percentage of the substance-abusing population than originally thought. In an unpublished survey of all patients attending a methadone maintenance center who were referred for psychiatric evaluation during a three-month period, 55 percent were diagnosed with bipolar spectrum disorders.

According to a study by Dr. Kathleen T. Brady, the clinical director of the Center for Drug and Alcohol Programs at the Medical University of South Carolina, and Dr. Susan C. Sonne, those patients with substance abuse disorder and bipolar disorder have a much earlier age of onset of the mood disorder. The average age of onset for bipolar abusers is 20, whereas the average age of onset in nonusers is 27. Other studies have found that substance-abusing bipolar patients are more likely to have dysphoric (irritable, paranoid) episodes of mania, rather than the elated kind. They are also more likely to relapse, have 50 percent more hospitalizations, and are less likely to respond to lithium.

This brings up the question of how these patients should be treated. Because there is a higher rate of mixed states and rapid cycling among substance-abusing bipolar patients, experienced clinicians have noted a higher success rate with divalproex sodium (Depakote) than with lithium. Not only does it decrease the affective symptoms, but there is some thought that it may reduce withdrawal symptoms and craving in these dually diagnosed patients.

But medication choice is just part of the treatment. Patients need to be informed and counseled that anyone with bipolar disorders (particularly bipolar I patients) will more likely become addicted and suffer a worse course of illness if he or she begins using either stimulants or alcohol. Patients with a dual diagnosis need not only medication and psychotherapy, but placement in groups and programs that address the substance abuse. According to the American Psychiatric Association's *Guideline for the Treatment of Patients with Bipolar Disorder,* "treatment for substance abuse disorder and mood disorder should proceed concurrently, to the extent possible. The treatment of one disorder may have effects on the treatment of the other."

9

HOW TO GET GOOD TREATMENT

The last few chapters indicate the importance of a combined medical and psychological treatment approach to affective disorders, but a patient doesn't usually just fall into an ideal treatment program administered by ideal treatment providers. There is a confusing array of mental health providers out there—psychiatrists, psychologists, social workers, and therapists, all with different orientations—and it will take serious investigation by the patient and family members to seek out the treatment best suited to their needs. The quality and amount of treatment a person receives will also be determined by the kind of practitioners available in the area, the type of insurance policy the patient has, or the amount of money the patient or family can afford to pay.

The first and most crucial step is the diagnosis. A medical doctor is the only person who can rule out diseases that might be masquerading as an affective disorder (such as multiple sclerosis, hypo- or hyperthyroidism, vitamin B_{12} deficiency, temporal lobe epilepsy, and other brain disorders). Should the problem prove to be an affective disorder, a psychiatrist is the only professional trained to treat these disorders with medications and electroconvulsive therapy and able, if need be, to admit the patient to a psychiatric unit.

WHAT TO LOOK FOR IN A DOCTOR

One survey estimated that 54 percent of adults with psychiatric disorders in the United States are treated by internists or family practitioners, and that there is a resistance to seeking out or receiving treatment from a psychiatrist. (No doubt stigma and limited insurance coverage for mental health services do much to produce this resistance.) In some situations, when the illness is mild and the doctor is knowledgeable about and interested in affective disorders, treatment by a nonpsychiatrist may be sufficient. But in the case of severe depression where there is a possibility of suicide, or where there are bipolar or psychotic symptoms, the patient should be cared for by an experienced psychiatrist.

A patient needs a psychiatrist who has had experience with the full range of affective syndromes, one who is adept in diagnosis and very familiar with the use of such medications as lithium, antidepressants, MAOIs, antipsychotics, and anticonvulsants (see Chapter 5). The psychiatrist should be affiliated with a good hospital and be able to deal with patients who may experience psychotic symptoms and require vigorous intervention or protection, sometimes against their will. The doctor should also be able to explain thoroughly what is known and what is not known about the disorder and the medications, and speak frankly with the patient about what he or she may expect.

But a patient should look for more than a diagnostician/pharmacologist. The doctor should have an empathic understanding of a person's experience during a state of depression, hypomania, or mania. He or she can then help the patient determine which aspects of behavior, wishes, or decision making are induced by the episodic mood swings and which arise out of personality, background, or everyday life situations.

Because depressive, hypomanic, and manic episodes can dramatically change the way in which a person relates to the peo-

ple closest to him or her—a spouse and other family members—
and because a family member's misunderstanding of the illness
can lead to conflict and estrangement, it might be advantageous
to choose a psychiatrist who, if necessary, will involve the family
members in the treatment. Some psychiatrists, however, feel that
couple or family treatment violates the patient's contract of confidentiality. If it's important that the family have the option of
meeting the psychiatrist to discuss their attitudes and feelings,
this should be discussed before treatment commences. (Naturally
it is difficult to "doctor shop" during a crisis, and we do not intend
to downplay the time element and judgment problems to be considered when someone is in an acute state.)

Patients who had been treated by a number of psychiatrists were very emphatic about what constituted a good doctor. They advise looking for someone who:

- "has basic qualifications: medical knowledge, pharmacological knowledge, psychological knowledge. I
  would advise someone to look for honesty. By this I
  mean a doctor willing to tell the patient the truth. I had
  a number of doctors who were very evasive for one reason or another."
- "gives details and talks to you like an intelligent person
  (doesn't patronize). Someone who lets you know what
  to expect and what to prepare yourself for, with the illness and the medications."
- "is not one-track-minded, like a psychopharmacologist.
  Someone who does not pressure you to hurry what
  you're saying. Preferably someone who appreciates the
  benefits of talking therapy."
- "shows genuine concern for your well-being, is available
  during emergencies, stays current with new alternative
  drugs and research, is willing to change medications if
  necessary and conducts psychotherapy as a useful
  adjunct."

HOW TO FIND A DOCTOR

There are several avenues to explore in finding the right doctor. Ask your personal physician for a referral. Or, if you live near a university-affiliated teaching hospital, you can call the department of psychiatry and ask to speak to the chief resident or the admissions director or the clinical director, and tell the person with whom you speak that you are looking for the names of psychiatrists who have expertise in the area of mood disorders. It is always a good idea to get two or three names so that you can not only seek a "second opinion," but also decide with whom you feel most comfortable. Trust your instincts.

Another source is Appendix 4 of this book, where you can find the telephone numbers of the nation's two leading patient support groups. When you call the office listed, tell the person you reach what it is you need. The patients and families who belong to these organizations have had firsthand experience with many of the psychiatrists in your area and they are often in a good position to steer you toward a highly competent physician. Of course, if you are enrolled in a managed care program, you will be referred to one of the psychiatrists on its panel.

Once you have the referral, make a telephone call. Just give your name, mention the name of the doctor or person who referred you, and tell the psychiatrist that you would like to schedule an appointment for a consultation. This is not the time for a long, detailed discussion—all of that will be handled in the consultation session.

THE CONSULTATION

The first meeting is simply a conversation between you and the doctor. The psychiatrist gets a complete picture of the specific symptoms that are troubling you by asking questions about mood, appetite, sleeping, and daily activity levels, as well as about relationships at home and at work. Because there is a genetic component to mood disorders, and because other illnesses can produce the symptoms of a mood disorder, the psychiatrist will ask about your family and medical history. As the doctor begins to get an impression of the current episode or problem, he or she explores the possibility that there may have been episodes of mania, hypomania, depression, or mood changes in the past.

Most people are uncomfortable telling a virtual stranger intimate things about themselves, their feelings and their behavior, and a sensitive psychiatrist expects and understands this. But since, as we mentioned before, there are no established laboratory tests that can confirm or refute a diagnosis in psychiatry, knowledge of the symptoms, behavior patterns, history and course of illness are essential for a correct diagnosis. It is quite possible that two or three sessions will be needed in order for the doctor to understand the problem and make appropriate recommendations for future treatment.

If the diagnosis of a mood disorder is made, and if the symptoms are now acute, it is likely that the psychiatrist will want to attenuate the symptoms with a medical intervention— one of the medications mentioned in Chapter 5. Before writing and explaining a prescription, however, the doctor should ask the patient to visit an internist for a complete physical examination, including routine blood tests and an electrocardiogram. The psychiatrist looks at the results of the physical exam, considers the course of the disorder and which drugs the person, or his or her family members, may have responded to in the past (medication response and side effects can be heritable), and decides on a medication trial. The patient should be informed as to why the drug was chosen; what laboratory tests, if any, will be required while taking it; and what short- and long-term side effects might be expected.

Because medications address only certain problems caused by a mood disorder, and psychotherapy addresses others, the patient and prescribing physician should talk frankly about the advantages of an adjunctive psychotherapy. This may necessitate a referral to another mental health professional because it is not always the case that the physician provides both the medications and the psychotherapy. And here's where things get confusing—an unfortunate polarization currently exists in the treatment of major affective disorders.

There are so-called "biological" psychiatrists and "psychodynamic" psychiatrists. Biological psychiatrists focus principally on precise diagnosis and medical treatment, and although they pay lip service to the need for the talking therapies, few make use of this body of knowledge in their approach to treatment. (A study by Drs. Frederick Goodwin and Kay Jamison of patients treated with lithium found that 50 percent of the patient group considered psychotherapy to be important in lithium compliance, while only 27 percent of the clinicians regarded psychotherapy as important. This observation may indicate a tendency for physicians to estimate the potency of a drug so highly that they underestimate the psychological aspects of the illness.) Conversely, while many psychiatrists with a psychodynamic or psychoanalytic orientation recognize biological contributions to the treatment of the symptoms, many do not make use of the knowledge in practice, and may believe that psychological treatments alone are adequate or even preferable. These real biases have contributed to a fragmentation in the field and in the care of patients that reflects the training and indoctrination of the psychiatrist rather than the current knowledge of the nature and course of the disorder.

Part of the problem is that there has been such a rapid accumulation of knowledge in the field. Discoveries constantly occur after the formal training of any professional and require a constant updating of knowledge through continuing education programs and careful attention to scientific and clinical journals. Because there are still gaps in our understanding of the causes and treatment of these disorders, and because physiological factors may predominate in some cases of depression while psychological factors predominate in others, there has been no uniform standard of treatment.

As a result, a patient is presented with a confusing array of practitioners whose conceptualization of the illness may include:

1. A view of the disorder that focuses on the treatment of some underlying deficit (presumed to be at the level of transmission between nerve cells) with medications. Psychological conflict, stress, or interpersonal issues may be seen as arising from the disorder or are considered unimportant.

2. A view of the disorder that focuses on the resolution of psychological conflict as the primary goal of treatment and precludes the conception that there may exist an underlying deficit at the level of neurotransmission. (Neither of these views has been proven.)

3. A view of the disorder that explains the symptoms as a reflection of interpersonal conflict occurring between family members. The focus of the treatment would be to reveal and modify this conflict.

4. Integrated, commonsense approaches, combining pharmacological and psychological methods, which we support.

During the consultation, patients and family members have every right to inquire about the mental health professional's orientation and clinical views, and such questions as "Do you believe drugs are important in treating the illness?" and "Do you feel psychotherapy is an important supplement to the medical treatment?" will reveal the orientation of the practitioner. The psychiatrist should help a patient decide if an adjunctive psychotherapy is indicated, and if the psychiatrist does not provide it, he or she should make a referral.

COSTS

Beyond the question of the psychiatrist's training and orientation is the question of whether or not the patient can afford frequent psychotherapy with that psychiatrist. Many patients who recognize the need to address the psychological aspects of their situation seek out less expensive mental health professionals to conduct the psychotherapy (this may be a psychologist, social worker, or nurse practitioner). The psychiatrist, then, manages the medical aspects of the treatment on a less frequent basis.

But a note of caution should be injected here also: if the professional who manages the psychotherapeutic aspects of the treatment does not have a solid understanding of the disorder, its course, and medical treatment, it is possible that aspects of the patient's behavior, mood, and thinking may be misinterpreted. For example, if a patient suddenly begins planning an exotic trip abroad and the therapist assumes that the behavior is motivated only by a wish to avoid the intensity of the therapy or some other unpleasant situation, and does not think to inquire about the presence of other symptoms (such as decreased sleep, changes in libido and appetite, etc.), the advent of a manic episode could be missed. Teasing apart motivations that arise from personality and background from those propelled by an impending episode of illness can be exceedingly difficult. However, the patient is best served when all things are considered, and this requires a comprehensive view of the person and the disorder.

How much would treatment with any of these different professionals cost? As this book goes to press, typical fees per session are:

Psychiatrist	$100–175
Clinical psychologist	$85–120
Social worker	$65–110

Some clinical psychopharmacologists may charge $150–500 for a comprehensive consultative assessment. Psychological testing may cost approximately $300–500. A follow-up visit to a psychiatrist for medication management may take 20 to 30 minutes and will probably cost about $100–140. Many mental health professionals have a sliding scale for fees based on an individual's ability to pay.

CLINICS

Anyone scanning the private fees listed above quickly realizes that the long-term medical and psychological treatment of these disorders costs a great deal of money or requires a very comprehensive insurance policy. Fortunately there are other alternatives: in most areas there are clinics that provide treatment based on a patient's income and ability to pay. As with any service, the quality of treatment varies.

In certain areas of the country there are major affective disorders clinics—usually attached to the departments of psychiatry in academic centers—and their interests often include research into the nature of the disorders and their treatment. The medical leadership of such clinics is usually sophisticated in the diagnosis and pharmacological treatment of the disorders, but not all of them assess the psychological and social ramifications of these illnesses with equal vigor and skill, or make patient education one of the primary goals.

Another kind of outpatient setting is the university-affiliated teaching clinic. Here the patient is seen by a resident who may have good training and supervision (although limited experience), but who will be in the clinic for only a limited period of time. The patient has a long-term disorder; the doctor may change every year or less. Should a close collaborative relationship develop, the patient suffers a loss when the resident rotates off the service. Then a new doctor–patient relationship has to be formed, and the new doctor will not have a level of training higher than the last.

More common is the publicly funded community mental health or catchment area clinic that serves a specific locality. Again the quality and level of sophistication varies from clinic to clinic. Affective disorders are not the only psychiatric conditions treated, and funds are limited. Very commonly a patient sees a doctor only for initial evaluation, medication renewal or adjustment, or to deal with a crisis. If psychotherapy is offered, it is almost always administered by a nonmedical therapist.

Few, if any, of these kinds of clinics actively involve the family, and this just doesn't make sense. In many instances the family is the only support the patient has during periods of illness and recovery, assuring the patient's adherence to medication and recognizing symptoms early. Moreover, given that there is a genetic vulnerability in families (see page 55), involving family members and educating them about the symptoms, course, and available treatments provides a measure of preventative treatment, assisting in the early recognition and treatment of the disorder should it appear in other family members.

THE IDEAL COMPREHENSIVE CLINIC PROGRAM

It is obvious that there are positive aspects as well as pitfalls in the current organization of psychiatric care and other mental health services. So, what constitutes an ideal approach to treatment that could be developed in an outpatient treatment setting? Let us draw a picture of how a good program can effectively address the needs of patients and families. Such a clinic would serve as a diagnostic, medical treatment and education center. It would assess the psychological impact of the illness on both patients and families and offer supportive services for long-term management of the disorder.

In this ideal arrangement, a patient is seen individually by a psychiatrist for several sessions. During these hours, a history of past episodes is spelled out and their frequency and duration documented. The family history is explored, as are previous treatments, their effects and side effects. The doctor then orders a complete medical evaluation, including a physical exam, in order to exclude other medical causes for the symptoms and to guide treatment.

Once the diagnosis has been clearly established, the patient and family are invited to participate in a workshop where the nature, course, possible causes, and treatments of the disorder are reviewed. The "psychoeducational" approach described in Chapter 6 is explained, and the family has the option of entering into several sessions of family counseling.

Then a recommendation for follow-up treatment is made. While a psychiatrist follows each patient individually for long-term medical treatment, some patients may also opt for individual psychotherapy, and some families may wish to continue in a family-centered treatment or join a multiple-family group. Attached to the clinic is a manic-depressive and depressive support group run by patients and family members (see pages 349–352).

Research into the nature and possible causes of these disorders is rapidly moving in the direction of identifying a genetic marker that would identify those at risk. These clinics could serve as a resource for this kind of research, perhaps contributing to a better understanding of the disorders and better treatments in the future.

Unfortunately, such a comprehensive program is not commonly available. Nevertheless, institutions responsible for the delivery of medical care in this country are becoming more responsive to consumer needs. If patients and family members come together and work with the leaders of such clinics, they can sensitize them to the services they need and want, and thus forge a better system. A group of people bound by ideas, commitment, and strong resolve could have their say and effect change.

THE PATIENT'S ROLE
IN OBTAINING GOOD TREATMENT

Now that we've alerted patients and family members to the possible pitfalls in psychiatric care, we want to close this chapter with a discussion of the patient's role in a good treatment plan. For there are two parts to the equation: a skilled, empathic doctor and a patient who realizes that he or she also shapes the outcome of treatment. Success very much depends on the ability of the patient to take an active part in and make a commitment to the treatment alliance.

First the patient must accept that it is not uncommon for there to be a trial-and-error period of drug selection and adjustment. Some people respond dramatically to lithium and antidepressant treatment and have few, if any, problems; others have a more difficult time of it. Either the response is not a complete one or the side effects are intolerable. Should this be the case, a period of new medication trials is initiated. During this time of uncertainty, which may last months or even a year, the patient is often frustrated, angry, and demoralized. A patient who understands the realities and the potential difficulties inherent in treating these conditions may be more willing to give the psychiatrist the time it takes to initiate and assess the medication trials and may feel more comfortable in the time preceding stabilization.

It is important that the patient report the side effects accurately to the physician. If there are considerations about changing the medication or adding a medication to counter the side effects, an open dialogue between the doctor and patient regarding the risks and benefits of alternate courses of action must take place. Naturally, it is the physician's responsibility to inform and educate the patient at each juncture of pharmacological treatment, but because there are these varying alternatives, the patient should expect to be part of the decision-making process.

Even though the psychiatrist and patient may initially concern themselves with the pharmacological treatment, any care-taking relationship rekindles earlier conflicts around dependency, attachment, and intimacy. Some patients are fearful of becoming dependent on the psychiatrist and may express these feelings by wanting to control the management of the medications entirely. They may either discontinue the medications or adapt their own regimes without consulting the doctor. Other patients have highly unrealistic expectations of the psychiatrist and can become disappointed and angry when these expectations are not met. These issues, which can interfere with the establishment of a therapeutic alliance, often have less to do with the illness than with specific personality problems. Although these conflicts and issues are foreseeable, they add to the complexity of the medical treatment and could cause the patient to terminate therapy. However, a good psychiatrist recognizes that just as patients respond differently to medications so they have variable responses to their having to take the medications and to the practitioner who prescribes them. These issues can be resolved, but only if the patient stays in treatment, discusses his or her feelings openly, and is able to work through the fears, unrealistic wishes, and positive and negative feelings toward the psychiatrist/therapist.

THREE

LIVING WITH THE ILLNESS

10
THE FAMILY
AND THE ILLNESS

When a relative experiences recurrent episodes of depression or mania, there is a profoundly disruptive and disorganizing effect on family life. The other members of the family are faced with the challenge of looking after and providing for the needs of their relative while at the same time maintaining their other responsibilities at work and at home—often within an atmosphere of confusion, isolation, embarrassment, anger, and guilt. Before long, the individual needs of all the family members are ignored as each tries to grapple with the tension and uncertainty that accompany these disorders.

It is probably not possible to calculate the degree of pain and the exhaustion such families feel. With guidance and encouragement, however, families can gain a better perspective and organize themselves so as to expend energy most effectively. There may still be bad feelings and even emotional storms, but the family doesn't have to weather them without the life preservers of knowledge, understanding, and practical coping strategies.

There are stages of recognition, adjustment, and adaptation to illness, and each family travels through the stages in its own time and in its own fashion. Many factors influence the family's initial response to the onset of the illness: some members need to protect themselves with the cloak of denial;

almost all invent theories or take responsibility in an attempt to explain the changes in behavior. When the symptoms are mild, and if they are interspersed with periods of functioning well, it is not difficult to attribute them to external events, personal circumstances, or personality quirks. Some families are more able or willing than others to tolerate behavior that deviates from the norm. Sooner or later, though, if the symptoms become more severe and disruptive, the patient and the family members may seek professional advice and find a name for their problem. Then a new period of adjustment and regrouping can take place within the family.

Each family is actually a caretaking system that over time has established rules, expectations, and basic assumptions about caring for each other. Illness of any kind has an impact on this caretaking system and necessitates shifts in the interactions among the members. It is vital that all the members seek a common perspective about the nature of the illness, its course, the limitations it imposes on the patient and what they can expect during acute episodes and over the long term in which there may be recurrences of illness and sustained disability.

The first change that confronts the family is the loss of functioning of the ill member. Since he or she is no longer able to fulfill usual responsibilities within the family, someone else must take on the tasks, and time must be devoted to caring for the person who is ill. In the case of a patient who is the principal wage earner and/or organizer of the home, severe disruption of ordinary family life may occur until effective role shifts have taken place.

When the patient is a young person in the family, parents suffer the anguish of watching their child in pain, and fear for the quality of his or her future. Hopes and expectations may have to be modified and mourned, and the child may grow into an adult who needs more attention, caretaking, and financial support than had previously been planned for, which sometimes causes anger and guilt.

Many families search for the blame among themselves and feel shame in having their relatives, neighbors, or colleagues know that there is mental illness in their home. Sadly, these worries deplete them all the more.

A host of problems and questions arise for each family, and the answers will vary from patient to patient and family to family. There is no typical scenario, but there are common problems and emotions that emerge in every family's attempt to cope with a major mental illness. The following pages examine a few of these.

ONE FAMILY'S RESPONSE TO DEPRESSION

When a person is feeling depressed and helpless, it is common for loved ones to assume that attention, assistance, and assurances will restore that person's capacity to respond. Most family members offer this kind of help and provide what seems to be required by the situation. But a person suffering depression usually feels fatigue, lack of energy, loss of appetite, and a general loss of ability to care for himself, and may respond negatively to well-wishers the harder they try to motivate him. A vicious cycle develops: the family members who have extended themselves conscientiously, and to no avail, may feel frustrated, resentful, angry, or despairing, and this further compounds the sense of isolation, guilt, or hopelessness the ill relative already feels.

One family's experience of this cycle began every morning as they tried to rouse their severely depressed mother. All the children would gather at her bedside offering positive statements and encouragement, impressing upon her the need to eat. As the day wore on her mood seemed to brighten somewhat, and in the late afternoon she actually got out of bed, joined the family at the dinner table, and shared in one of a string of jokes her son told to ease the tension and entertain her. The children, although exhausted, felt a great sense of relief and pride at night, thinking their efforts had done much to lift her spirits. They fully expected that each day would bring further improvement.

The following morning their mother was again unable to eat and did not want to get out of bed. She was irritable and seemed annoyed by the children's attention to her condition. The family, in turn, felt increasingly ineffectual and irritated with their mother. Their good intentions and best efforts had made no lasting impact and even seemed to make matters worse.

And therein lies the cruel hoax of depression. There is typically a daily variation in the intensity of symptoms called a *diurnal mood variation.* The person may feel awful in the morning, but as the day progresses, the mood brightens. This pattern continues day after day, dashing the hopes and expectations of family members—in some ways mocking their efforts.

The children consulted their mother's psychiatrist, and after informing them that the antidepressant she was taking would take at least two or three weeks more to work, the psychiatrist helped them devise a method of coping with the situation. They set up a schedule of two-hour shifts among themselves to ensure that someone was always in the house and nearby, but they stopped pressuring her to make immediate gains. They simply expressed confidence that time would pass and she would recover.

This family coped with the vicious cycle of tremendous effort, fluctuating hopes, exhaustion, and resentment by modifying their expectations. While their mother needed to know of their continued concern and support, the children realized that their best efforts would not permanently restore her disposition. In some ways they were doubly burdening her with their wishes for early improvement. She experienced this as an impossible demand with which she was unable to comply and about which she felt increasingly guilty and frustrated.

By modifying their natural tendency to expect immediate

results and improvement, the children lessened the demands they placed on themselves and on their ill mother, and they increased their stamina and capacity to endure.

SUICIDAL BEHAVIOR

Few things in life are more threatening than a relative (or patient) who expresses suicidal thoughts or behavior. When a person is overtly suicidal, most families recognize the necessity of immediate professional help. However, suicidal intentions are often expressed in more subtle and ambiguous ways. Most families are not prepared to judge the seriousness of the threat, and the lack of a plan of action or response raises their anxiety level to such a degree that the family is unable to act effectively and in a timely fashion.

If relatives even suspect that the patient is thinking about suicide, they should call the treating psychiatrist immediately and alert him or her to that fact. Depending on a variety of factors, hospitalization may be indicated. Suicide is often an impulsive act: the patient can be having coffee in the kitchen with someone one minute, retire to the bedroom, and leap from an open window. It happens that fast; it happens that unexpectedly. The myth that people who threaten to commit suicide never do so is a dangerous one to subscribe to. People often carry out their threats, particularly if they are ignored.

The family may have to resort to involuntary commitment to prevent the patient from killing him or herself. Family members who have a severely depressed relative should first consult with a psychiatrist. If the patient's condition warrants hospitalization, the family members should discuss with the psychiatrist the procedure for admission to a psychiatric unit. Chapter 11, on hospitalization and commitment, should help to clarify this process.

What are the common warning signs of suicidal intention?

- feelings of worthlessness or hopelessness
- preoccupation with morbid topics or death
- withdrawal from previous activities or relationships and estrangement from family and friends
- increased risk-taking behaviors (for example, driving too fast, drinking heavily, handling knives or guns)
- sudden brightening of mood or increased activity in someone who has been seriously depressed
- putting one's affairs in order (for example, writing a will, giving prized possessions away, saying goodbye to people)
- feelings of anguish or desperation
- voices that are commanding the patient to hurt himself or other irrational experiences
- actually thinking about a plan to take one's own life

People with a family history of suicide are at particular risk. Others before them have used suicide as a solution to a problem and they may use that self-destructive act as a model. Moreover, there is evidence to suggest that for some there is a genetic predisposition to suicide. Biological studies conducted in the late 1970s by Drs. Herman van Praag in Holland and Marie Asberg in Sweden revealed that certain suicide attempters had a decreased level of the metabolite of the neurotransmitter serotonin in their spinal fluid (5-hydroxyindoleacetic acid or 5-HIAA). Individuals with these lower levels of 5-HIAA were more likely to attempt suicide in an impulsive and violent manner. Some researchers believe that this finding may one day lead to a biochemical test to predict who is at risk for suicide.

In the meantime, once the family suspects the patient's suicidal potential and has located and consulted a psychiatrist, there are some practical steps that the family can take to limit the expression of the impulse:

1. Remove access to knives, guns, medications, automobiles, and other potentially lethal instruments.

2. Monitor the taking of medications, first to ensure that the patient is taking them (thus limiting the time that he or she suffers with suicidal depression), and also to guard against an overdose. Antidepressants or lithium and some sleeping pills (especially if taken with alcohol) can be fatal if taken in too large a dose.

3. Let the patient talk about suicidal thoughts without the family's expressing shock and condemnation. If the family understands that suicidal thoughts and impulses are not unusual in severe depression, and conveys this understanding, the patient may feel less guilty and isolated. The patient is not forced into secrecy, and such open communication may allow both the family and the patient to better judge when protective hospitalization is necessary.

COPING WITH MANIC BEHAVIOR

Coping with a relative who is in a manic state can be exhausting and demoralizing also. A person experiencing depression is usually so fatigued and tentative that, unless he or she is suicidal, there is little likelihood that he or she will make rash and impulsive decisions that would have an impact on other family members. In mania, just the opposite is true. The patient has boundless energy, unshakable drive, but little capacity to appraise the consequences of his actions realistically. It is common for individuals in a manic episode to engage in reckless buying sprees. Huge and unreconcilable debts can be incurred, and our legal system often holds families accountable for their relative's financial mismanagement. Judgment and insight can be so impaired in the manic state that patients may flout all authority and become so intrusive and demanding as to harass others and violate social and sexual mores. At the worst, they may become irritable, aggressive, or even assaultive, leading to the involvement of the police and legal authorities. The family is often placed in the unenviable position of having to set limits on someone who refuses to acknowledge the family's responsibility and concern or who becomes openly hostile when challenged.

Once an episode has reached a certain pitch and the patient cannot be reasoned with, it is both protective of the patient and expedient to move quickly toward hospitalization. Because the patient's mood can fluctuate—ranging from mild euphoria to extreme irritability—and because the patient may speak logically and coherently for periods of time, it is often difficult for families to know when to force this issue. These lucid intervals can be deceptive, however. Unless the patient is being treated aggressively with antipsychotic or mood-stabilizing medications (and the patient is taking the medication), it is unlikely that the manic episode will end safely without hospitalization. Thus the hospitalization should be viewed as a positive step as it will serve to limit the damage that people in a manic state could do to themselves, their social network, and their family.

Therefore, should the family observe the following behaviors and be unable to convince the patient to see his or her psychiatrist and take the necessary medication, arrangements should be made for immediate hospitalization:

- sleeplessness for several nights with frequent shifts of mood, pacing and agitated behavior and no acknowledgment on the part of the patient that anything is wrong
- reckless and impulsive decisions or actions that may lead to financial ruin or social ostracism
- threatening, menacing, or assaultive behavior
- the presence of delusions or hallucinations

THREATS AND ASSAULTIVE BEHAVIOR

When someone is experiencing mania or acute psychosis, his or her mood may shift rapidly from excitement to irritability. Some manic patients become exceedingly hostile and angry. The fear that the ill person will lose control and not be able to contain aggressive impulses paralyzes those around the patient. Family members, afraid to anger their relative or inflame an already volatile situation, often step back, trying to placate or mollify their agitated relative. Not knowing what to do or how to act, most families tend to wait it out and hope the mood will shift back to reasonableness and equanimity.

This is rare. Mania in most cases continues long after the family's patience and stamina have been exhausted. It is in no one's interest to tolerate threats and assaultive behavior. When faced with threats, the family should confront them directly. For instance, if a patient tries to intimidate a relative by saying, "I'll get you for doing this to me," the family member can respond by identifying the statement as a personal threat and refusing to accept it. He or she may say something like: "I take what you're saying to be a threat and I can't accept that. This kind of behavior shows me that you are out of control because when you are not ill, we're able to resolve our differences without threatening each other." Often, people experiencing mania are frightened by their loss of control, and a firm stance may help to establish temporary boundaries. They may be dangerous, however, and family members should not place themselves in a situation from which they cannot withdraw easily.

If this is not a first episode, and the patient has a psychiatrist, the family should naturally call and consult with the doctor. The questions most in need of answering are: How dangerous is the situation and how quickly must an intervention be made? The answers to these questions often depend on the answers to the following questions: Has the patient ever been assaultive before? At what point in the episode did this occur, and is he or she approaching that point? Has the patient been taking street drugs or drinking alcohol? Is the patient severely irrational and misperceiving or distorting events?

EMERGENCY INTERVENTION AND ITS AFTERMATH

Delusional thinking and misinterpretation of events can lead to violent or assaultive behavior. Therefore, when an ill relative expresses delusional thinking in the context of a manic episode (when the control of impulses may be lost), it is imperative that the family act quickly to consult the psychiatrist and initiate commitment procedures. The family may even have to call the police and ask an officer to take the patient to a hospital for an evaluation. The police are trained to work with people who are psychiatrically ill and can be a tremendous help. (See the next chapter for an explanation of the commitment procedure.)

Families who have been called upon to commit a relative in the past are sometimes loath to do it again as they feel the patient has never fully forgiven them. Something was ruptured in the relationship and both family and patient harbor fear and resentment. The family must overcome those feelings sufficiently to act responsibly, even if that requires involuntary hospitalization. Certainly it takes great courage to assume this responsibility and to see it through. Despite the toll that this exacts, there may be some consolation in knowing that you are protecting someone who is no longer able to judge the situation accurately.

The aftermath of an acute episode of mania poses another set of problems. Fearing that the least stress might set off another episode, the family lives with prolonged uncertainty and apprehension. In such an atmosphere, the patient's behavior and natural expressions of emotion—joy or sadness—come under close scrutiny or even suspicion. The family, in the position of being an "early warning system" of impending mood swings, can easily slip into the role of prosecuting attorney: the patient may be faced with seemingly endless questions and doubts and be asked to provide motives for almost every act. One woman with a history of mania told us that if she washed the dishes at midnight, she'd turn around to find her husband and children standing uneasily in the doorway, checking to see if this was a sign of sleeplessness or increased activity. They were afraid of another episode; she just wanted to clean up the kitchen and have some time to think quietly.

This is a corrosive atmosphere for everyone concerned: the patient's credibility and competence as a person are called into question by the sometimes unspoken suspicion of his or her motivations and emotions, and the family is placed under a terrible strain.

Thus, before the patient is discharged from the hospital it would be to everyone's advantage to meet with the psychiatrist to talk about the impact the episode has had on everyone and to develop a strategy for aftercare that is fair to the patient *and* the family. The idea is to help the patient understand what the family members went through in trying to cope with him or her during an episode, and encourage the patient to participate in an agreement that will help reduce the chances of a future hospitalization or establish guidelines if another hospitalization becomes necessary. (It is helpful for families faced with the wrenching situation of having to commit a relative to think back to that meeting and remember the patient's agreement to a future hospitalization.) A formulated plan establishes guidelines, reduces misperceptions, and relieves the family members of the onerous task of deciding if and when to hospitalize. An episode can be resolved more swiftly if there is less conflict over this decision.

Some of the questions that need to be worked out include: What behavior will constitute sufficient cause to call the psychiatrist and ask for an emergency intervention? Which family member will make that call? What will be sufficient cause for voluntary hospitalization or for involuntary hospital-ization? A family that attempts to deal with these questions beforehand can avoid becoming paralyzed with guilt and inde-cision when a crisis occurs.

Such a plan worked well for a family with an 18-year-old daughter. She had bipolar disorder, and had had two previous manic episodes. The episodes began with her staying out late for several nights, and with her becoming irritable and accusing her mother of not understanding her need to be independent. The daughter viewed her need to be out late at night as a nat-ural part of growing up and being on her own, and saw her mother's protestations of her violation of curfew as an example of rigid parental authority. The parents, not fully understanding the course of the disorder and feeling that there might be some truth to their daughter's accusation, did not press her to see her psychiatrist.

During the next few weeks, her sleeplessness and activity level increased, and she began playing her stereo at full volume late into the night and dancing in the hallway scantily dressed. Her accusations of her parent's rigidity progressed to delusional thoughts that her family was imprisoning her and controlling her behavior. A crisis ensued, requiring a late-night call to the police and an involuntary commitment to the hospital.

Several weeks later, when the daughter was stable and about to be discharged from the hospital, the entire family sat down with the psychiatrist. Everyone got a chance to explain his or her response to the onset of the symptoms. The patient's brother revealed how ashamed and embarrassed he felt by his sister's provocative sexual behavior. The mother was also very upset and stated that she thought her daughter had become a loose woman and had been taking drugs with an unsavory group of friends.

The patient described her experience of freedom during the hypomanic part of the episode and remembered that she had thought that others were envious of her and that her mother was "uptight and inhibited." However, after listening to their genuine concern and fears for her, she was more willing to acknowledge that her behavior may have been determined by the illness.

Prior to discharge, the patient and the family members, along with the treatment team at the hospital, worked out a written, step-by-step plan detailing how the family would manage a recurrence of the illness. The plan was as follows:

1. *The patient and family members would identify the specific list of symptoms that precede a manic episode.* For this patient they were: (a) sleeplessness for more than two nights; (b) increased socialization (for example, talking on the telephone excessively, defined as more than 45 minutes at a time, more than five times a night, for more than 3 nights); (c) pressured speech—talking so fast that on at least two occasions members of the family did not understand what she was trying to say.

   Irritable mood and accusatory statements to the mother were discussed but purposely excluded from the plan because they were tied to an ongoing conflict over independence and therefore potentially confusing. This issue was something that would be talked about in the daughter's psychotherapy and in the family therapy.

2. *The patient would choose someone in the family to inform her when the signs and symptoms of the disorder started to manifest themselves.* The daughter chose her father because she felt less threatened when he called attention to changes in her behavior and thus would more easily be able to cooperate with the plan.

   If the father did notice the signs of an impending episode, he would ask his daughter to call her psychiatrist and find out if a change should be made in her medication regimen. If the daughter refused to make this contact, the father would make the call and arrange an appointment with the psychiatrist.

If the daughter refused to follow through and the mania spiraled out of control, the following agreement was reached regarding guidelines the family would follow in order to initiate hospitalization:

a. The parents would ask the daughter to commit herself voluntarily to the hospital.
b. If the daughter refused voluntary hospitalization, and both parents felt hospitalization was necessary, the police would be called to assist in transporting her to the hospital. The father would sign the family application for commitment.

Parents who bring a newborn home from the hospital and follow the baby through every developmental stage, urging the child on with love and high hopes, never dream they might have to call the police and watch that child be wrestled into restraints and taken away to a psychiatric hospital. Those who have had to do it never forget the experience and the events that led to its necessity. But a few people who had been hospitalized involuntarily looked back on the experience and spoke of it differently. One woman summed up their feelings by saying: "If our families won't look after us and take over when we're out of control, who will?"

HOW THE FAMILY CAN HELP WITH MEDICATIONS

Family members who've been traumatized from a previous episode can be desperate that their relative remain symptom-free by taking the medications. They may start hovering over the patient and pressuring or cajoling him or her on the subject. A clash of wills may ensue.

This is a particular problem when the patient is an adolescent or young adult. Adolescence is a vulnerable time: a person is struggling to achieve independent functioning and move out of the orbit of parental supervision. There are concerns over the need to show oneself as capable, mature, and not in need of anyone's help. At this time in life, the idea of having a disability or needing medications to control it may be intolerable, and conflicts over independence may arise, particularly over the subject of medication.

Because of the potentially tragic effects of frequent episodes at this critical period in life, every effort should be made for the family as well as the patient to enter treatment to help the patient and family to separate conflict over issues of independence from the necessity to adhere to a medical regimen. Somehow the family must seek to strike a balance between legitimate concern and overprotectiveness and intrusiveness.

How else can family members help with the subject of medication? One way would be to keep a list of the drugs prescribed, the dosages, and the results and side effects. In the event of a relapse, they can give accurate information to the hospital physician and eliminate a lot of guesswork. Also, should the patient and doctor decide on a change in the medication regimen, the family members can act as an "early warning system" and report any symptoms or untoward side effects.

HOW BROTHERS AND SISTERS ARE AFFECTED

People tend to underestimate the effect that one sibling with a mood disorder has on other children in a family. After all, it's reasoned, they're the healthy ones; they're lucky to have escaped such problems.

Yes. But these healthy siblings suffer in subtle, often insidious ways that affect their sense of self-esteem and the quality of their lives. It is crucial that they be given careful consideration and that their needs not be overlooked by family members and professionals working with the family.

A host of conflicting emotions overwhelm the well siblings. Often love and admiration for the brother or sister who is diagnosed with an affective disorder are entwined with guilt and regret. The well brothers or sisters may be secretly triumphant that they escaped the illness and consequently feel anxious or guilty about their good fortune. If the brother or sister with the effective disorder is older, and if he or she begins to founder in life, younger siblings may find it distressing and uncomfortable to surpass their sibling and go on to fulfill ambitions and dreams.

Resentment and jealousy dog the footsteps of many well siblings because so much of the parents' attention and energy goes toward worrying over and solving the problems of the patient and because so much of the family resources are channeled into treatment and support rather than into the education and pleasure of the rest of the family.

Many siblings reported that they were frustrated with the way their parents denied the illness or attempted to deal with it. One sibling said: "Getting together with the family isn't fun anymore. There's always that tension about my brother's mental illness between us. I'm always angry at everyone for not dealing with the problem like I think they should." It is discomfiting for children to see their parents being ineffectual in the face of their sibling's depression or mania.

The well siblings are perhaps angriest that the patient has so disrupted family life and the good times all families should share. They may feel that they've been cheated. They also can become socially isolated. The turmoil and uncertainty that overtake the household often prevent children from inviting their friends home. They don't want others to be frightened by what their brother or sister may do, and begin to worry that others will conclude that they have a "touch of it" also. Children who don't feel proud of their family find it difficult to be confident socially. As one woman wrote: "The feeling that my family was different distanced me from other people."

Years later, the fear of the heritability of the disorder can again hover over the well siblings—this time as they have their own children. They may become apprehensive about any signs of shifting moods in their offspring, and may even question their decision to have children.

Other problems arise as the parents age and urge the well siblings to look after their ill brother or sister. The well children may not wish to be involved as they now have their own families to care for, and they may feel that their lives have already been too influenced by the problems the disorder has thrust their way.

It's not difficult to conclude that siblings suffer loss—the loss of the companionship of their ill brother or sister, the loss of their parents' attention and a unified family life and a loss of expectations. What can ease their burden and help dissolve the anger they feel? Education and understanding. Only by understanding that their brother or sister did not deliberately act to embarrass them or disrupt the family life can some sympathy be gained and some of the rancor be erased. One man described his stages of coming to terms with his sister's disorder thus:

> During the first few years of my sister's mental illness I was totally intolerant and unsympathetic. My reaction to mental illness was representative of the mainstream of our society today. I was embarrassed by my sister's unconventional behavior and style of dress. I was outraged by the disruption that mental illness caused within our family. I often felt angry about the entire situation.
>
> Eventually because of parental prodding I began to educate myself about mental illness. This is the second stage, the stage of learning. . . . I learned that the symptoms of this disease contributed to the malaise that characterized my sister's disposition. I learned the most important lesson of all: that my sister did not choose to lead a life of chaos lacking direction or continuity. I learned that this had all been imposed upon her life in a cruel and arbitrary fashion and that she deserved enormous credit for continuing her life and attempting to improve it.

Victoria Secunda has written a groundbreaking book that explores the profound impact of mental illness on all the members of a family. It's called *When Madness Comes Home: Help and Hope for the Children, Siblings and Partners of the Mentally Ill* and is published by Hyperion.

MOM AND DAD COUNT TOO

Having read the material in this chapter, the empathic reader will feel for the parents of children with mood disorders, or recognize themselves in the vignettes. Next to the patient, the parents carry the greatest burden. They trained at no special school, they have no experience to guide them, yet they are forced to deal with an illness that they *and* the professionals don't fully understand. If the emotions of the situation don't paralyze them, then the state laws or the cost of psychiatric treatment may. No matter what the parents do or don't do, say or don't say, it is likely that they will feel they're doing it wrong, saying it wrong, and that society and the rest of their family are holding them accountable.

Many of these parents begin to pull away from people rather than deal with the odd looks and questions. Sometimes they are just not ready to admit that anything is wrong, and they don't want their friends to recognize and comment on the problem first. Some parents find it agonizing to hear about their friends' healthy children and shut themselves off from the envy and anger by avoiding social situations. If their friends begin to avoid the subject of their child, or seem strained in his or her presence, the friendships will quickly unravel and the parents become all the more isolated.

Marriages are placed under a heavy strain. The exhaustion of trying to deal with the crises leaves a couple little energy for evenings out, and they may wake up to realize that almost every conversation centers around the problems of their ill child. It is difficult for parents to demand and reserve time for themselves and to develop a plan for their own needs and pleasures in life; yet if they don't, they'll have even less energy. As author Maryellen Walsh writes: "Self-sacrificers tend to burn out early; they haven't taken care of themselves. To be effective over the long run, to keep our psychic and physical tanks full, we parents *must* take care of ourselves."

Where can parents go to let off some steam, learn about some better ways to cope and gain the support and sympathy of others who've been through the same ordeal? Two groups come to mind. A manic-depressive support group that offers education, information, and emotional support to patients and their families, and any of the more than 700 nationwide family support groups affiliated with the National Alliance for the Mentally Ill (some of these family groups may have a majority of members whose child or sibling has schizophrenia, but they have programs that address the problems of families with manic-depression also).

Members of these support groups exchange information on doctors, hospitals, medications, and coping strategies and offer each other a sympathetic ear. Furthermore, families can band together to seek changes in commitment laws, lobby for better housing, or launch their own halfway houses. These two groups are committed to educating the public about psychiatric disorders, combatting stigma, and campaigning for increased research funding. Each family voice swells the ranks and makes a difference.

To locate a family group or manic-depressive support group near you, check Appendix 4 of this book. Because they are multiplying so rapidly, we advise you to call the headquarters of the National Depressive and Manic Depressive Association in Chicago, or the National Alliance for the Mentally Ill in Arlington, Virginia, for an up-to-date listing.

11

COPING WITH HOSPITALIZATION

Hospitalization—even for a happy occasion such as a birth—is attended by feelings of helplessness and fear. But mention a psychiatric hospitalization and you've got an even darker picture: the words conjure images of forgotten back wards with hapless and bizarre inmates subordinated by Miss Ratched-like nurses. Unfortunately, Hollywood and the press have sensationalized isolated stories and depicted fiction so realistically that the patient who needs hospitalization, and the family who must support and sometimes request the hospitalization, suffer immensely from the associations.

We're not trying to suggest that neglect and abuse never happen, but today there are so many advances being made in the treatment of psychiatric illness, so many laws protecting patients' rights, and so many quality assurance agencies surveying hospitals on a regular basis that the picture has radically changed. Today's psychiatric hospitalization ranges from an average of 6 to 14 days. The object is to diagnose, treat, and return the individual to family and community as quickly as possible. The doors of a psychiatric ward may lock; they also always open.

The majority of people with even severe mood disorders, if treated appropriately and in time, do not need hospitalization. But for those who do, we want to outline the procedures and introduce the professionals that a patient and family members encounter throughout the period of hospitalization.

WHEN HOSPITALIZATION IS WARRANTED AND WHAT IT ACCOMPLISHES

There are a variety of reasons for hospitalizing a person with acute symptoms of an affective disorder. A hospital is a protected environment where a team of professionals participate in the diagnosis of the illness, order and administer the medications and treatments, and observe any untoward side effects. Since suicidal thoughts and impulses often accompany moderate to severe depression, the patient is far better off in an environment where 24-hour monitoring is available.

The symptoms of depression—social withdrawal; poor concentration; lack of initiative; slowed-down movement, thought, and speech; disrupted appetite and sleep cycles— make it difficult or nearly impossible for the person to cope. The depressed person's lack of concentration and hopeless feelings about the future frustrate the family's attempts to help, and the depressed person may feel irritable and may experience shame when he or she cannot respond to the family's efforts. This may touch off a corresponding set of feelings in the family members. A professional staff taking over the caretaking responsibilities at this time eases the tensions for everyone.

The person experiencing an acute manic state has a spectrum of symptoms that may necessitate hospitalization for other reasons. A primary consideration is whether the patient can control his or her impulses. While sometimes the mood of a person who is in a manic state is euphoric, overconfident, and optimistic, it may deteriorate rapidly into irritability or anger. He or she may engage impulsively in activities that could be devastating to personal relationships and careers, such as buying sprees, sexual indiscretions, foolish business investments, or even violent behavior. Some manic patients suffer delusions that cause them to lose touch with reality.

In this case, hospitalization provides a badly needed brake on the impulsive behavior and checks the tendency to engage in the reckless, possibly ruinous activities that could endanger a livelihood or a life. The medications temper the agitation and impulsiveness, and the staff has the legal authority and physical capability to restrain the person who might do harm in an uncontrolled state.

The hospital is probably the only place where the unusual, often frightening behavior of these patients is tolerated without judgment and recrimination. Hospitalization has another function, however: it takes the individual who has temporarily lost control out of his work and social environment, thereby limiting the damage that could be done. Not only might the ill person scar or sever relationships during an acute episode, he or she often loses credibility and respect. This would very much complicate the person's return to society.

People who have been hospitalized during a depressed or manic episode report feeling in retrospect that the hospitalization was helpful for the following reasons:

- "I needed safety from myself and what I might do if depressed or manic."

- "It made me realize that I do have a problem, and that I don't have to live with the ups and terrible downs if I am compliant with treatment."

- "I was hospitalized following a serious suicide attempt. After recovery I had time to reevaluate life and conclude that there might be a better answer than suicide."

- "Isolation from the outside world."

- "Being out of your home when you can't function and into a place where you have only yourself to care about."

- "Being with people who were having like problems made me feel secure."

- "It was a safe place to pull myself together, regulate the medication, have constant supervision and scheduled activities. I didn't feel alone during my recuperation."

GETTING A PERSON INTO A HOSPITAL

Some patients sense their urgent need for more intensive treatment and express the wish to go to the hospital. It is vital that family members heed the cues and begin to act on them. Sometimes the patient can't actually spell out the need for hospitalization, but if family members are firm and positive about it, he or she may not argue and may depend entirely on the relatives' better judgment. In this case, the hospital commitment is by voluntary request. The patient signs into the hospital for a specified number of days and can walk out at any time. Some states, however, require the patient to write a request for release to the director of the hospital. The amount of time that a patient has to wait to be released varies according to state laws. A voluntary commitment can be converted to an involuntary one if the treating psychiatrist, after observing the patient, feels that a release would not be in the better interest of the patient or the community. However, he or she would have to initiate legal proceedings to convert the status of the patient.

But what if, as is so often the case, the patient does not recognize the need for treatment? The family and friends may be trying to reason with someone who not only does not grasp their point of view, but who also is rapidly beginning to view them as the enemy. The very mind that needs to be engaged and addressed is, as a result of the illness, misperceiving reality.

So now we enter the sticky but unfortunately necessary world of involuntary commitment with all its attendant legal terms, guilt, and furor. The family member who must take the responsibility and press for the hospitalization is in a very uncomfortable position. But this relative is probably the only person who stands between the patient and the dangers that exist during an acute phase of the illness. In fact, many family members tell us that once a patient stabilizes he or she is often grateful to the relative who took a stand.

The purpose of commitment laws is to enable persons who are mentally ill to be put forcibly into hospitals for treatment before they harm themselves or others. Each state enacts its own laws governing commitment.

These laws rest on two legal foundations: *parens patriae,* the right of the state to act as parent and protect the well-being of a citizen who cannot care for him or herself (this concept evolved from English common law, which held that the king was "father" of all his subjects); and the right of the state to protect its citizens from a person who is dangerous. This means that if a person is so disabled that he cannot recognize the need for treatment, cannot provide for his own basic needs, or may otherwise be dangerous to him or herself or to others, that person may be committed to a psychiatric treatment center for a specified period of time.

Since the 1960s, a movement in this country has focused attention on the civil rights of the psychiatrically ill, with the aim to amend the commitment laws. Today it is more difficult to commit a patient to a hospital against his or her will. Dr. Thomas Szasz, a vocal antagonist of involuntary commitment, states that "we should value liberty more highly than mental health no matter how defined" and "no one should be deprived of his freedom for the sake of his mental health." Bruce Ennis of the American Civil Liberties Union feels that the goal "is nothing less than the abolition of involuntary hospitalization."

Their respect for the individual and his or her civil rights is indeed admirable, but our feelings lie closer to those of Dr. Paul Chodoff, who took more into consideration in his article "The Case for Involuntary Hospitalization for the Mentally Ill":

It is obvious that it is good to be at liberty and that it is good to be free from the consequences of disabling and dehumanizing illness. Sometimes these two values are incompatible, and in the heat of the passions that are often aroused by opposing views of right and wrong, the partisans of each view may tend to minimize the importance of the other. Both sides can present their horror stories.

He concludes rather cogently:

We are now witnessing a pendulum swing in which the rights of the mentally ill to be treated and protected are being set aside in the rush to give them their freedom at whatever cost. But is freedom defined only by the absence of external constraint? Internal physiological or psychological processes can contribute to the throttling of the spirit that is as painful as any from the outside. Today the civil liberties lawyers are in the ascendancy and the psychiatrists on the defensive to a degree that is harmful to individual needs and the public welfare.

All voices sounding all views maintains a healthy balance, and no doubt the impassioned opponents of involuntary commitment have been responsible for the correction of many abuses, but in some states it is extremely difficult to get people who need treatment into a hospital. This has caused undue suffering for patients and family members and has thwarted psychiatrists who might otherwise treat the patients and protect them and others.

Recently, after almost two decades of restrictions, the pendulum is making a return swing: the national trend is toward making it easier to commit involuntarily patients with psychiatric illnesses. Addressing the issue, the American Psychiatric Association has devised a model commitment law that would allow commitments not only when patients are dangerous to self and others, but also when the patients are suffering and would be likely to deteriorate without treatment; in the presence of a major psychiatric illness that could be treated, provided that treatment is available; and when patients are mentally incapable of deciding for themselves. In the past few years several states have amended their laws and broadened the commitment criteria. (Arizona, Delaware, Hawaii, Iowa, Oklahoma, New York, and South Carolina changed their laws and made it easier to commit patients to a hospital.)

These laws (and the debators who aim to restrict or broaden them) directly affect the person struggling with mental illness *and* his or her family, and it's vital that everyone keep informed. The *Mental and Physical Disability Law Reporter* will accomplish this. It's published bimonthly by the American Bar Association, 740 15th St., NW, Washington, DC 20005. It is very expensive, however. At this writing, the yearly subscription cost is $229.

HOW TO HAVE SOMEONE COMMITTED

As a result of a 1975 U.S. Supreme Court ruling that a state cannot confine a patient who refuses voluntary hospitalization and can manage outside the hospital alone or with the help of family or friends, the states demand proof that a person is mentally disturbed and a danger to himself or herself or others. Each state varies somewhat in its wording of its grounds for commitment and the standard of proof required. Some states allow a little flexibility and do not rely strictly on "dangerousness" criteria— the *parens patriae* rationale we spoke of earlier still plays a part. For instance, the state of South Carolina says that a person can be committed if "he is mentally ill, needs treatment and because of his condition (1) lacks sufficient insight or capacity to make responsible decisions with respect to his treatment, or (2) there is a likelihood of serious harm to himself or others." The chances of getting a commitment in a state like this are greater than in New Hampshire, whose law states starkly that a "person must exhibit dangerousness to self or others."

The standard of proof is another murky area; if a man *says* he'll kill someone, is that admissible evidence proving dangerousness or does he have to injure that someone first? The least stringent level of proof is "clear and convincing evidence," while the "beyond a reasonable doubt" level of proof demanded by California, Kentucky, Massachusetts, New Hampshire, and Oregon makes it more difficult to get a commitment. This of course does not take into consideration a judge's interpretation of the law, which is also governed by personal bias and the feelings of the community at a particular time.

It all sounds dry and legal on paper, but living with the law is another matter. Consider the case of one mother in California whose son had a bipolar disorder. He stopped taking his lithium and she began to see signs of mania. When she suggested that he see a doctor and continue with his lithium, he told her she was crazy and stormed out. Because of the stringency of California law, she was powerless to do anything and had to stand by and let the illness run its course. Three days later, after he'd wrecked his apartment and threatened his girlfriend, the police found him wandering the streets and were able to convince him to go to the hospital.

The procedure for initiating a commitment is also dictated by state law, and each state varies somewhat. We'll explain how a person could be committed in the state of New York, and then direct readers how to check the procedure in their area.

Should a family member or responsible adult see that a person is exhibiting conduct that is dangerous to self or others, there are two ways they could try to get the person to the hospital: the police can be called, or the family can go to the State Supreme Court and file a petition for commitment. The patient must have either made a suicide attempt or have acted in a menacing fashion, such as punching people or harboring a weapon such as a knife; or the patient must be dazed or confused and seem unable to take care of himself or herself. If the responsible adult calls the police and they don't come to check out the situation (they most often do), the responsible adult must go to the Supreme Court and file a petition, an affidavit with the court, setting forth the reasons why this person needs to be hospitalized and why the person is a danger to self or others.

If the judge is convinced by the argument, a warrant is issued. The police can then find the patient and bring him or her to the emergency room of a hospital for an evaluation. In order for the person to be hospitalized, the evaluating psychiatrist must decide that the person is a danger to self or others. Within 72 hours, a second doctor must confirm that opinion or the person is released. If the second doctor does confirm that the person needs hospitalization, the person is held under an emergency commitment status, not to exceed 15 days. At the end of that period, the person must be released unless the director of the hospital or the family petitions the court for longer-term commitment. In practical terms, this simply means signing commitment papers provided by the hospital with a statement documenting the reasons the family member is requesting commitment. To complete the commitment procedure two psychiatrists are required to evaluate the patient and sign the certification document stating that in their opinion the patient's mental state warrants involuntary commitment. The patient can then be kept in the hospital for a period not to exceed 60 days (if there was an emergency 15-day commitment initiated beforehand, the long-term commitment lasts for no longer than 45 days).

At any time, the patient can go to court and contest the commitment. A mental health information lawyer is available to represent the patient at a hearing held before a judge, usually within chambers in the hospital. The patient, family members, and examining psychiatrist testify at the hearing, where normal judicial rules of evidence and due process apply.

Perhaps it would be easier to go over this in context. The following case happened in and proceeded according to the laws of New York State:

Jonathan was a 25-year-old man suffering from a bipolar disorder. He lived at home with his mother and two younger sisters, and was being treated by a psychiatrist. Frequently, however, Jonathan would not comply with treatment and he would refuse to take his medications. This time, two and a half weeks after he stopped the drugs, he stopped sleeping at night. He began pacing around his room and began to see himself as a religious figure destined to save the world.

His mother urged him to see his psychiatrist and go back on his medications, but he responded with irritable anger and outright threats. One afternoon, after a particularly upsetting confrontation, Jonathan reached out and scratched his mother's face.

She then called the psychiatrist he'd been seeing. The doctor questioned her at length to determine the symptoms and agreed to make a house call and talk to Jonathan. At the house, he was able to see that Jonathan was indeed behaving bizarrely and he decided that, at this point, hospitalization was indicated.

The psychiatrist wrote a letter to the local police stating that Jonathan had a well-documented mental illness with recurrent relapses. He went on to describe Jonathan's delusional ideas, the aggressive incident with the mother, and indicated that Jonathan might be a threat to himself or others. The doctor closed the letter with the request that Jonathan be taken to a psychiatric emergency room by the police and that he be evaluated there.

Jonathan's mother took the letter to the police station, and two policemen came to the house and asked to speak to Jonathan. After viewing his unusual and idiosyncratic behavior, the policemen decided to bring him to the emergency room of the city's public hospital.

Once there, Jonathan was evaluated by a staff psychiatrist who noted that he was experiencing auditory hallucinations. Jonathan began to discuss his conversation with Jesus the night before. Jesus told him about the special role that only Jonathan could fulfill. The doctor recommended that he enter the hospital on a voluntary basis, but Jonathan refused and kept stating that his mother just wanted to put him away.

The emergency room psychiatrist decided to pursue an involuntary commitment on an emergency basis. This kind of commitment lasts for 15 days. Unfortunately, at the end of that period, Jonathan was still delusional, and the staff decided to convert Jonathan's status to a commitment that lasts for 60 days. It requires a three-part petition: two certificates signed by two examining psychiatrists, and a form on which a family member or person living with the patient signs his name and outlines the reasons for requesting the commitment. In this case, Jonathan's mother signed the petition.

Jonathan became extremely upset when he heard this, and demanded to see the patient-advocate lawyer (all patients are given the phone number of this professional, who is not hired by the hospital and whose business is to assist and protect the patient).

The lawyer, after talking to Jonathan, agreed to take the case to court. The hospital had a room that was a judge's chambers and Jonathan, his lawyer, the treating psychiatrists, and his family participated in the hearing. Because his family was afraid to have him back in the condition he was still in, the judge asked where he would go if he were released. Jonathan really had nowhere else to go, and finally agreed to stay in the hospital for the remaining period of the long-term commitment.

Naturally every case is different. Jonathan's family was lucky in that he had been seeing a psychiatrist who was willing to make a house call and there was a documented history to support the claim that he needed help. If a family member is faced with a first episode and hasn't the name of a psychiatrist, he or she can call the family doctor and ask for help or for a referral to a psychiatrist who might make a home visit. Also, by calling the admissions office of the nearest psychiatric hospital (or emergency room) a person can obtain some information as to the procedures for commitment in that state. The police can fill you in, too. One more suggestion: We spoke to a leader of a state AMI who said that her group not only gives a family member the number to the DA's office for help and direction, but they put him or her in touch with another family who's been through the very same commitment procedure and who can act as coach and comfort. (See Appendix 4 for the number of NAMI headquarters, whose personnel will put you in touch with your state AMI.

WHICH HOSPITAL IS BEST?

Years ago, the person in need of psychiatric treatment in a hospital went one of two places: a state facility, or a private—and very expensive—sanitorium. But today there are more options. Community hospitals (public and private) are carving out psychiatric inpatient services for short-term care, and they generally deliver a satisfactory level of service. University-affiliated teaching centers have excellent reputations that are largely dependent on their clinician/researcher teaching staff; on the other hand, it is the residents and interns—the least experienced members of the department—who tend to the patients (see pages 307–308 for a discussion of this type of hospital). Private psychiatric hospitals range in quality from those that offer excellent treatment to those whose unsoothing under-the-breath mantra is "money first, patient next." If the patient is a veteran, an admission to a Veterans Administration hospital is a possibility, but criteria for admission are becoming more stringent. In some cases patients are accepted for treatment only if the condition is considered service-related. Another possibility is that the patient may live in a catchment area that is serviced by a Community Mental Health Center with an inpatient service. Finally, there are the state hospitals. Most people cringe at the mention and see the state hospital as a last and desperate resort, but there are some state hospitals that offer excellent care, as well as those that too closely resemble the Bedlam of old.

But don't let private rooms and fancy facilities be the assurance of quality. The diagnostic abilities and the treatment philosophy of the psychiatrist running the unit are far more important. Admittedly, these are difficult matters to assess, but the doctor and/or staff members should be willing to explain the evaluation procedure and the goals and objectives of the hospitalization.

In Chapter 2, we outlined the diagnostic criteria for affective disorders and discussed the dilemmas that face the psychiatrist in establishing a diagnosis—particularly in the acute state (see pages 42–46 on misdiagnosis). Although DSM-IV is not infallible, if it is not being used in the diagnostic process, chances are the patient is not receiving up-to-date medical care. The following checklist of questions should aid a family in assessing the quality of care their relative is receiving:

- Has the family been invited to the hospital to expand on or explain the history of the patient's disorder?
- Has the family history been explored? (If not, this may be an indication that rigorous diagnostic procedures are not being observed.)
- Is there an adequate number of nurses and aids to oversee the depressed patient who may be suicidal? What is the procedure for this? (See page 309 on constant observation.)
- How will the manic patient be dealt with? What is the policy and procedure for seclusion and restraint? (See the discussion later in this chapter.)

- How frequently is the patient seen by a staff psychiatrist?
- What are the arrangements for medical consultation? Are there an internist and neurologist assigned to the service? How are other specialists seen?
- Is there an attempt to educate and inform the patient and family members as to the nature of the disorder and the benefits and risks of short- and long-term treatment?

An important assurance of hospital quality is accreditation by the Joint Commission on Accreditation of Healthcare Organizations. JCAHO, as it's called, is an outgrowth of the Hospital Standardization Program established by the American College of Surgeons in 1918. A hospital invites a survey team from the Commission to visit and evaluate the hospital's performance and safety features. The team also examines the therapeutic environment, the number and quality and credentials of the staff, the record keeping, and the administration. Hospitals that pass the inspection receive a three-year accreditation.

Any hospital that does not have a JCAHO certificate should be given a wide berth. Medicare and Medicaid actually specify that the hospitals participating in their programs must be certified by either JCAHO, or the Health Care Financing Administration, and most insurance companies do not reimburse bills from a hospital that does not have a JCAHO accreditation. Look in the lobby or entranceway for the certificate, or ask someone in the hospital's administration office to tell you where it is. Also, you can call the Joint Commission on Accreditation of Healthcare Organizations in Illinois at (630) 792-5000 or write to them at One Renaissance Boulevard, Oakbrook Terrace, IL 60181.

An excellent way to check out the quality of care in the hospitals in an area is to call the local chapter of a manic-depressive support group or family organization (which you can find by calling one of the national headquarters listed in Appendix 4). They can give you the names and numbers of family members who've had experience with the area's mental health hospitals and who are in a position to warn and advise. Also, you will no doubt gain support and a sympathetic ear.

ADMISSIONS PROCEDURES

We've discussed voluntary and involuntary hospitalizations, and we've outlined the different choices on the hospital horizon, but the specific, concrete steps that lead from an episode of illness to a person's actually walking into a psychiatric unit for treatment may seem a bit blurry and confusing. The two situations that follow should help clarify the hospital admissions procedures.

Adam McDonough is a 35-year-old advertising executive who became increasingly withdrawn and irritable. He found himself unmotivated at work and began to spend hours sitting at his desk accomplishing little. His wife noticed that he wasn't sleeping at night, and that at times he became very teary. She called their family physician, who, after examining Adam, referred him to a psychiatrist. Adam was very resistant about going to see a "lunatic's doctor," but his wife was able to press the point and he did keep the appointment.

Adam described his symptoms to the psychiatrist and began to discuss his feelings of worthlessness. He admitted haltingly that he'd had thoughts of taking his own life so that his wife could be free of him. He hadn't the energy to fight through his feelings.

The doctor realized that Adam was experiencing a major depression and felt that as there was a possibility of suicide, he should be treated on an inpatient service. The psychiatrist called the director of a private teaching ward and asked if there was a bed available. He presented the case and the director agreed to admit Adam. He asked that Adam's wife call the administrator of the hospital so that the insurance policy could be checked.

After the phone call, Mrs. McDonough was asked to

bring Adam to the admissions office of the hospital. There, he was met by the resident assigned to him. The resident spoke to Adam and asked him to fill out several forms: one was a voluntary commitment form, and others authorized general treatment at the hospital. He was then escorted to his room.

Diane Polisi is a 22-year-old receptionist at a design firm. She is high-spirited and fun-loving, so when she began coming into work in the morning enthusiastically describing her "all-nighters" at the discos, her coworkers commented on the energies of youth and didn't notice that anything was wrong. By the end of the week, though, she began to talk faster and faster and she began embarking on several self-appointed projects such as straightening all the files in the storeroom and rearranging all the furniture in the conference room. She then began to call client after client, as she felt she should "drum up some business." The manager of the firm walked in and overheard her exhorting a client into a fanciful promotion and realized something was very wrong. She spoke calmly to the now-agitated Diane and told her she was calling her sister who worked nearby. Her sister drove her to the emergency room of the public hospital.

At the hospital, the resident on duty interviewed Diane and her sister and made note of some of the manic symptoms. He felt that Diane should be hospitalized for further evaluation and treatment. Since Diane's firm had a Blue Cross/Blue Shield policy, and as the beds for a public hospital were really intended for people not covered by private insurance, the resident asked the social worker in the emergency room to call the local private hospitals and arrange for a bed for Diane. In the meantime, he gave Diane a physical exam and an injection of haloperidol to diminish the level of agitation she was experiencing and to reduce her racing thoughts. Six hours later she was transferred by ambulance to the private hospital.

Adam's wife and Diane's sister had little experience with mental illness and were totally unfamiliar with the subjects of public versus private hospitals, but these experiences taught them that there are professionals who deal with this all the time and who will help people steer through the system and obtain appropriate medical attention.

WHAT TO BRING TO THE ADMISSIONS OFFICE

A telephone call to the admissions office of the hospital will fill you in on what's required for the admitting procedure. In all probability you need to bring and to know the following:

- Patient's insurance card (or cards if he or she has several policies); a Medicare and/or Medicaid card if the patient has one
- Social Security card or number of the person who will bear the responsibility for the bill
- Name, address, and telephone number of the patient's employer and of his or her spouse, if any
- Name, address, and telephone number of the person to be notified in case of an emergency
- Information about the patient's military service (only if he or she is seeking admission to a Veterans Administration hospital)
- A checkbook or credit card (some hospitals require deposit)

INSURANCE AND COSTS

There's an unpleasant reality here: a hospital is a business—the administration seeks reimbursement for the services provided. Therefore, the extent of the patient's insurance coverage is very important. How many days in a psychiatric hospital are covered? Are psychiatric hospitals covered at all or is the policy intended for a psychiatric unit in a general hospital? Will the insurance company reimburse if the hospital has no JCAHO accreditation? Is there a ceiling to the dollar amount reimbursed? How much of the doctor's fee is covered? What is the deductible? Granted, the small print on policies is difficult to understand (see Chapter 12 for a more complete picture of insurance policies), so you should ask the insurance agent or the person responsible for employee benefits to translate and clarify the coverage. If you have several policies, you'll need to know when and whether one picks up for the other. If your coverage is inadequate, the business office may be able to initiate a Medicaid application, help arrange a bank loan, or negotiate another payment mechanism. Families should be aware that there is a form of hospital "catastrophic medicaid" that covers patients who are not currently Medicaid recipients and whose expensive inpatient hospital care exceeds 25 percent of their annual income. This coverage is valid for only six months from the date of application and only inpatient care is covered. The more information you have going in, the more secure you will feel when the issues of money and insurance are raised.

What would two weeks of psychiatric hospitalization cost? The charges of a city, county, or state public hospital vary according to the patient's income, but a patient admitted to a private, nonprofit (university-affiliated) hospital in the New York City area in 1996 would incur bills for this period of about $23,100. Additionally, the patient might be billed for selected services that are separate from the hospital bed rate. Charges for specific treatments would approximate these:

Electrocardiogram (EKG)	56.00
MRI brain scan (with contrast)	1,500.00
ECT (10 treatments)	5,000.00
Therapy fees (individual medical psychotherapy)	1,200.00
Consultation fees	300.00
Psychological testing	400.00

Thus, fees approximating $32,000.00 should provide powerful motivation for anyone to look into his or her insurance situation. If a person does not have coverage and lacks financial resources, a public hospital will take care of the treatment and initiate a Medicaid application.

AFTER ADMISSION

After the patient signs authorization-for-treatment papers, he or she is escorted to the unit. The family or friend may go along and help the patient settle in. In most situations, the nursing staff handles the orientation and intake procedure. During this discussion, the patient is informed about the daily schedule, the hospital rules, the therapy programs, meal schedules, and visiting hours (to the extent his or her clinical status permits them). Most hospitals provide a brochure that explains these matters. Items that are sharp, breakable, heavy, and potentially dangerous to the patient or anyone else on the unit are usually returned to the family or held for the patient.

Next the nurse takes a medical and psychiatric history and begins to explore the relationships the patient has with his or her family members. The care plan that the nurse writes outlines how much watching the patient needs and reports medical problems that need attention. The nurse's intake not only helps orient the patient to his or her new surroundings, it also gives the people who are working most closely with the patient a chance to get to know him or her. In many ways it is not only an assessment, but a valuable personal introduction.

Once the intake is complete, the psychiatrist responsible for the patient begins a medical and psychiatric work-up. In some hospitals the private psychiatrist who admitted the patient to the unit will be his or her private attending physician, and will thus be very familiar with the patient's history; but in the case of a unit that assigns its own staff to each new patient, the work-up requires the assembling of many facts. If the patient is unable to assist the doctor with this admittedly extensive amount of information, the accompanying family member should be prepared to give details about the following:

- What was the patient like before the problem arose?
- What was the development of the problem? What changes did anyone notice in the patient's behavior?
- What kind of medications or treatments did the patient have prior to this hospitalization? What side effects did he or she experience? Were there any prior hospitalizations? When?
- Are there any existing medical problems? Does the patient have any allergies?
- Is there a history of learning disabilities, social adjustment problems, drug, or alcohol abuse?
- Is there a history of mental illness in the family? Is there a history of alcoholism in the family? (These two questions could possibly help pinpoint the diagnosis of an affective disorder—as painful as it is, try to give the doctor very detailed information about any other family members with psychiatric or alcohol problems.) If anyone in the family has been treated for a similar condition, what medications did he or she respond to? (Response to medication is often genetic, so this information is extremely important.)

The psychiatrist explores the "mental status" of the patient by asking questions and then assessing his or her mood, emotional state, and thought processes. The doctor determines whether the patient knows the day, the month, the year, who he or she is, to whom he or she is talking, and the name of the place he or she is in. The patient's memory, concentration, and ability to think abstractly are also tested.

The patient's history of illness, the current symptoms, the previous episodes of illness, and the mental status exam lead the psychiatrist to a list of possible diagnoses. Further information and history, possible psychological testing, and the results of the physical examination and laboratory tests lead to a more conclusive diagnosis.

THE PHYSICAL EXAMINATION

All patients who enter a hospital are given a physical exam and certain routine screening tests such as blood tests, urinalysis, and a chest X-ray. The findings of these tests may point to a physical origin of the psychiatric problem, or may unearth a coexisting medical problem, but will definitely guide the physician in the choice of psychotropic medications. For instance, a patient with kidney dysfunction may be unable to take lithium and the psychiatrist may instead prescribe carbamazepine (Tegretol); a patient with a history of grand mal seizures is prescribed a neuroleptic that would have less of a potential for lowering the seizure threshold (all neuroleptics lower it to a certain degree). Depending on the clinical picture, the psychiatrist may call for a medical consultation with a neurologist, an endocrinologist, or a cardiologist.

Once the diagnosis is established, the treatment begins. Under the psychiatrist's direction, a team of other professionals—psychologists, social workers, nursing staff, and occupational and activities therapists—continuously review, discuss, and treat the patient.

THE HOSPITAL TEAM

Who are the different professionals and other staff members who treat the patients in a psychiatric hospital? What kind of training do they have? How can they help? The following brief descriptions should answer these questions.

The *psychiatrist* is a medical doctor who specializes in the diagnosis and comprehensive treatment of mental and emotional illnesses. After completing four years of medical school, he or she completes a four-year residency training program in psychiatry (at least six months of the first year is spent in general medicine). The residency is situated in a hospital approved by the American Board of Psychiatry and Neurology and the resident is supervised by experienced psychiatrists while learning differential diagnosis and specific approaches to the treatment of major psychiatric disorders. The education encompasses medical treatment approaches as well as psychotherapeutic approaches—individual, family, and group. A psychiatrist, as a physician, is the only mental health professional who can prescribe medications and perform electroconvulsive therapy.

The *clinical psychologist* is also called "Doctor," but here the title refers to a Ph.D. degree in clinical psychology. The psychologist not only completes three years of course work, but also an internship in a psychiatric hospital or mental health clinic. In addition, most programs require a dissertation on a research topic. While a psychologist cannot prescribe medications, he or she is trained to do psychological testing, psychotherapy, and research.

The *psychiatric nurse* is a registered nurse who has been specifically trained to work with people who have psychiatric disorders. He or she is the professional who spends the most time with the patient. Not only does the nurse dispense the medications ordered by the psychiatrist, but he or she closely monitors side effects. The nurse's daily report gives the rest of the treatment team valuable information about the patient's medical and mental status. Some nurses have Master's degrees, and some are nurse practitioners trained to do psychotherapy.

The *psychiatric social worker* can be invaluable to the family as well as the patient. After four years of college, the psychiatric social worker completes a two-year course with an internship in a psychiatric setting and is awarded the degree

Master of Social Work (M.S.W.). Not only can this professional conduct psychotherapy sessions, but he or she assesses and coordinates the needs of the patient and the family during and after hospitalization. The social worker may arrange a place in a group home or halfway house if the patient requires it; or the social worker may initiate disability, SSI, Medicaid/Medicare applications where they are appropriate. If the initials A.C.S.W. appear after a social worker's name, it means that he or she has met the requirements of and is certified by the Academy of Certified Social Workers.

The *occupational therapist* (O.T.) has specialized training in evaluating an individual's employment and social skills and his or her ability to conduct the commonplace activities of daily living. The O.T. organizes structured activities and group tasks that aid concentration, socialization, and living skills. Some of these group and individual activities focus on job interviews, writing skills, cooking skills, and the running of a household. An occupational therapist completes either a four-year undergraduate program leading to a Bachelor of Science with a major in occupational therapy or a Master's degree program in occupational therapy with six months of supervised clinical experience. An O.T. with either of these degrees may become registered by passing an examination administered by the American Occupational Therapy Association.

Many psychiatric units also have *activities therapists* who may specialize in art therapy, dance or music therapy, or recreational therapy. They are graduates of accredited bachelor's or master's programs that emphasize the therapeutic application of the art or physical education. The activities programs are devised to encourage self-awareness and the exploration of feelings as well as to provide the patient with an opportunity to engage in a structured, shared leisure activity that promotes socialization and the improvement of interpersonal skills. The activities therapist understands the treatment goals for each patient and attempts to reinforce them through the projects undertaken.

In addition to the professionals just mentioned, the patient comes into close contact with other hospital personnel: the physician's assistant who may do physical exams, mental health aides, and nursing aides. In a good hospital, these people not only do their jobs but also offer patients encouragement and reassurance.

THE STAFF-IN-TRAINING ON A TEACHING WARD

In a nonacademic hospital setting, the staff psychiatrist usually directs the evaluation and treatment of the patient, but on university-affiliated training units, there are fellows, chief residents, residents, and medical students who may have a more direct day-to-day involvement with the patient and the family. There are advantages and disadvantages to this system. John McPhee, in an article for *The New Yorker,* cites the advantages:

> The hospital's quality as a congregation of working doctors has been elevated by the presence of the residency in part because, as a teaching hospital, it is a place where more questions are going to be asked than would be asked if the residency were not there. In teaching rounds, scheduled conferences, and other forms of interaction, the residents engender a running dialogue that tends to draw specialists together.

McPhee goes on to quote a residents' teacher, Dr. Alan Hume: "If someone asks me a question and I don't know the answer, I come back tomorrow with an answer. This makes me a better doctor, and the patient gets better care. The resident is a built-in audit."

The disadvantage is that the least experienced staff member has the most contact with the patient.

A psychiatric fellow is someone who has completed a psychiatric residency and has elected to specialize in an area of clinical activity or research under the tutelage of a senior psychiatrist. He or she often provides valuable expertise in diagnosis and treatment.

The chief resident on a unit is in the final year of residency and is chosen from among his or her peers to assist in the administration of the unit and in the teaching of less senior residents.

A resident on an inpatient service may be in his or her second, third, or fourth year of training. On a university-affiliated training ward, the resident is the primary therapist and is chiefly responsible for the management and care of the patient. The director of the unit, the staff psychiatrists, and the chief resident supervise the resident's work.

A medical student does a clerkship on a psychiatric unit during the third year of medical school. He or she usually becomes very involved with one or two patients. Although the least experienced member of the medical team, the student can be a valuable ally who has the time to gather a detailed and possibly revealing history of the patient and the illness. This can help the staff to develop a better therapy formulation and treatment plan. A good medical student can listen well and offer support and the human touch.

THE DAILY AND WEEKLY SCHEDULE

Treatment for depression or mania should begin with an integrated plan to ameliorate the symptoms of the illness, help the patient reestablish a sense of self-esteem, educate the patient and the family as to the nature of the illness, and develop a practical outpatient treatment that will serve to prevent rehospitalization. The many meetings, medical rounds, and social and therapeutic interactions during the hospital day are aimed at accomplishing this agenda.

Typically each morning the staff assembles for "rounds." This is the medical vernacular for the nurses' report on the medical and behavioral status of the patients on the unit. If there are any questions about changes in the treatment plans, or concerns about a response to medication or a family visit, they are brought up at this time. The residents may report on their patients as well.

Many inpatient services divide the patient responsibilities into two teams. Detailed discussions of each patient are conducted in team meetings several times a week. Should a problem arise concerning a diagnosis or psychiatric medication, a psychiatrist with an expertise in these areas is called in for a consultation. In addition, supplemental medical rounds are conducted for patients experiencing neurological or medical problems.

Individual, group, and family meetings are scheduled throughout the week, and the occupational and activities therapists offer recreational, skills, and various art groups. Naturally, there are hours set aside for grooming periods, meals, and visiting hours. (An example of a weekly schedule appears on the next page.)

WHEN CONSTANT OBSERVATION IS NEEDED

Some patients are watched more closely by or have more contact with the nursing staff. This is because the medical staff has determined that the patient is suicidal or aggressive toward other patients, or is so confused and disorganized that the patient cannot take care of his or her own needs without close contact. Part of the treatment plan, then, is a period of time under close or even constant observation. Constant observation usually means that a nurse or assistant is assigned to stay within an arm's length of the patient at all times and make frequent eye or verbal contact with that patient.

	Monday	Tuesday	Wednesday	Thursday	Friday
8:00	Breakfast	Breakfast	Breakfast	Breakfast	Breakfast
9:00	Community meeting	—	—	—	Community meeting
10:00	Patients meet with their primary therapists	Group therapy	Patients meet with their primary therapists	Group therapy	Patients meet with their primary therapists
12:00	Community lunch	Community lunch	Community lunch	Community lunch	Community lunch
1:00	Expressive writing workshop	Art therapy	Social skills group	Recreational therapy	Social skills group
2:00 to 5:00	Visiting hours	Visiting hours	Visiting hours	Visiting hours	Visiting hours
4:00 to 5:00	Family meetings	—	Family meetings	—	Family meetings
6:00	Dinner	Dinner	Dinner	Dinner	Dinner
6:00 to 8:00	Visiting hours	Visiting hours	Multiple family group visiting hours	Visiting hours	Visiting hours

THE SECLUSION ROOM AND PHYSICAL RESTRAINT

The fast ideas become too fast and there are far too many . . . overwhelming confusion replaces clarity . . . you stop keeping up with it—memory goes. Infectious humor ceases to amuse—your friends become frightened . . . everything is now against the grain . . . you are irritable, angry, frightened, uncontrollable and trapped in the blackest caves of the mind—caves you never knew were there. It will never end. Madness carves its own reality.

This patient's description of a manic episode should help people understand that a person experiencing psychosis can be overwhelmed by noises, environmental stimuli, and people. A normal conversation may sound like artillery fire, and anything can be interpreted as a direct threat. The patient may feel the need to hide or retaliate as protection. The patient may hear voices encouraging suicide, and may become so frightened that only a quiet and protected room will help remove the painful stimuli, help the patient feel safe, and protect him or her from hurting anyone. That is why most psychiatric units have a room where a patient can be isolated until he or she is calm and able to be with people. It's called a seclusion room.

Physically it is a room stripped of any sharp or heavy objects that could be used by the patient to hurt him or herself or the staff. The walls may be covered with padding, and there is a mattress on the floor for the patient to rest and sleep on (a bedframe has too many sharp angles). The door locks, but a window in it allows staff members to observe the patient. The seclusion room often does more to lock the world out than to lock the patient in, and its use is governed by many regulations.

The seclusion room can be used only to prevent a patient from hurting himself or others, and only when other therapeutic treatments are ineffective. A doctor must write the orders for seclusion, the patient's behavior must be observed and documented frequently, vital signs (blood pressure, pulse, respiration rate, and temperature) must be taken periodically, and if the patient is not sleeping, he or she must be released, walked around, and taken to the bathroom every two hours.

The nursing staff is instructed to greet the patient, tell him or her why the seclusion time is necessary, and listen to the patient's response. The intention is to explain what is happening and allay the patient's anxiety.

If a patient is very manic and out of control, it is not easy for the staff to monitor his or her physical state or administer medications. If the patient was given an antipsychotic medication, the blood pressure and pulse are monitored. In such situations, aides and security guards may be summoned to restrain the patient. One member of the staff talks to the patient and explains what they intend to do, and assures the patient that he or she will not be harmed, nor will the patient be allowed to harm anyone else.

There may be times when additional restraints are necessary until medication calms the extremely agitated patient. Psychiatric units are allowed to use wrist and ankle restraints as well as straitjackets if their use is deemed appropriate, but again, state law demands justification of restraints and regulates their use. However medieval and inhumane the physical restraints appear to the onlooker, they are sometimes necessary and serve to limit the patient's impulse to hurt himself or herself or others. Restraints are often only necessary for a few hours and are removed as soon as the patient is in control again.

In the event that a patient refuses medication, typically the clinical director of the unit and the patient advocate are informed, and a decision is made concerning involuntary medication of the patient. Most states allow single dose involuntary medication without a court order if the situation is judged an emergency.

The family members who view what seems like the locking away of their relative have a very difficult time coming to terms with the idea of a seclusion room. A 16-year-old girl described what it was like to watch her older brother secluded on the unit:

> My brother was sitting in the corner, on a mattress on the floor. His face looked scared and tense and yet

sedated. He looked at me as if he didn't know me, as if I were the enemy.

How could locking a human being up alone in complete solitary confinement be a good thing? How could this work? The whole thing sounded like a cruel joke.

My mother broke down and sobbed and I just cringed, I felt so guilty. I knew he'd never forgive us. We were abandoning him to some sort of hell and we didn't know if the doctors and nurses were right or if we should rescue him from there or what. But how could we handle him in that state? It was a nightmare.

The uneasiness and guilt and confusion the family members feel are very understandable, yet when we spoke to a young woman who was secluded in a quiet room for two days during a manic episode, she recalled how it felt for her on the "inside":

I had been running around trying to do a thousand things and my mind was going a million miles a minute. I was exhausted, and the room seemed a quiet and simple place for me. The pressure was off, I didn't have to accomplish anything, I could just slow down and rest. I'm sure a seclusion room must enrage or frighten some people—it's all so individual—but for me, those two days were a retreat. It seemed an appropriate place for me to be at that time.

WHEN YOU VISIT

Few people like to visit patients in hospitals—patients are in pain, the surroundings are rarely attractive, and it doesn't take long before you think: that could be me. So we realize that a visit with someone on a psychiatric unit is not just unpleasant—it can be downright frightening at first. Even mental health professionals report an insecure feeling the first time they visit a locked unit and hear the door close behind them. Don't worry; it passes. But we do think a discussion about what you'll see and how to act and interact with staff, family members, and the other patients on the unit will do much to alleviate anxiety.

We've all passed people on the street who seem strange or out of touch with reality, but a psychiatric unit certainly has a concentrated population of such people and you won't be able to avoid coming face to face with someone like this as you make your way through the unit. The big questions that come to mind are: How do I act? Should I smile and say hello? What do I do if someone approaches me?

Most of the apprehension people feel when confronted by a person acting strangely comes from the fear that the individual will harm them. In fact, you are probably safer on a psychiatric floor than on a city street. Many mentally ill psychiatric patients are frightened themselves—of external stimuli, of sounds, of you. So treat people naturally and gently and respond to them directly. If a patient in a confused state asks, "Are you my grandmother?" you could help establish reality by answering the truth, "No, I'm here to visit my sister." If someone does bother you, simply tell the nurse on duty and politely disengage yourself from the situation.

A lot of emotions are dredged up when you visit your relative in a hospital, but if you understand how the illness is affecting the patient's ability to communicate, the visit can be more constructive and helpful—it will also be less painful for all concerned.

It is often the case that a person in a depression responds to questions or conversation remarkably slowly. It may take quite a while for the patient to respond to the question, "How are you feeling today?" Most relatives view the long pauses as a sign that the patient does not wish to be with or communicate with them. Anyone who must wait a prolonged period for a simple response feels embarrassed, frustrated, devalued, and angry. But this thought latency is a classic sign of depression—a slowing down of biological processes. It might be helpful to acknowledge to the patient that you understand that it is taking him or her time to respond. This may lessen the patient's burden when trying to communicate with you.

Another common feature of severe depression is a loss of appetite; your relative may stop eating. Rest assured that your relative is being watched closely for weight loss (he or she will be weighed several times a week), and if it becomes too pronounced, a naso-gastric tube will be inserted to maintain the vital functions until the medications have a chance to restore normal appetite.

One more thought: a gentle sense of humor is a blessing at a time like this, but don't attempt to turn into a comedian in front of the patient. You probably won't be able to raise your relative's spirits with jokes and chipper phrases, and he or she may read other things into your attempt at humor or feel you are making him or her the butt of the joke. Just be constant, positive, warm (but not intense), and firm in the knowledge that the depression will pass in time.

If your relative is in a manic phase and was recently hospitalized, it might be advisable to call the unit staff and find out when you should visit. There may be a dramatic improvement in several days, but people respond variably to medications and the primary symptoms of mania may linger for several weeks. If this is the case, natural conversation is difficult because the patient is flooded with ideas and may want to involve you in a lot of unrealistic plans. The patient may also insist that he or she doesn't belong in the hospital. You may feel overwhelmed or angry.

Most family members react to the patient's energy level and tell him or her to calm down. Rarely does this have any effect. One possible intervention, though, is to express your feelings to the patient. Tell him you are overwhelmed by the rapid speech, you are confused, and you are having trouble following what he is saying. If you cannot communicate with the patient, tell him or her that you'll return soon and that you hope you can talk more then. Reassure him that you will visit regularly.

The patient may be very angry with you for helping to hospitalize him, and this is very hard to deal with. You might say something like "I brought you here because you were unable to control your impulses and I thought it was best for you and me. I also understand that you feel on top of the world, but I feel you need treatment now." Don't expect to win back friendship immediately—no matter what you say. Give it some time and keep in mind that you took a stand because you realized that your relative was in a very precarious position. The picture will change as soon as the manic phase is under control.

WHO CAN YOU CALL TO CHECK ON YOUR RELATIVE?

Naturally you'll want to check in and ask the staff how your relative is feeling; you'll also want to "test the waters" and determine if a visit is advisable that day. The nursing staff has close contact with your relative and is in the best position to answer your questions. Find out which nurse on which shift is assigned to the care of your relative and ask him or her when would be the best time to call. Elect one family member to make the call so as not to overburden the nurse.

THE COLD SHOULDER TREATMENT?

If you feel you are getting the cold shoulder from any of the staff members, or are not satisfied with the treatment you see administered to the patient, speak up. Perhaps there's been a misunderstanding or a lack of communication. If you receive no satisfaction, make an appointment to speak to the director of clinical services. He or she should be able to resolve the situation, but if not, consult the admissions brochure you were given at the beginning of the hospital stay and look for the name of the patient representative. This person is a direct link to the hospital's administration and should be able to help find a solution to the problem.

COMING HOME: DISCHARGE AND AFTERCARE

Once the acute symptoms of the affective episode resolve, the staff meets to determine a discharge plan and date. The social worker evaluates the situation in the community to which the patient will return. Most often the patient has a family or apartment; in the event that the patient has neither, the social worker will attempt to find a group home or halfway house and make the necessary application after discussing it with the patient.

Most people leave the hospital on a medication that requires regular visits with a physician. If the patient did not have a private psychiatrist before entering the hospital, or cannot afford a referral to a private psychiatrist, he or she will be referred to a community mental health center or a local clinic. Clinics normally charge a sliding-scale fee based on the patient's ability to pay. The social worker at the hospital makes the first appointment, and the patient is asked to sign a release form so that the record of hospitalization can be transferred to the clinic.

This transition from the closely supervised hospital setting to a normally overcrowded clinic can be an uncomfortable one for the patient. Unfortunately, the quality and organization of aftercare services are not always what they should be. Ideally the patient should be evaluated and treated by the same doctor, one who has an expertise in the treatment of affective disorders. The treating team, whether it includes psychiatrists, psychologists, social workers, or other mental health professionals, offers a coordinated treatment plan.

This is all too rare. A more common scenario is that the patient sees a doctor who comes in from time to time to renew the medications prescription (but who may not be following the patient closely). Meanwhile, the patient is seen more frequently by a mental health professional, who may have no training in the neurosciences and little understanding of the course of the disorder and its medical treatments.

In the event that a patient is unhappy with the referral he or she received, a call to the referring doctor who treated the patient in the hospital may encourage the doctor to call that clinic and intervene, or arrange for a referral to another kind of clinic.

It should be obvious from all of the above that there is little if any follow-up of the patient's care once he or she leaves the hospital, prescription and appointment in hand. The reality is that no one at the hospital will know what happens to the patient unless he or she stops taking the medication and eventually returns to the hospital. It is vital, then, that the patient have the support of family members who can ensure that medications are taken and appointments are kept. They can also help the patient critically assess the quality of the aftercare. When no family is around to be involved, a patient's participation in a support group may make all the difference.

A man who had been hospitalized with a bipolar disorder wrote and urged us to stress several points that would help people with the illness avoid hospitalization. He outlined three, and we quote his words:

1.   Patients must come to accept the fact that no one in the world can do them any good if they fail to help themselves.
2.   The family and the patient must work together with the doctor. Most patients—more than they want to admit—need family or a close friend, to help monitor their taking the medication and their going to see their therapist.

3. This is important: try to admonish patients that because of the precarious and tricky nature of manic-depressive illness, the patient must be ready to accept advice—if necessary make a contract with a family member or friend—to be warned when "danger signals" are in evidence. For example, when the patient is saying or doing inappropriate things; when the patient is taking unreasonable risks, or manifesting abnormal behavior of any sort. At this point the medications can be altered and a full-blown episode (and thus the probability of another hospitalization) can be avoided.

Sound advice from one who's been there.

12

UNDERWRITING THE ILLNESS: THE WORLD OF INSURANCE

Between the interaction of the professional and the patient between the admission to a hospital and the release lies the bill. Yes, money hovers over and tracks silently behind the receipt of mental health care.

We don't know many people who could specify what their coverage would be in the event of hospitalization, or many people who realize that mental health coverage is far less than that for a "physical" illness—there is no parity—or that it's mostly earmarked for inpatient, not outpatient, care. Therefore, this chapter is really a minicourse on insurance and the economic realities of the mental health marketplace.

THE HISTORY OF PRIVATE INSURANCE

The health insurance movement in this country began just before the Great Depression when Justin Kimball of Baylor University offered prepaid hospital protection to the public school teachers of Dallas. For three dollars each semester, the teachers were covered for up to 21 days of hospitalization. It didn't take long for this novel concept to catch on, and other cities soon began to offer similar plans. An organization in Minnesota first began to use the now-familiar Blue Cross name and symbol, and in 1939 the state of California initiated a plan that was to become the prototype of Blue Shield—the insurance that covered doctors' bills. These two organizations merged and are referred to as Blue Cross/Blue Shield.

Most people are covered by group plans through their place of employment, professional association, or union, and these group policies are more generous (and cheaper) than individual ones, but not always when it comes to psychiatric coverage. An employer usually has a choice as to how comprehensive the psychiatric benefits will be, but the standard policy typically covers 20 to 30 days per year of a psychiatric hospitalization, along with about $1,000 for outpatient consultation or counseling. Most of the payments for outpatient therapy visits come from the employee's own pocket.

If a person is unemployed or self-employed and cannot purchase group insurance through a professional association, he or she should purchase an individual policy, but keep in mind that individual policies cost quite a bit more and are less generous with benefits. The psychiatric coverage will most likely be very limited (with no option of increasing the coverage) and there will no doubt be a form/questionnaire to fill out that examines closely the psychiatric history of the would-be policyowner and his or her family. One application we looked at asked, "Have you or any named dependent within the past five years had any mental or physical disorder?" Answering truthfully does not guarantee a turndown for coverage; it does make matters a bit more complicated, and as with certain preexisting physical illnesses, benefits may be eliminated for a certain period of time. Psychiatric coverage may be denied completely.

A person with a history of mood disorders who leaves a job that offers a group plan and has not yet found another may be able to sidestep such a preexisting illness clause, but he or she must act in a timely fashion. Once the person leaves the job, coverage ends after a specified grace period, but he or she has the option to convert the group policy to an individual or family policy *without a physical examination or any questions asked.* It is important to make that conversion and pay the premiums on the now-converted individual policy. If not, the person with a history of manic-depression may find it next to impossible to get access to mental health insurance until he or she is employed again and enrolled in another group plan.

As one explores the world of insurance more thoroughly, one hears the terms "first-dollar" coverage and "deductibles, copayment and coinsurance." These terms determine how much out-of-pocket expense a patient will have in the event of treatment. "First-dollar" coverage will have a higher premium and may not cover the same amount of services as a policy that has a deductible and coinsurance, but once the premium is paid, the patient can stop worrying about paying other expenses. A "deductible" is the specific dollar amount the insured person must pay before the policy takes effect; "coinsurance" refers to the percentage of all costs that the insured individual must pay. A plan with a deductible has a lower premium, and tends to deter a person from running to the hospital for nonessential treatment. Many of these plans pay 80 percent of the bills, while asking the insured party to cover the remaining 20 percent.

Everything we've written up to this point has described the traditional way in which health care was financed in this country in the private sector. A corporation or individual subscribed to a "fee for service" plan in which a patient selected the doctor of his or her choice, and the bill was paid by the insurance company with certain limitations imposed by the policy.

For persons with serious mental illnesses, insurance carriers limited their risk by capping the dollar amounts of annual and lifetime mental health benefits; requiring preadmission certification for hospitalization; limiting services covered, often with incentives for inpatient care; charging higher copayment and deductible amounts; and excluding coverage for certain disorders. Because of these discriminatory practices, people with serious psychiatric disorders were denied sufficient coverage and were forced either to obtain treatment from public mental health services or—in the worst case scenario—to go entirely without treatment.

Despite such efforts at cost containment, however, medical costs skyrocketed in the 1980s and 1990s. In 1992, spending for American health care exceeded $800 billion, more than 12 percent of the gross domestic product. Corporations like AT&T reported that one-third of their operating costs were devoted to health care expenditures. In the public sector, an equally daunting figure was tallied: state Medicaid budgets in 1991, 1992, and 1993 rose faster than any other state program costs, exceeding state spending on higher education. In 1993, Medicaid expenditures increased 29 percent over those of 1992.

Some of the factors contributing to this alarming rise in health care costs were the increasing use of sophisticated medical technology; our inability as a nation to ration health care, particularly in the last six months of life; burgeoning malpractice litigation that resulted in the defensive (and thus expensive) practice of medicine; and abuses in the fee-for-service reimbursement system: some doctors and hospitals charged unreasonable fees for services and overutilized technology and procedures.

Clearly the run-away costs of medical care had to be corralled. An experimental model formulated in the 1980s promised to provide efficiency and cost containment. Enter the world of managed care.

MANAGED CARE: A RADICAL CHANGE IN THE DELIVERY OF HEALTH CARE

Managed care is a system of organizing, financing, delivering, and evaluating services that deliberately seeks to control costs while promising to deliver high-quality health care. There are several models of managed care programs, but most fall into the category of a health maintenance organization (HMO).

Traditionally, an insurance company underwrote some of a patient's health care, but it was up to a patient to find the medical personnel to supply it. Then he or she had to file the claims and hope the treatment was within the bounds of the policy. The idea behind the HMO is that the health insurance and the health services are provided by the same organization, and there is the promise of follow-through and integration of treatment. An emphasis is also on preventive care. A member pays a fixed monthly or quarterly premium and receives health care from a team (or teams) of doctors, nurses, technicians, and other health professionals—often under one roof—but there are no deductibles, few if any copayments, and absolutely no forms to send in to the insurer. All medical records are kept in a central office, and the emergency room services are available 24 hours a day. (Out-of-area emergency room services are also generally covered.)

The model described, in which all services are provided under one roof, is one used by a company like Kaiser Permanente on the West Coast. It's referred to as a clinic or staff model. But many, many managed care organizations are networks of independent physicians—*providers*—who direct the patient's treatment with guidelines set by the managed care company, and who are reimbursed with a fee structure also set by the managed care company. The enrolled members can choose from a list of providers or accept the physician recommended by the *PCP—the primary care physician* to whom they are assigned. These PCPs are family practitioners or internists who function as "gate keepers" to a network of specialists.

What does this mean? In the fee-for-service system, if a patient is troubled by headaches, he or she could wake up one morning, get the name and number of a neurologist, and make an appointment to see that physician (a specialist). It was not unlikely that the specialist would charge a significant fee for the consultation or order expensive MRI and other tests.

Managed care companies make the argument that such a patient initially should see a generalist—a primary care physician—who should first explore whether the headaches might be stress-related or masked depression, and so on. And only then should the patient be referred to the appropriate specialist—a psychiatrist or a neurologist—thus better matching the patient's problem with the more appropriate and least costly intervention.

This is a reasonable approach and likely to be effective in regulating some of the excesses in the system, so long as the profit incentives do not impede appropriate and timely referrals.

So quickly did the idea of managed care catch on in corporate America that by 1996 over 75 percent of all employees were covered by health benefits provided by managed care organizations. And now managed care companies are moving into the public sector and vying for Medicare and Medicaid contracts. Champus, the Civilian Health and Medical Program of the Uniformed Services—the insurance plan that covers members of the armed forces and their families—now provides health care totally within a managed care model.

We are in the midst of a huge paradigm shift in the delivery of medical care in this country. There are new models, new methods, and a new vocabulary that accompany them. Understandably, the changes have provoked significant anxiety and a fair amount of turmoil. The dust has yet to settle. Let us discuss the vocabulary first and then touch on a few of the bigger issues.

Managed care companies build the profit incentive into the system with a concept known as *capitation*. This means that the doctor will receive a fixed amount of money and once he or she accepts that money, he or she agrees to provide a range of services to a group of patients. If the doctor provides the range of services the patient needs and it amounts to less than the capitation received, the doctor can keep the difference. If the range of services costs more than the capitation, the doctor underwrites the difference. (While medicine should not be practiced with a "sky's the limit" mentality, many are concerned about this front-and-center position of dollar signs in the vital decision-making process a physician must conduct and by the fact that managed care companies do not necessarily place the interest of the patient above the motivation for profit.)

Patient choice is another arena of anxiety. People are loyal to and comfortable with their own doctors, and they do not like to be assigned a doctor not of their own choosing or to be forced to leave their group of doctors in order to receive reimbursement. Many managed care plans, however, offer what is called a *dual-option* plan or *point-of-service* option. This means that a employee is allowed to seek care outside the managed care network at any time, but must pay deductibles, copays, and so on, as with any traditional insurance plan.

Managed care plans have benefit limits just as traditional plans do. In psychiatry, most plans cover 30 days of inpatient care a year, with about 20 annual outpatient psychotherapy visits. This is inadequate for people with mood disorders, but a senior staff psychiatrist at Kaiser Permanente told us that under their auspices medication visits are unlimited, and that they are very aware that if they don't treat a psychiatric problem intensively, it will show up in the inappropriate and more expensive medical sector.

A few companies such as U.S. Healthcare offer what is called a *conversion of benefits.* A patient can choose to convert inpatient days for outpatient psychotherapy visits as well as aggregate visits for family therapy. For instance, if a family thinks that family therapy is the most appropriate use of outpatient visits, they can utilize 20 visits of one family member, and then the 20 visits of the next, and so forth. In our conversations with U.S. Healthcare's senior medical directors, several said that they believed that if a patient is not treated in an appropriate and timely manner, then the problem will ultimately engender more medical problems in family members caring for that inadequately treated patient. They mentioned how often they see those closest to the patient suffering from stress-related illnesses. (These cost-effective philosophies that inform the policies of managed care organizations may actually benefit some people with psychiatric disorders.)

Doctors have yet to get comfortable with this model, however. The concentrated effort to reduce costs has shifted the balance of power in treatment choice from the physician to the insurer. Doctors we spoke with resent the frequent calls they receive from employees of health care companies—*the case managers*—who have nowhere near the physician's level of training or experience questioning the physician about his or her treatment plans. Also, the managed care companies reimburse the physicians at rates far below their customary fees (and a noted authority in his or her field with years of experience is often paid the same fee as a doctor fresh out of a residency training program). There is a tremendous amount of paperwork and request forms, and a few doctors admitted that they were afraid they would be "deselected" from the network if they made too many referrals or requests. Their contracts would not be renewed. And confidentiality, an important aspect of the treatment agreement between doctor and patient (especially in the psychiatric setting), is totally abrogated because managed care organizations require frequent record reviews.

Many physicians who work at university teaching hospitals also have serious concerns about the viability of these academic centers. Because these hospitals are traditionally more expensive than nonacademic institutions, managed care companies tend to steer contracts away from them, and these important centers of research and graduate education are in jeopardy.

Any major change brings losses as well as opportunities, and while we've mentioned a few of the concerns about managed care, it is now the dominant force in health care delivery. It is a young and unregulated industry, however, and it is still evolving. Legislation that protects the rights of patients is currently being enacted, and the National Committee for Quality Assurance (NCQA) in Washington, D.C., has recently issued behavioral health (psychiatric) guidelines against which a managed care company can be measured and accredited. This will be an especially important credential to have when businesses make decisions as to which managed care company they contract with. The NCQA lists the credentialed managed care companies on the internet under http://www.ncqa.org.

In the meantime, if patients or family members feel they are being denied access to care, each managed care company has a phone number to call and a procedure for initiating an appeal. Consumers and physicians sit on the grievance committees, so it is likely that an appropriate request will be granted in the appeals process. Managed care companies are very concerned about customer satisfaction because if a valued employee is not happy or returned to health and good functioning, then the employer paying for the benefits is going to be dissatisfied and prone to switch managed care companies when the contract expires.

The National Alliance for the Mentally Ill (NAMI)—the nation's largest patient-advocacy group—is watching the managed care revolution intently. A special committee has been established whose mission is to educate their state affiliates to the intricacies of managed care as well as to influence the managed care company's guidelines for psychiatric treatment and reimbursement. Dr. Laura Lee Hall, NAMI's deputy director of policy and research, is spearheading this effort and has observed that there are significant risks in managed care, but opportunities as well. She outlined what she viewed as the opportunities in this new form of health-care delivery.

> Managed care is bringing to bear the tools of science to psychiatric treatment. We have excellent data about effective treatment for severe mental illness. There are new medications and specific methods of psychotherapy that work; there are interventions like supportive employment that we know can be extremely effective and improve quality of life. We have sound data and we will look to managed care to apply proven therapies to the people who need them.
>
> Another plus we see is that these companies have huge computer systems. With sophisticated data capacities they are in a position to analyze the effectiveness of various services and to develop profiles on the effectiveness of providers.

In addition, she noted that moving managed care into the public sector—Medicare and Medicaid—may put an end to the two-tiered system that has always existed in this country: patients in the private sector are treated differently than those relying on the public safety nets. For the first time, the same player will be in both fields, so to speak, and they will undoubtably transfer proven models from one to the other.

Dr. Hall's committee is looking carefully at each managed care company and its policies and has recently published a three-part *National Report Card*. This study, funded in part by the Ittelson Foundation, provides a national snapshot of managed care policies and practices in the U.S. public mental health system and their impact on people with severe mental illnesses and their families. The first section will provide a summary of state policies underpinning the move of managed care into the public mental health system; part two directly probes consumer and family member perceptions and experiences of managed care; and part three focuses on the policies and practices of managed care organizations themselves. This resembles a mental health care report card, and it focuses on the largest managed behavioral health care organizations, and details information on product lines and practices, treatment guidelines, family and consumer involvement, the comprehensiveness of services, and approaches to outcome management.

These publications as well as an excellent primer on managed care written by Michael Malloy and entitled *Mental Illness and Managed Care* are available from NAMI, 200 N. Glebe Road, Suite 1015, Arlington, Virginia, 22203-3754 (703) 524-7600.

PUBLIC INSURANCE

The federal government (through state programs) provides two main forms of public health insurance, Medicare and Medicaid, and two forms of disability insurance, Social Security and Supplemental Security Income. Members of the armed services and their dependents are covered by a third form of public insurance.

Medicare

Medicare is the program administered by the Health Care Financing Administration (HCFA) for people over 65, for some younger people who are disabled, and for people of any age with permanent kidney failure.

To be eligible for Medicare you must be one of the following:

1. Sixty-five or older and eligible for Social Security or the qualified railroad retirement system.
2. Not eligible for Social Security or railroad retirement benefits, but of age 65 before 1968. Or of age 65 after 1967, with a certain minimum number of quarters of Social Security coverage.

3. Sixty-five or older, a United States citizen or lawfully admitted alien who has continuously resided in the United States for at least five years.

4. Under 65 and have received either Social Security or Railroad Retirement disability payments for at least 24 months.

5. In Federal employment for a minimum length of time and meet the requirements of the Social Security disability program.

6. In Federal employment since January 1, 1983, and not otherwise covered.

There are two parts to the Medicare package: Part A, also referred to as HI (Hospital Insurance); and Part B, Supplementary Medical Insurance (SMI), which helps pay for outpatient care.

Part A is financed by Social Security contributions from employers, employees, and the self-employed. (If an employee has received a weekly paycheck, he or she is familiar with the Federal Insurance Contribution Act [FICA] deduction.) This hospital coverage is then free to anyone eligible. Part B is financed partially by the monthly premium paid by those who wish to buy it. If a person is over 65 but has not worked long enough to be entitled to the hospital insurance provided by Medicare, he or she can buy into Medicare, so to speak, but will have to buy Parts A and B. In that instance, there is no option of not paying for Part B.

Medicare is a safety net, but a net with many holes. There are deductibles, coinsurance, items and services that are not covered and certain limits on how much Medicare will reimburse. In addition, benefits are not covered unless Medicare says they are "medically necessary" and they are furnished by providers certified or approved by Medicare. Medicare pays 80 percent of "responsible charges" for lab tests, but does not pay for prescription drugs. Thus, lithium levels or thyroid function studies will need 20 percent financing by the patient. However, Medigap policies (see below) may help with the prescription drugs.

The hospital insurance of Part A limits its coverage to 190 days of inpatient psychiatric hospital care *during the entire lifetime of a beneficiary.* An outpatient may receive psychiatric services from a physician, a comprehensive outpatient rehabilitative facility, a physician's assistant, or a psychologist, but this treatment is subject to a special payment rule. In effect, Medicare pays only 50 percent of approved charges for these benefits. Hospital outpatient treatment to include partial hospitalization psychiatric programs of mental illness is not subject to this limit (in other words, 80 percent of the approved charges is covered).

No one can afford to rely on Medicare to cover the costs of treatment today, and most people do buy some sort of private Medigap policy to fill in where Medicare leaves off. A policy such as this may pay some or all of the deductibles and coinsurance, or extend the hospital days and pay for some prescription drugs. Many insurance policies that cover people before they are 65 can be converted to a Medigap policy, and this should be investigated.

You apply for Medicare at your local Social Security office, and you can keep current on the law by reading the most recent Social Security Handbook. Every Social Security office has it and also a supply of pamphlets that will guide you through the labyrinth of Medicare.

Medicaid

Medicaid is a form of public assistance for low-income persons—the medically indigent. The program is financed by federal, state, and local taxes and administered by local public assistance offices.

The Medicaid patient is not responsible for deductibles

and coinsurance, and all inpatient or outpatient hospital care, doctors' fees, lab tests, X-rays, and skilled nursing home care and transportation are covered. Sometimes adult daycare and prescription drugs are covered also (the benefits vary from state to state). But while Medicaid covers all charges from qualified providers, it reimburses the professionals and the facilities with sums well below their standard fees. Consequently, many doctors and hospitals do not accept Medicaid patients.

Some people qualify for both Medicaid and Medicare, and anyone receiving the Supplemental Security Income discussed below is automatically covered by Medicaid. To find out if you're eligible, contact your local public assistance office. Look in the telephone book under City Government Departments and scan down the sublistings until you find Social Services.

Disability

The Social Security Administration disability program provides monthly cash benefits for disabled workers (and their dependents) who have contributed to the Social Security trust fund through the FICA tax on their earnings. These people have an "earned right" to disability insurance benefits. You may qualify if a physical or mental condition prevents you from working for at least 12 months.

The years of work credit needed for disability checks depend on your age when you become disabled:

- *Before 24.* You need credit for 1½ years of work in the 3-year period ending when your disability starts.
- *24 through 31.* You need credit for having worked half the time between 21 and the time you become disabled.
- *31 or older.* You need the amount of credit shown in the following chart.

Born after 1929, disabled at age	Born before 1930, disabled before age 62	Years of work credit needed
31–42		5
44		5½
46		6
48		6½
50		7
52	1981	7½
53	1982	7¾
54	1983	8
55	1984	8¼
56	1985	8½
57	1986	8¾
58	1987	9
60	1989	9½
62 or older	1991 or later	10

If you are a disabled worker 31 or older, generally you must have earned at least 5 years of work credit in the 10 years immediately before you become disabled. *Exception:* If you are disabled by blindness, the required credit may have been earned at any time after 1936; you need no recent credit.

If you are disabled, certain members of your family may receive benefits from Social Security also: unmarried children under 18, disabled children 18 or over if they were disabled before the age of 22 and a spouse if he or she is 62 or older or has an eligible child in his or her care. A divorced individual is entitled to a former spouse's benefits if he or she was married to the worker for 10 years prior to the date the divorce became final.

How to Apply for Benefits

The Social Security Administration regards a mental illness that results in "marked constriction of activities and interests, deterioration in personal habits or work-related behavior, and seriously impaired ability to get along with other people" as a disabling condition. Applications for disability benefits may be made by telephone or mail, or in person at the Social Security office and should be made as soon as a person becomes disabled. If a patient cannot manage his or her own affairs, the application can be completed by a spouse, parent, other relative, friend, or legal guardian. (A toll-free number that allows you to talk to someone about disability benefits is (800) 772-1213 Monday through Friday during normal business hours. To avoid a busy signal, try calling early in the morning or late in the afternoon.)

In order to complete the application and process a claim, you will need the following:

- The Social Security number and proof of age for each person eligible for payments.
- Names, addresses, and telephone numbers of doctors, hospitals, clinics, and institutions that treated you and approximate dates of treatment. (Be as complete and correct as possible to avoid delays in processing your claim.)
- A summary of where you worked in the past 15 years and the kind of work you did.
- A copy of your W-2 (Wage and Tax statement), or if you are self-employed, your Federal tax return for the past year.
- Dates of military service, if any.
- Dates of any prior marriages if your spouse is applying.
- The claim number of any other benefit you receive (or expect to receive) because of your disability.
- If you are applying for benefits as a disabled widow or widower, the worker's death certificate and proof of marriage.
- If you are applying for benefits as a disabled surviving divorced wife or husband, bring proof that the marriage lasted at least 10 years.

You should also bring your checkbook or savings passbook in the event that you choose for your checks to be deposited directly into your bank account. Otherwise, you can receive your checks through the mail.

Once an application is completed, the Social Security office reviews it and decides if the applicant has met the requirements of the law. If so, the office sends the application to the Disability Determination Services (DDS) office in the patient's state.

A physician and a disability evaluation specialist in that office then consider all the facts of the case. Often they request other medical evidence from the physicians, hospitals, and clinics or institutions who have treated the patient, but the government pays for any medical reports that it requests. Doctors are asked to supply a medical history of the condition: What is wrong? When did it begin? How does the condition limit activities and what treatment has been provided?

It is not unusual for a person applying for disability to be asked to take a special or consultative medical or psychiatric examination, but Social Security pays for this and for certain travel expenses that the patient incurs.

It generally takes two to three months to process a disability claim. The Social Security Administration contacts you with a written notice. If your claim is approved, the notice will indicate the amount of your benefit and when the payments will begin (monthly benefits generally start with the sixth full month of disability. There is, however, no waiting period for a person disabled before age 22 who qualifies on the Social Security record of a parent).

The amount of monthly disability benefits is based on a worker's lifetime average earnings covered by Social Security. The average monthly benefit for a disabled worker in 1996 was $682.00, and the average payment to a disabled worker with a family was $1,148.00.

What If Your Claim Is Denied?

You have the right to appeal an unfavorable decision on your claim. There are four appeal levels. The first is a reconsideration, which gives you an opportunity to submit any new evidence not previously considered. You have about 60 days after receiving notice to file an appeal. If you then disagree with the reconsideration decision, you can request a hearing before an administrative law judge. The third and fourth levels of appeal are a review by the Appeals Council and, finally, a civil action in a Federal court. In 1996, the reversal rate of disability claims at the second level of appeal was about 70 percent. This should greatly encourage people to press on through the system.

Disability Reviews

Under Social Security law, all disability cases must be reviewed periodically. The frequency of review can range from six months to seven years, depending on the expectation of improvement. A review occurs after you receive a notice. Someone then interviews you in person or on the telephone. During this interview, you will be asked to provide information about medical treatment and any work activity and you will be asked to describe how your condition affects you. Your updated case folder than goes to the state agency that makes disability decisions on behalf of Social Security. The process starts again, and again, if you disagree with the findings of the review, you can initiate an appeals process. If you are no longer disabled and are returning to work, you will receive a benefit for the last month of disability and two additional months.

SSI

Supplemental Security Income (SSI) is a federal program designed to provide a floor of income for the aged, blind, or disabled who have little or no income and resources. It is administered by the Social Security Administration and is financed by general tax revenues. There are no periods of work required—a person qualifies solely because of need. Medicaid medical insurance is provided also. As with disability, a determination and review of the claim is made by a special committee.

In order to apply for SSI, a person must not have countable resources in excess of $2,000 (individual), or $3,000 (as a couple). Certain resources, however, are excluded when determining whether one is eligible for SSI: the home you live in and the land it is on are not counted; your car usually does not count. A person applies for SSI at the local Social Security office by filling out some forms. The personnel at the office will need to see proofs and documents that would show the applicant's assets, such as bank books, insurance policies, paycheck receipts, other proof of income, and car registration.

People on SSI are paid at different monthly rates. The levels are determined by whether an individual lives alone, lives with others but pays his or her own expenses, or lives in the household of others and receives support and maintenance. These payments are not large. In 1996, a recipient who lived alone in the state of New York received a monthly SSI check for $556, one who lived at home supported by his or her family received a check for $336.* Other states pay more or less. If the person gets a job, the payments are reduced or cut. Being eligible for SSI means that the person is also eligible for Medicaid and may be eligible for housing programs, vocational rehabilitation, and food stamps.

Those who are truly disabled and believe they are entitled to the benefits of SSI are going to need a lot of persistence. Sometimes a claim is not hard to document and is very apparent. Other claims may be denied for many reasons. The law defines a disability as "the inability to engage in any substantial

---

*These figures increase every year.

gainful activity by reason of any medically determinable physical or mental impairment which can be expected to result in death or has lasted or can be expected to last for a continuous period of not less than 12 months." The problem phrase here for psychiatric disabilities is the one that stresses "medically determinable physical or mental impairment." Because it is extremely difficult to count the days or assess the outcome of a mental disorder, an applicant for SSI or the representative making the claim for him or her should know about the appeals process.

Should an applicant receive a denial, he or she has 60 days to submit a request for reconsideration to the district office. A Legal Aid service lawyer can help prepare this (the law provides for payment of legal fees in an amount up to 25 percent of the award approved for Social Security claims). If the claim is then denied at the reconsideration level, a request should immediately be made for an administrative law judge hearing. In 1996, a very significant number of the claims heard by a judge were allowed despite their having been denied twice before the hearing. Keep all this in mind to bolster your defense.

Patients and family members should know that Social Security has several provisions that may help the person who has been ill and who has been receiving monthly disability or Supplemental Security Insurance checks return to work. Counseling and guidance services are available, as are job training and placement. The patient receives full disability benefits for up to nine months while testing his or her ability to work.

We just want to state that on a good day we're often confused by the ifs, ands, and buts of the policies and plans, the bureaucracy and the rapid change in laws. How then, we wondered, could someone in a disabled state sort all this out? Well, with a lot of help. Your best bet is to talk to a social worker, either at the hospital before discharge, or at a clinic or community mental health center. These professionals are aware of the laws and programs and know how to initiate petitions for Medicaid/Medicare, disability, and SSI. If you're fortunate enough to have a family member, friend, or advocate who will help you negotiate the system, with patience and time you'll get where you need to go and get what you need to have.

FOUR

COMING FULL CIRCLE

13

RECOVERY AND
THE WORLD OUTSIDE

When a person with a mood disorder obtains information and treatment, and comes to accept what has happened to him because of the illness, he has added very necessary ballast to his life. Much of the initial phase of stabilization and education involves a member of the mental health profession. But the next phase finds the patient turning outward and interacting with his or her family members, office colleagues, and social networks. The details of the disorder, and perhaps also an absence from the home and workplace, must be explained. How will my spouse and I explain it to our children? Should I tell my boss? How do I repair and rebuild? Where do I go from here? These are just a few of the questions to which answers must be found.

Now we come full circle—the patient who was very much in need of information is now the person who must decide who to inform and in what way. Here are some ideas that may ease the tensions surrounding these issues.

HOW TO TELL A CHILD

It is difficult enough for a husband or wife to deal with an ill spouse, but when there are children in the home the strain and the complexity of the situation multiply. Most parents have a tendency to want to shield children from the unpleasant realities of life—"There's time enough for that when they're older" is the rationale. But most people underestimate children's extreme sensitivity to a parent's mood and their capacity to imagine things more terrible than reality. When a depressed parent becomes silent and inactive, no longer able to care for the children or look after the household, the children are bound to become confused and anxious; if the parent suddenly begins to act in a wild and erratic way, with explosive emotional outbursts, the children will become skittish, filled with fear and resentment. Unfortunately, children also have a huge capacity for guilt and self-blame. They may assume they caused the parent's problem. They can't understand what has happened to the parent they knew and counted on, and they no longer feel secure, protected, and loved.

A simple explanation from the well parent would do much to help the child deal with the fears and replace untoward imaginative fantasies with firm and guilt-free facts. A mother in St. Louis told us that she explained everything to her children at the beginning of what was to become a series of hospitalizations for their father, who was manic-depressive. She wrote to us recently and summarized the responses of her 14-year-old son, Tim, to his father's illness:

> Tim is extremely bright and knowledgeable about manic-depressive illness. He said that in his earlier years he was very afraid of his father when he was in a manic mood and he felt great relief when his Dad was depressed as he slept most of the time and didn't bother the children very much. As he got older and was better able to understand the information about the illness that I had been constantly feeding him, his response became less that of dread and more of loving concern for his father's welfare. Remember, though, that as Tim was getting older, his father was becoming more stabilized and Tim's understanding combined with his Dad's stability helped immensely in establishing a very good rapport between

both of them. Some of Tim's comments are that he doesn't fear his Dad anymore. Because of his constant education about the disorder, he regards the illness as no more complicated than any other medical problem he may encounter. Being fully aware of the genetic factors involved, Tim is firmly convinced that under no circumstances would he fight treatment if he experienced an onset of manic-depression. He has seen first-hand the devastation this illness creates and wants no part of it. He has also witnessed the massive change in his father's whole personality because of stabilization and he is extremely proud of his Dad's accomplishments under oftentimes great duress.

Children who share their parents' joys *and* sorrows often develop strength and a sense of self-worth.

Author Helene Arnstein, in *What to Tell Your Child About Birth, Death, Illness, Divorce and Other Family Crises,* offers some fine phrases for telling even a very young child what is going on. She relates how a father helped his five-and-a-half-year-old, whose mother was hospitalized for depression by saying:

Tommy, Mommy cried a lot before she went to the hospital, and she didn't seem to pay as much attention to you as she used to. She just felt tired and sick. Feelings sometimes get sick just the way bodies do. Do you remember the time when you had the measles? You didn't *seem* to love anybody because you felt so bad. Well, Mommy loves you but she cannot show it because *she* feels so sick. When she feels better again and comes home, Mommy will be able to play with you and hug you, and you'll know she has never really stopped loving you and me.

After explaining the situation, a parent should wait patiently for the child to ask questions, and answer them honestly. It should not be assumed that a lack of questions or curiosity implies that the child is too young to understand, or that there is not turmoil churning within. In fact, the silence may be the clue as to how upset the child really is.

A child who witnesses a parent's being forcibly removed from the home and taken to a hospital will be terrified (this scene is a searing one for an adult witness also). Ms. Arnstein advises a conversation something like this:

> Daddy (or Mommy) didn't know just then what was best for him. He didn't know that the hospital is the safest and most comfortable place to be in while he is getting well. You know, there were times when you too had to do things you didn't want to, but which we knew were good for you. It was that way with Daddy, too. Other people needed to decide what was best for him.

Teenagers have other concerns. They may fear bad blood in the family and ostracism from classmates and dates; their shame and embarrassment may keep them away from friends. Because teenagers find it particularly embarrassing to discuss emotional problems with parents, it might be best if they spoke to an informed doctor, social worker, or other adult who understands the illness and can listen and respond well to an adolescent boy or girl.

If a child with a hospitalized parent can imagine what the hospital looks like, can envision some of the personalities of the staff working with the mother or father, and can understand what the parent does during the day, he or she will feel reassured that the parent is being cared for, will get well, and will return home again. This is not to suggest that the child visit the hospital, but when the well parent actively describes the hospital setting, the child is usually more comfortable with the temporary changes in the home life. When the patient does return, however, the child is going to have a lot of mixed feelings: relief, anger, anxiety, and embarrassment. The well parent should not insist it be a joyous reunion unless the child attempts to make it one, and the child should be warned that the recovering parent needs a lot of rest and time to adjust to the homecoming. Everyone needs some time to get used to each other again and to let the harshness of the preceding crisis fade a bit.

TO TELL OR NOT TO TELL AN EMPLOYER

People who have mood disorders react differently. Some people, once treated, are able to function well; others experience recurrences that cause problems when they return to work. Much depends, of course, on the employer's attitudes concerning illness. Does the employer generally react with suspicion or understanding when an employee becomes ill?

For the most part, an employer is concerned with productivity. He or she prefers employees who come into work every day, work hard, and take a minimum of sick days (employees who utilize insurance benefits raise the company's premiums). But there are employees who may understand a worker's problems, especially if the worker has been valuable to the company. Recently more companies are becoming enlightened, and some are sponsoring programs to deal with alcoholism, drug abuse, and emotional problems.

A person with a recurrent disorder must weigh all the factors and decide either to make a full disclosure or no disclosure at all. There is little value in minimal disclosure as it leaves open the possibility of the employer's assuming that the situation is worse than it is. The employer may also link unrelated aspects of work performance to problems with the disorder. It's unfortunate, but there are risks to disclosing information about psychiatric disorders—stigma is not a thing of the past. No one can offer blanket advice about the best course of action, and we caution you to proceed thoughtfully.

If a person wishes to inform an employer, he or she

should make an appointment at a time that will ensure privacy and attention. The employee can say that he or she has an affective disorder, a medical illness that affects sleep, activity level, and concentration—and that it is treated with medication. The employee might add that he or she is in treatment with a physician who is administering the medication, and while no one can guarantee that there won't be brief periods where these functions aren't disturbed, for the most part the doctor and the employee are closely monitoring the problem. No doubt the employer will have questions, and the employee should do his or her best to answer them in a straightforward manner.

Naturally, if there is a sudden hospitalization, a family member or friend will notify those in charge at the workplace. Early in the episode, many details (such as what will happen and how long it will be before the patient can return to work) are unknown. Perhaps it is wisest not to say too much before some facts and progress are known. The friend or family member should simply say that Mr. D. has not been well lately, has been hospitalized, and is being evaluated and that the employer will be kept informed. As soon as the picture is clearer, the employer should, if possible, be told when to expect the employee back at work.

Many people who have dealt with the problem of whether or how to tell an employer wrote to us. They received varying responses to their disclosures:

- "I had to explain where I had been for a month, so I told them. They took it well. It seems someone told them already."
- "I told them and apologized for my illness. They responded with understanding but I resigned, and my resignation was accepted."
- "I did tell them and their response was very positive. They bent over backwards to help. Everything possible was done to make my job easier."

- "I didn't tell my employers but they seemed to know. Insurance payments through the firms are not 'secret.' There have been three lay-offs in the past five years in which I have been included."

- "After I was diagnosed I was terminated. I was told they couldn't take a chance with me (I might commit suicide). I am very careful not to reveal anything on future applications."

- "I said, 'I need to clue you in on something. I have an illness called manic-depression and it sometimes interferes with my concentration. I take medication—lithium—and I do not consider it a handicap. I just want you to know.'" (The employer's reaction was to caution the employee to write things down so she wouldn't forget them.)

- "I told my employer largely in medical terms and I stressed the analogy to high blood pressure or diabetes. My employer was sympathetic and reestablished my job. I later received a promotion."

- "I told them I had manic-depression, that I took medications for it, and that I should be able to work without difficulty. With two exceptions, the response has always been negative. When job hunting, the mention of this topic seems to provide a sure guarantee for not getting a job."

- "I never mentioned it before I was hired. After that, I gradually made remarks about my past and let them know I had been hospitalized. Employers have never hesitated to hire me back after a bout in the hospital or after I had my children. I must be a productive worker in spite of the disorder."

SUPPORT GROUPS

One of the greatest boons to people suffering with manic-depression and depression is the recent proliferation of support groups. They offer individuals with a chronic or recurring psychiatric illness *and* their family and friends information, assistance, acceptance, and a chance to join forces with others to lobby for better research and legislation. Many groups are developing antistigma campaigns in order to improve public understanding of the serious psychiatric disorders. The National Depressive and Manic Depressive Association, the National Alliance for the Mentally Ill, and Recovery, Inc., are the three major support organizations, with affiliates throughout the country.

Although they all offer education and support, there are differences among the organizations. The National Depressive and Manic Depressive Association, with almost 300 affiliates across the United States, is an organization of individuals who have been diagnosed as having mania, depression, or both, and their family members. Monthly meetings feature lectures by experts in the fields of depression and mania, as well as "rap" sessions where people can talk about their problems and share information about the solutions they've found.

The National Alliance for the Mentally Ill (NAMI), soon to celebrate its twentieth anniversary, has over 1100 affiliates. This organization has become a powerful force with state governments and in Washington, and members testify before congressional hearings quite often. Their affiliates, or Alliances for the Mentally Ill (AMIs), consist mostly of family members of schizophrenic patients, but their programs do include patients and families with affective disorders.

Recovery, Inc., founded in 1939, is the oldest of these organizations. It was begun by a Chicago-based psychiatrist, Dr. Abraham Low, for formerly hospitalized psychiatric patients. Today nearly one thousand chapters worldwide serve anyone with emotional problems. The weekly meetings, led by former patients, are based on a method of temper control, behavior modification, and cognitive reconstruction. Recovery, Inc., is the only support group where diagnosis, medication, and treatment are not discussed at meetings. However, cooperation with the treating psychiatrist is encouraged.

A newcomer to the list of support groups is Depressives Anonymous: Recovery from Depression. This organization uses a self-help method originated by Dr. Helen De Rosis, which involves specifying particular problem areas in a person's life that can be broken down into manageable units and overcome by applying a four-step approach. Depressives Anonymous offers a course for health professionals and lay people who wish to start a group of their own.*

People who have joined support groups speak enthusiastically about the benefits. One member said: "There is a great deal of comfort in finding other people like you with the same experiences and problems. We learn from one another and are a great comfort to each other during crisis situations." Many people find it therapeutic to share what they've learned and to offer encouragement and support to others. It raises a person's self-esteem. Another member put it this way: "Helping someone with the same disorder helps me lessen my dislike of my own disorder. It's better to be active than passive."

Most of the groups publish regular newsletters that keep members informed of monthly schedules and meetings, report on areas of research and legislation pertinent to the membership, and review books that are thought to be helpful.

These are all ample reasons for seeking out a support group, but even greater possibilities exist when people join together in advocacy of research, destigmatization, and better services and support. There is power in numbers, and until recently people with psychiatric disorders were among the

*Addresses of the National Depressive and Manic Depressive Association and the National Alliance for the Mentally Ill are to be found in Appendix 4. The national headquarters of Recovery, Inc., is located at 802 North Dearborn Street, Chicago, IL 60610 (312) 337-5661. Depressives Anonymous: Recovery from Depression may be contacted at 329 East 62nd Street, New York, NY 10022 (212) 689-2600.

least powerful. Because they had no voice, they were at the mercy of by-the-whim decisions about funding and legislation. One out of every four hospital beds in this country is occupied by someone with a psychiatric disorder and the cost of mental illness to the American economy exceeds $36 billion in direct costs *per year,* yet the dollar amount allocated to mental illness by the Federal government is about the same as that for tooth decay. This money is allocated by Congress and administered through the National Institute for Mental Health.

CHANGING THE PUBLIC'S ATTITUDES

Unfortunately, public spending is quixotic and generally mirrors the support and spending trends of the private sector. Of the more than 22,000 private foundations in America, only a handful—namely, the MacArthur Foundation, the Ittleson Foundation, the Scottish Rite, the Schizophrenia Foundation, the Van Ameringen Foundation, and the Brain Research Foundation—donated significant funds for psychiatric research.

The patient and family advocacy groups mentioned began to address this pitiful state of private and public funding for mental health care and research. In 1986, the National Alliance for the Mentally Ill (NAMI) announced the newly founded National Alliance for Research on Schizophrenia and Depression (NARSAD).* NARSAD's aim has been to launch a public funding arm for research in the field of mental illness. The foundation is admirably fulfilling its mandate. In its first 10 years of grantmaking, NARSAD awarded $43 million in grants to scientists on the faculty or staff of over 100 institutions throughout this country, Europe, and Canada. NARSAD is dedicated to the idea that all of the funds solicited go exclusively for research

---

*The address of NARSAD is: NARSAD, 60 Cutter Mill Road, Suite 404, Great Neck, NY 11021 (516) 829-0091.

grants. In other words, a dollar donated is a dollar spent on scientific research (several families have come forward and underwritten all of the organization's operating expenses).

In the early 1990s, the Theodore and Vada Stanley Foundation joined with the National Alliance for the Mentally Ill and began to donate significant funds for research directly related to the causes or treatment of bipolar disorder and schizophrenia. Today, the Stanley Foundation supports the Neurovirology Lab on Schizophrenia and Manic-Depressive Disorder at Johns Hopkins University, six research centers in Europe, and a multisite Bipolar Disorder Treatment Outcome Network. Each year, some 50 researchers are granted awards to initiate or continue important research in these areas.

So, thanks to concerned families, the lack of research funding for severe psychiatric disorders is being remedied. Meanwhile, NAMI advocates lobby in Washington and talk with legislators, testify before subcommittees, offer seminars, and make the case for increased government spending for research.

NAMI has also targeted the areas of stigma and public education. This organization has enlisted the help of actors such as Kirk Douglas to film public service announcements whose aim is to reduce stigma and encourage people to seek help. In a country where fewer than 1 in 3 people with a clinical depression seek treatment of any kind, and fewer than 1 in 10 visit a mental health specialist, this kind of attention to the problem is urgent. The commercial shows Mr. Douglas straight-on, sitting in a chair. He says:

> It's been troubling me. Now, why is it that most of us can talk openly about the illnesses of our bodies, but when it comes to our brain and illnesses of the mind we clam up and because we clam up, people with emotional disorders feel ashamed, stigmatized and don't seek the help that can make the difference. Now let's start now, talk openly about mental illness, help us change those attitudes.

This commercial, and others like it made by other celebrities, are simple and effective. They urge people not to let stigma keep them from getting the help they need.

The National Alliance for the Mentally Ill has launched a "media watch" campaign whose aim is to reduce stigma. When television commercials, talk show hosts, or movies make jokes about mental illness or portray mental illness incorrectly, broadcasters and filmmakers hear about it from NAMI members. Usually one rational and polite letter does much to educate and alert media personnel to the disservice they are performing, but sometimes the one letter fails to enlighten. For example, a giftware company in Southern California was manufacturing a coffee mug that said: "Kiss me twice—I'm schizophrenic!" Chuck Harman, public relations director of NAMI, wrote to the company that

> schizophrenia and other brain diseases are not laughing matters to the thousands of families who have joined our organization to receive support and to advocate for their mentally ill relatives. Would your company print similar words about other diseases, such as cancer or diabetes? I think not.
>
> I request that you immediately suspend production of the mug and remove those already distributed. The turmoil that patients and relatives of the mentally ill experience is bad enough. Stigma compounds the problem.

The giftware company, after conferring with its lawyers, responded that they were protected by the First Amendment and said: "Our plans are to continue the 'Kiss me twice—I'm schizophrenic' mug throughout the next season." They added that the "good taste of our products has never been questioned in the past."

Mr. Harman wrote back and acknowledged that they had every right to use the First Amendment argument, but so did members of his organization. One of the members of an AMI, a father with two ill sons, called the president of the company and told him what it was like to live with mental illness and the harm that products like this cause. After that phone conversation, the company decided to suspend manufacturing of the mug.

Business leaders can be crucial in educating people and working to lessen stigma. For example, the executives at Allegheny Ludlum circulated the following letter to their employees and helped establish an atmosphere in which people could talk about problems and seek help.

Dear Employees, Retirees, and Friends:

You have all heard people say they feel "depressed," and you may even have that "blue feeling" from time to time. But experts say when the sad feelings linger on for weeks at a time, clinical depression may develop.

Current knowledge says depression costs our nation over $36 billion each year. About 1 in 20 Americans now suffer from a depressive disorder. It is estimated that over the course of a lifetime fully one-fifth of the population will suffer a major depressive episode.

Because of these findings and our concern with your health, Allegheny Ludlum is participating in the Depression/Awareness, Recognition, and Treatment (D/ART) Public Education Campaign to inform you about clinical depression and its treatment.

Take the time to read the enclosed brochure, *Depression: Define it. Defeat it.* We can defeat the myths about depression by learning more about it, and we can obtain effective assistance for those suffering from clinical depression by recognizing the symptoms of depression, offering our support, and suggesting ways to get help.

If you have additional questions or feel you need help after reading the brochure, *call the toll-free Depression Line number listed inside.* By becoming better educated and working together, we can defeat depression.

Sincerely,
Harry P. Hanley
Director, Employee Benefits

In the 1990 gubernatorial race in Florida, former Senator Lawton Chiles ran against the incumbent Governor Bob Martinez. During the primaries, the press revealed that Senator Chiles had been treated for depression the previous year. Senator Chiles spoke forthrightly about his battle with depression and his use of Prozac to overcome the illness. His opponents suggested quietly that perhaps Senator Chiles lacked the energy to govern the country's fourth most populous state.

Senator Chiles continued to campaign and ran a race viewed by many as an experiment in American politics. Announcing that he wanted to shut out the influence of big money and special interest groups, Senator Chiles limited campaign contributions, spent his time away from evening news "photo opportunities," and concentrated on walking the state, talking to people, and finding out which programs worked.

Apparently his constituency liked his ideas and his former work and did not hold his depression against him. Chiles won the election and referred to the campaign as "one of the most glorious times" of his life. He proved brilliantly that there is indeed life and work and joy after depression.

Certainly the winds of change are stirring. The National Institute of Mental Health continues its major educational campaign to publicize the mental health professions' increasing ability to treat depression of all kinds. Coming after two decades of productive research on the biology, epidemiology, and treatment of affective disorders, D/ART—for Depression/ Awareness, Recognition, and Treatment—came into existence when the NIMH realized that too many people who suffer from depression do so needlessly. As many as 80 to 90 percent of persons with depression can be treated successfully; however, current evidence suggests that depression is poorly recognized, undertreated, and inappropriately treated by the health care system.

D/ART aims to improve the identification, assessment,

treatment, and clinical management of depressive disorders through a national educational campaign focused on three major target audiences: the general public, primary care providers, and mental health specialists. The program reaches the public through the media and through the initiatives of private businesses, as seen in the preceding letter; special materials have been developed for physicians and mental health specialists. It is an ambitious and exciting project in that it seeks to link the scientific leadership and expertise of the NIMH with the resources and knowledge of health education groups, professional organizations, private foundations, unions, insurance companies, and the media for the common purpose of improving the early identification and treatment of depression.

Another organization was formed recently, is rapidly growing, and is making a difference. The National Mental Health Consumers' Self-Help Clearing House is concerning itself with legislative, judicial, and social issues affecting present and former mental patients. It is a broad-based self-help and advocacy organization that intends to improve the quality of life of people with psychiatric illness and empower them to speak for themselves. The NMHCA operates a national clearinghouse that provides information and referral services to individuals and groups around the country.*

Ten years ago, a press conference and congressional reception on Capitol Hill announced the establishment of the National Depressive and Manic Depressive Association (NDMDA). This was an important milestone in the history of mental health advocacy. For the first time, a group of patients had banded together to form a national organization. Their message? "We suffer from a treatable medical illness, not a character flaw." The national organization's mission has been to:

---

*To contact the NMHCA, write or call: 1211 Chestnut Street, Suite 1000, Philadelphia, PA 19107 (215) 751-1810 or (800) 553-4539.

- improve the way society perceives this disorder and treats those suffering from it, especially in terms of medical insurance coverage and employer attitudes
- stimulate further research on affective disorders
- promote public and professional education about depression
- provide support for people with depressive illness and their families

Local affiliates can continue to do much to improve the situation and services allocated in their part of the world to people with manic-depression and depression. Some ideas might include:

- Surveying clinics and hospitals to find out if an integrated up-to-date treatment approach is being utilized (compile a list of such places for members).
- Compiling lists of doctors in the area who use a modern, integrated treatment approach and passing the names on to people who need them.
- Organizing a speakers' bureau and booking dates with local organizations and clubs. Educating the community.
- Inviting the press to meetings, writing articles about depression and manic-depression, and arranging interviews with researchers and psychiatrists about new findings or studies.
- Developing antistigma campaigns and Public Service Announcements for radio and television.
- Pinpointing which state legislators might be sympathetic to the issues and arranging meetings with them. Inspire them to raise the issues in Congress and vote for better legislation, for research, insurance issues, and commitment laws.

That evening in May at the congressional reception, Senator Paul Simon of Illinois opened his remarks by reminding the guests that he was from the same state as the most famous man who suffered from depression, Abraham Lincoln. He spoke of the fact that Lincoln had been so tormented by the illness that from the ages of 32 to 34 he had contemplated suicide. "What a loss that would have been for the nation," said Senator Simon. There was a long pause, and then he asked quietly: "Would there have even *been* a nation?"

It's time now. We have the treatments, we have the talented researchers, we have a democratic nation that depends upon its constituency and listens to its concerns. The only thing that can stop the groundswell for change is indifference. Everyone—patients and family members—can play a part. First by seeking the proper treatment and by learning about the illness, then by giving support to others and joining together to foster research, fight stigma, and promote public education.

This generation can do what none before had the knowledge or treatments to do. The suffering, neglect, and stigma surrounding these disorders can be ended. The cycle *can* be broken.

APPENDIXES

APPENDIX 1

CYCLE CHART

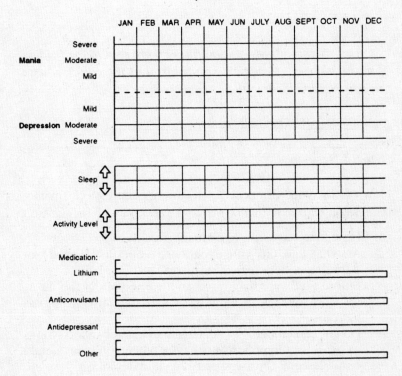

Cycle Chart

APPENDIX 2

THE AFFECTIVE DISORDERS QUESTIONNAIRE

Copies of this questionnaire were sent to the leaders of manic-depressive support groups around the country, who then distributed them to their membership.

Age _____ Marital Status _____
Sex _____ Ages of Children _____
State of Residence _____

How were you diagnosed? (recurrent depression, manic-depression with hypomania, manic-depression with mania, etc.)

1. How long have you had an affective disorder?
2. At what age did you experience your first episode of depression, hypomania, or mania?
3. Before you were diagnosed and learned about the disorder, how did you attempt to explain the early symptoms to yourself?
4. Do you remember experiencing unexplained mood swings or periods of hyperactive behavior when you were a child or adolescent? (Please specify age and describe.)
5. How often in a one-year period do you experience a depressive or manic episode?
6. What is the usual duration of each episode?
7. Does anyone else in your family have an affective disorder? What relationship are they to you?

8. With whom did you first consult—family practitioner, social worker, psychologist, or psychiatrist?

9. Who made the diagnosis of an affective disorder?

10. Were you ever misdiagnosed? What diagnosis were you given?

11. How did you find the health professional who made the correct diagnosis?

12. What kind of treatment was prescribed—medications, individual therapy (supportive or insight-oriented), family therapy, a combination of medications and a form of therapy?

13. What medications do you take, and what are the daily dosages?

14. Was your response to the medications partial or complete?

15. What side effects did you or do you experience? (List medication first, then corresponding side effects.)

16. Did you ever go off the medications? Why?

17. What is your opinion about the medication you are taking?

18. Did your doctor explicitly describe the nature of the illness, the medications and their side effects?

19. What, in your opinion, constitutes a good doctor? What would you advise someone else to look for?

20. What has your experience been with individual psychotherapy, family therapy, and group therapy?

21. What were the approximate monthly costs of treatment? Medications $ _____ Therapy $ _____

22. How did you pay for it?

23. How did you tell family and friends about the disorder?

24. Did it change their perception of you and your behavior, even during periods of well-being?

25. Did people ever urge you to try vitamins or nutritional therapy? Did they ever chide you for using medications? How did you respond?

26. Did you ever tell your employer about the disorder and how it affects you? How did you phrase the explanation?

27. What was the response?

28. How has the disorder affected your employment? In what field are you employed?

29. How has your social life been affected?

30. After the diagnosis and prescription of medication, did you ever consider pregnancy?

31. Understanding that medications are potentially harmful to a fetus, how did you and your doctor handle the management of medications during the period of conception and gestation?

32. During pregnancy, if no medications were used, did you experience mood swings?

33. What about the postpartum period?

34. Were you ever hospitalized?

35. In what kind of hospital? (private, city, state, VA hospital, community mental health center?) For how long?

36. What was the most helpful aspect of the hospitalization?

37. Was there any attempt to involve family members and educate them as to the nature of the disorder?

38. If not, would this have been helpful?

39. What kind of follow-up program was recommended after discharge?

40. Do you receive Supplemental Security Income (SSI)? Who helped initiate the application?

41. Can you give a descriptive account of how your thinking, mood, and behavior change during the period of time in which you are depressed?

42. Can you give a descriptive account of how your thinking, mood, and behavior change during the period of time in which you are hypomanic or manic?

43. What are the most enduring and problematic aspects of having this disorder?

44. Do you feel more creative without medications?

45. What books have you read about the disorder? What did you think of them? What journals or magazines do you read to keep current on the subject?

46. Do you find a support group helpful? Why/why not?

47. What do you think can be done about the stigma that people with psychiatric disorders face? Have you made any efforts in addressing the problem?

48. Is there anything you would like to say to us, or any issue you hope will be covered in this book?

49. About manic-depression and depression: What do you know now that you wish you had known when the illness first manifested itself?

If you have a written account of your personal experience with manic-depression or depression, we hope you'll send it to us for possible inclusion in the book.

If we found a phrase or description on this questionnaire that we thought would help explain the disorder to others or help make a particular point, would it be acceptable to you if we quoted it from an anonymous source? _____ Yes. _____ No.

APPENDIX 3

ORGANIZING AND PUBLICIZING A MANIC-DEPRESSIVE SUPPORT GROUP

Should you decide that a manic-depressive support group would be helpful to you and the people in your community, contact the National Depressive and Manic Depressive Association, 730 N. Franklin St., Suite 501, Chicago, IL 60610, (312) 642-0049, for start-up materials and suggestions.

We also recommend that you get a copy of a booklet published by the National Alliance for the Mentally Ill, *First Steps in Starting a Local NAMI Support and Advocacy Group*. It offers advice on how to contact other families, it gives a fledgling group directions for becoming incorporated and obtaining tax-exempt status, and it also includes sample by-laws, a sample newsletter, and some ideas on how to structure a meeting (including some topic suggestions).

Once the preliminary organizational logistics are worked out, you will need to inform the general public about the group. There are several ways to go about this: you can design a flyer and distribute it through mental health clinics, psychiatrists, psychologists, and social workers; and you can write a press release and mail it to local newspaper editors and radio and television broadcasters. These editors and broadcasters may then list the date of the meeting in the daily community events column, write an article about the new organization or announce your upcoming meeting over the air.

WRITING A PRESS RELEASE

An entire communications network that needs ideas and information exists in each community in this country. The editors—the people who receive the notices—*will* view you as a reporter in the field, but there are contact formats and skills that one must understand in order to gain coverage. If you send a correctly constructed, properly worded press release, you increase the chances of obtaining publicity for your organization and spreading the message to the public.

The press release is the announcement of your new organization, its intentions, and information concerning its first meeting. It should basically follow the format shown on page 371, but there is plenty of room for variation in the body of copy. Tell the editor what is happening—when, where, and why. Then follow this information with some background or facts.

The person who is listed as the contact in the upper right-hand corner should be accessible, available, and able to speak articulately about the group and the disorders if an editor should call for more information or for an interview.

If your new group has letterhead stationery, the release should be typed double-spaced on it; if not, a plain bond paper will do as well. It can be duplicated by photocopying or offset printing. The release is usually mailed six weeks before the scheduled meeting, but it's always a good idea to check the deadline requirements for each publication.

To compile a list of the editors and announcers you should contact with the release, call the switchboards of the newspapers and radio and television stations (check your local Yellow Pages under "Newspapers," "Radio" and "Television—Cable"). Explain that you wish to publicize the starting-up of a manic-depressive support group and that you need to know who handles articles on health-related topics and who handles calendar listings for community events. Send each of these people a copy of your press release. But don't let it rest there. Follow up with a telephone call to see if that person received the release and to find out if he or she needs any further information. You can be warmer and more immediate on the telephone, you can tune the editor in, and you might just stir up enough interest to persuade the editor to do an article about your group. This would be a great coup as many people in the community who might really benefit from your efforts can read about the group in the paper, call you and get involved. Interested physicians and mental health professionals will also know how to get in touch with you and might offer their services to help launch the group.

Contact: Jackie Hauger
(202) 555-4321
FOR IMMEDIATE RELEASE
March 25, 1997

MANIC-DEPRESSIVE SUPPORT GROUP TO HOLD
FIRST MEETING—MAY 7, 1997

A newly formed manic-depressive support group will hold its first meeting in the auditorium at St. Luke's Hospital, 230 Maple Avenue, at 8:00 P.M. on Tuesday, the 7th of May, 1997. The public is welcome and encouraged to attend.

Manic-depressive illness (bipolar disorder) or recurrent depression currently affects more than 20 million Americans. Although the disorders have afflicted humankind since its beginnings, today there are new treatments and medications that can do much to attenuate the mood swings and help a person salvage career and relationship networks.

The manic-depressive support group intends to provide information, referrals, emergency aid, and support to patients, their families, and friends. Monthly lectures will feature psychiatrists, researchers, and health professionals who will provide the most current information about the disorders. In addition, there will be smaller "rap" sessions in which patients and families can tell their own stories, trade information, and give and gain support. Eventually, the group will join with the National Depressive and Manic Depressive Association in order to promote research and antistigma campaigns in this country.

For further information about the group and the meeting, please call (202) 555-4321.

APPENDIX 4

SUPPORT ORGANIZATIONS

Manic-depressive support groups are starting up all over the country. The National Depressive and Manic-Depressive Association presently lists 275 affiliates across the United States with an average of five added each month. To find out if a group exists in your area (or to get help in establishing a support group in your locale), contact the national headquarters:

National Depressive and Manic-Depressive Association
730 N. Franklin Street, Suite 501
Chicago, IL 60610
(312) 642-0049/FAX 312-642-7243
(800) 82-NDMDA

The National Alliance for the Mentally Ill, or NAMI as it is known, currently has over 1,000 affiliates around the country and continues to grow rapidly. To find the organization nearest you, contact the national headquarters:

National Alliance for the Mentally Ill
200 N. Glebe Rd., Suite 1015
Arlington, VA 22203-3754
(703) 524-7600/FAX 703-524-9094
(800) 950-NAMI (6264)

BIBLIOGRAPHY

CHAPTER 1

Bosworth, Patricia. *Diane Arbus: A Biography.* New York: Alfred A. Knopf, 1984.

Bowers, Malcolm B. *Retreat from Sanity.* New York: Human Sciences Press, 1974.

Cavett, Dick. Interview on "The Larry King Show," radio station WOR. November 19, 1985.

Cherry, Laurence. "The Good News About Depression." *New York Magazine,* June 2, 1986.

Clayton, Paula J. "The Epidemiology of Bipolar Affective Disorder." *Comprehensive Psychiatry* 22 (January/February 1981):31–43.

DSM-III: Diagnostic and Statistical Manual of Mental Disorders, 3rd ed. Washington, DC: American Psychiatric Association, 1980.

Gallagher, Winifred. "The Dark Affliction of Mind and Body." *Discover,* May 1986.

Goldstein, Michael J., Bruce L. Baker and Kay R. Jamison. *Abnormal Psychology.* Boston: Little, Brown and Company, 1980.

Hamilton, Ian. *Robert Lowell: A Biography.* New York: Vintage Books, 1982.

Havens, Leston. *Making Contact.* Cambridge: Harvard University Press, 1986.

Kaplan, Bert. *The Inner World of Mental Illness: A Series of First Person Accounts of What It Was Like.* New York: Harper & Row, 1964.

Knauth, Percy. *A Season in Hell.* New York: Harper & Row, 1975.

Lickey, Marvin E., and Barbara Gordon. *Drugs for Mental Illness.* New York: W. H. Freeman and Company, 1983.

McGhie, Andrew, and James Chapman. "Disorders of Attention and Perception in Early Schizophrenia." *British Journal of Medical Psychology* 34 (1961): 103–16.

Millet, Kate. *The Looney Bin Trip.* New York: Simon & Schuster, 1990.

Rovner, Sandy. "Down but Not Out." *Washington Post,* February 12, 1986.

Styron, William. *Darkness Visible.* New York: Random House, 1990.

TUCKER, JONATHAN B. "The Scary Ups and Downs of Manic-Depression." *Cosmopolitan,* April 1985.

U.S. DEPARTMENT OF HEALTH AND HUMAN SERVICES. *Mood Disorders: Pharmacologic Prevention of Recurrences* (Consensus Development Conference Consensus Statement). Volume 5, April 1984.

VONNEGUT, MARK. *The Eden Express.* New York: Holt, Rinehart, & Winston, 1975.

WALSH, MARYELLEN. *Schizophrenia: Straight Talk for Family and Friends.* New York: William Morrow, 1985.

WHYBROW, PETER C., HAGOP S. AKISKAL and WILLIAM T. MCKINNEY, JR. *Mood Disorders: Toward a New Psychobiology.* New York: Plenum Press, 1984.

YANCEY, BERT. Lecture for the New York Manic-Depressive Support Group. July 5, 1990.

CHAPTER 2

AKISKAL, HAGOP S. "The Bipolar Spectrum: New Concepts in Classification and Diagnosis." In *Psychiatric Update: The APA Annual Review,* Volume 2, 271-92, ed. Lester Grinspoon. Washington, DC: APA Press, 1983.

AKISKAL, HAGOP S., ARMEN H. DJENDEREDJIAN and RENATE H. ROSENTHAL. "Cyclothymia Disorder: Validating Criteria for Inclusion in the Bipolar Affective Group." *American Journal of Psychiatry* 134 (1977):1227-33.

ANDREASEN, NANCY. "Affective Flattening and the Criteria for Schizophrenia." *American Journal of Psychiatry* 136 (July 1979):944-47.

ANDREASEN, NANCY. *The Broken Brain.* New York: Harper & Row, 1984.

BLEULER, EUGEN. *Dementia Praecox or the Group of Schizophrenias.* New York: International Universities Press, 1950.

BROCKINGTON, I. F., and J. P. LEFF. "Schizoaffective Psychosis: Definitions and Incidence." *Psychological Medicine* 9 (1979):91-99.

CARLSON, GABRIELLE A., and FREDERICK K. GOODWIN. "The Stages of Mania." *Archives of General Psychiatry* 28 (February 1973):221-28.

COHEN, STEPHEN M. et al. "Relationship of Schizoaffective Psychosis to Manic-Depressive Psychosis and Schizophrenia." *Archives of General Psychiatry* 26 (June 1972):539-46.

DISALVER, STEVEN C., and KERRIN WHITE. "Affective Disorders and Associated Psychopathology: A Family History Study." *Journal of Clinical Psychiatry* 47 (April 1986):162-69.

DSM-III: Diagnostic and Statistical Manual of Mental Disorders, 3rd ed. Washington, DC: American Psychiatric Association, 1980.

DSM-IV: Diagnostic and Statistical Manual of Mental Disorders, 4th ed. Washington, DC: American Psychiatric Association, 1994.

DUNNER, DAVID L., and RONALD R. FIEVE. "Clinical Factors in Lithium Carbonate Prophylaxis." *Archives of General Psychiatry* 30 (1974):229-33.

DUNNER, DAVID L., and NORMAN E. ROSENTHAL. "Schizoaffective States." In *The Psychiatric Clinics of North America,* Volume 2. Philadelphia: W. B. Saunders Company, 1979.

ENDICOTT, JEAN, and ROBERT L. SPITZER. "Use of the Research Diagnostic Criteria and the Schedule for Affective Disorders and Schizophrenia to Study Affective Disorders." *American Journal of Psychiatry* 136 (January 1979):52-56.

FEIGHNER, JOHN P., ELI ROBINS, SAMUEL GUZE et al. "Diagnostic Criteria for Use in Psychiatric Research." *Archives of General Psychiatry* 26 (January 1972): 57-63.

HARROW, MARTIN, LINDA S. GROSSMAN et al. "Thought Pathology in Manic and Schizophrenic Patients." *Archives of General Psychiatry* 39 (June 1982): 665-71.

HATSUKAMI, DOROTHY K., JAMES E. MITCHELL and ELKE D. ECKERT. "Eating Disorders: A Variant of Mood Disorders?" In *The Psychiatric Clinics of North America,* Volume 7. Philadelphia: W. B. Saunders Company, 1984.

HIMMELHOCH, JONATHAN. "Mixed States, Manic-Depressive Illness, and the Nature of Mood." In *The Psychiatric Clinics of North America.* Volume 2. Philadelphia: W. B. Saunders Company, 1979.

JAMPALA, V. CHOWDARY. "Anorexia Nervosa: A Variant Form of Affective Disorder?" *Psychiatric Annals* 15 (December 1985):698-704.

JOYCE, PETER R. "Age of Onset in Bipolar Affective Disorder and Misdiagnosis as Schizophrenia." *Psychological Medicine* 14 (1984):145-49.

KENDELL, R. E. "Reflections on Psychiatric Classification—for the Architects of DSM-IV and ICD-10." *Integrative Psychiatry* 2 (March-April 1984):43-47.

KENDELL, R. E., J. E. COOPER et al. "Diagnostic Criteria of American and British Psychiatrists." *Archives of General Psychiatry* 25 (August 1971):123-30.

KLERMAN, GERALD L., GEORGE E. VAILLANT et al. "A Debate on DSM-III." *American Journal of Psychiatry* 141 (April 1984):539-53.

LICKEY, MARVIN E., and BARBARA GORDON. *Drugs for Mental Illness.* New York: W. H. Freeman and Company, 1983.

LORANGER, ARMAND, and PETER M. LEVINE. "Age of Onset of Bipolar Affective Illness." *Archives of General Psychiatry* 35 (November 1978):1345-48.

MAJ, MARIO. "Evolution of the American Concept of Schizoaffective Psychosis." *Neuropsychobiology* 11 (1984):7-13.

MELLOR, C. S. "First Rank Symptoms of Schizophrenia." *British Journal of Psychiatry* 117 (1970):15-23.

POPE, HARRISON G. "Distinguishing Bipolar Disorder from Schizophrenia in Clinical Practice: Guidelines and Case Reports." *Hospital and Community Psychiatry* 34 (April 1983):322-28.

POPE, HARRISON G., and JOSEPH F. LIPINSKI, JR. "Diagnosis in Schizophrenia and Manic-Depressive Illness: A Reassessment of the Specificity of 'Schizophrenic' Symptoms in Light of Current Research." *Archives of General Psychiatry* 35 (1978):811-22.

POPE, HARRISON G., JOSEPH F. LIPINSKI, JR. et al. "Schizoaffective Disorder: An Invalid Diagnosis? A Comparison of Schizoaffective Disorder, Schizophrenia, and Affective Disorder." *American Journal of Psychiatry* 137 (August 1980):921-27.

PRIEN, ROBERT F., JONATHAN M. HIMMELHOCH and DAVID J. KUPFER. "Treatment of Mixed Mania." *Journal of Affective Disorders.* 15 (1988):9-15.

PROCCI, W. R. "Schizoaffective Psychosis: Fact or Fiction?" *Archives of General Psychiatry* 33 (October 1976):1167-77.

ROTH, M. "Classification of Affective Disorders." *Pharmakopsychiat* 11 (1978):27-42.

ROY-BURNE, PETER P., RUSSELL T. JOFFEE, THOMAS W. UHDE and ROBERT M. POST. "Approaches to the Evaluation and Treatment of Rapid Cycling Affective Illness." *British Journal of Psychiatry* 145 (1984):543-50.

SCHNECK, JEROME M. *A History of Psychiatry.* Springfield, IL: Charles C. Thomas, 1960.

SPITZER, ROBERT L., and JANET B. W. WILLIAMS. "Classification in Psychiatry." In *Comprehensive Textbook of Psychiatry,* 4th ed., ed. Harold I. Kaplan and Benjamin J. Saddock, 591-613. Baltimore: Williams & Wilkins, 1985.

SPITZER, ROBERT L., JEAN ENDICOTT and ELI ROBINS. "Research Diagnostic Criteria." *Archives of General Psychiatry* 35 (June 1978):773-78.

SPITZER, ROBERT L., JANET B. W. WILLIAMS and ANDREW E. SKODEL. "DSM-III: The Major Achievements and an Overview." *American Journal of Psychiatry* 137 (February 1980):151-64.

TAYLOR, MICHAEL A., and RICHARD ABRAMS. "Manic-Depressive Illness and Good Prognosis Schizophrenia." *American Journal of Psychiatry* 132 (July 1975):741-42.

TAYLOR, MICHAEL A., and RICHARD ABRAMS. "The Phenomenology of Mania." *Archives of General Psychiatry* 29 (October 1973):520-22.

TORREY, E. FULLER. *Surviving Schizophrenia.* New York: Harper & Row, 1983.

WHYBROW, PETER C., HAGOP S. AKISKAL and WILLIAM T. MCKINNEY, JR. *Mood Disorders: Toward a New Psychobiology.* New York: Plenum Press, 1984.

CHAPTER 3

BARON, MIRON, NEIL RISCH, RAHEL HAMBURGER et al. "Genetic Linkage Between X-Chromosome Markers and Bipolar Affective Illness." *Nature* 326 (March 1987):289-92.

BARON, MIRON. Telephone conversation with Demitri Papolos, February 1, 1991.

BERRETTINI, WADE H., LYNN R. GOLDEN et al. "X-Chromosome Markers and Manic-Depressive Illness." *Archives of General Psychiatry* 47 (April 1990):366-73.

BLACKWOOD, DOUGLAS H. R., LIN HE, STEWART W. MORRIS et al. "A Locus for Bipolar Affective Disorder on Chromosome 4p." *Nature Genetics* 12 (April 1996).

BYERLEY, WILLIAM, and CHARLES MELLON. "Mapping Genes for Manic-Depression and Schizophrenia with DNA Markers." *Trends in Neuroscience* 12 (1989):46-48.

DEL ZAMPO, M. A. BOCCHETTA et al. "Linkage Between X-Chromosome Markers with Manic-Depressive Illness." *Acta Psychiatra Scandinavia* 70 (September 1984):282-87.

EGELAND, JANICE A. "Amish Study, III: The Impact of Cultural Factors on Diagnosis of Bipolar Illness." *American Journal of Psychiatry* 140 (January 1983):67-71.

EGELAND, JANICE A. "Amish Study, V: Lithium-Sodium Countertransport and Catechol O-Methyltransferase in Pedigrees of Bipolar Probands." *American Journal of Psychiatry* 141 (September 1984):1049-54.

EGELAND, JANICE A. "Bipolarity: The Iceberg of Affective Disorders?" *Comprehensive Psychiatry* 24 (July/August 1983):337-44.

EGELAND, JANICE A. "Genetic Studies of Affective Disorders among Amish." National Institute of Mental Health Grant Application, February 1986.

EGELAND, JANICE A., and ABRAM M. HOSTETTER. "Amish Study, I: Affective Disorders among the Amish, 1976-1980." *American Journal of Psychiatry* 140 (January 1983):56-61.

EGELAND, JANICE A., DANIELA S. GERHARD, DAVID L. PAULS et al. "Bipolar Affective Disorders Linked to DNA Markers on Chromosome 11," *Nature* 325 (February 26, 1987):783-87.

EGELAND, JANICE A. Lecture at the Albert Einstein International Conference on the Genetics of Affective Disorders. November 9, 1990.

EGELAND, JANICE A. Telephone conversation with Janice Papolos, January 27, 1991.

EGELAND, JANICE A., JAMES N. SUSSEX, JEAN ENDICOTT et al. "The Impact of Diagnoses on Genetic Linkage Study for Bipolar Affective Disorders Among the Amish." Presented in part by the senior author at the First Congress for Psychiatric Genetics, Cambridge, England, August 3, 1989.

EZZELL, CAROL. "New Genetic Linkages for Manic Depression." *The Journal of NIH Research* (May 1996).

FREIMER, NELSON B., VICTOR I. REUSS, MICAELA A. ESCAMILLA et al. "Genetic Mapping Using Haplotype, Association and Linkage Methods Suggests a Locus for Severe Bipolar Disorder (BPI) at 18Q22-q23." *Nature Genetics* 12 (April 1996).

GERSHON, ELLIOT S., and J. I. NURNBERGER, JR. "Inheritance of Major Psychiatric Disorders." Amsterdam: Elsevier, North-Holland Biomedical Press, 1982.

GERSHON, ELLIOT S., JOEL HAMOVIT, JULIET J. GUROFF et al. "A Family Study of Schizoaffective, Bipolar I, Bipolar II, Unipolar, and Normal Control Probards." *Archives of General Psychiatry* 39 (October 1982):1157-67.

GINNS, EDWARD I., JURG OTT, JANICE A. EGELAND et al. "A Genome-Wide Search for Chromosomal Loci Linked to Bipolar Affective Disorder in the Old Order Amish." *Nature Genetics* 12 (April 1996).

HODGKINSON, STEPHEN, ROBIN SHERRINGTON et al. "Molecular Genetic Evidence for Heterogeneity in Manic-Depression." *Nature* 325 (February 26, 1987): 305-6.

HOSTETTER, ABRAM M., JANICE A. EGELAND and JEAN ENDICOTT. "Amish Study, II: Consensus Diagnosis and Reliability Results." *American Journal of Psychiatry* 140 (January 1983):62-66.

KELSOE, JOHN R., EDWARD I. GINNS, JANICE A. EGELAND et al. "Reevaluation of the Linkage Relationship Between Chromosome 11p Loci and the Gene for Bipolar Affective Disorder." *Nature* 342 (November 16, 1989):238–43.

KELSOE, JOHN R., JANICE A. EGELAND, ABRAM M. HOSTETTER et al. "Studies Search for a Gene for Bipolar Affective Disorder in the Old Order Amish." *Psychiatric Times,* June 1990.

KIDD, KENNETH K., JANICE A. EGELAND et al. "Amish Study, IV: Genetic Linkage Study of Pedigrees of Bipolar Probands." *American Journal of Psychiatry* 141 (September 1984):1042–48.

KOLATA, GINA. "Manic-Depression: Is It Inherited?" *Science* 232 (May 2, 1986):575–76.

LACHMAN, HERBERT M., JOHN KELSOE et al. "Linkage Studies Support a Possible Locus for Bipolar Disorder in the Velo-Cardio-Facial Syndrome Region on Chromosome 22" (submitted for publication).

LACHMAN, HERBERT M., YUE-MIN YU et al. "A Codon 158 Mutation Leading to a Valine to Methionine Substitution Is a Common Polymorphism in the Catechol-O-Methyltransferase Gene." *Pharmocogenetics* (June 1996):243–50.

LACHMAN, HERBERT M., BERNICE MORROW et al. "Association of Codon 108/158 Catechol-O-Methyltransferase Gene Polymorphism with the Psychiatric Manifestations of Velo-Cardio-Facial Syndrome." *American Journal of Medical Genetics* 67 (1996):468–72.

MAUGH, THOMAS H. "Is There a Gene for Depression?" *Science* 214 (December 1981):1330–31.

MENDLEWICZ, JULIEN, and JOHN D. RAINER. "Adoption Study Supporting Genetic Transmission in Manic-Depressive Illness." *Nature* 268 (July 1977):327–29.

NADI, SUSAN N., JOHN I. NURNBERGER, JR. and ELLIOT S. GERSHON. "Muscarinic Cholinergic Receptors on Skin Fibroblasts in Familial Affective Disorder." *New England Journal of Medicine* 311 (July 1984):225–30.

NURNBERGER, JOHN I., and ELLIOT S. GERSHON. "Genetics of Affective Disorders." In *The Neurobiology of Mood Disorders.* Baltimore: Williams & Wilkins, 1984.

PAPOLOS, DEMITRI F., GIANNI L. FAEDDA et al. "Bipolar Spectrum Disorders in Patients Diagnosed with Velo-Cardio-Facial Syndrome: Does a Hemizygous Deletion of Chromosome 22q11 Result in Bipolar Affective Disorder?" *American Journal of Psychiatry* (December 1996).

ROBERTSON, MIRANDA. "False Start on Manic-Depression." *Nature* 342 (November 16, 1989) 222.

SCHAEFFER, PHYLLIS. "Molecular Genetics to Help Understand Psychiatric Illness." *Clinical Psychiatry News* (November 1985).

SCHLESSER, MICHAEL A., and KENNETH Z. ALTSHULER. "The Genetics of Affective Disorder: Data, Theory, and Clinical Applications." *Hospital and Community Psychiatry* 34 (May 1983):415–21.

SCHMECK, HAROLD, M. "Defective Gene Tied to Form of Manic-Depressive Illness," *The New York Times,* February 26, 1987.

SCHMECK, HAROLD M. "Scientists Now Doubt They Found Faulty Gene Linked to Mental Illness." *The New York Times,* November 7, 1989.

TSUANG, MING T. "Genetic Counseling for Psychiatric Patients and Their Families." *American Journal of Psychiatry* 135 (December 1978):1465–74.

TSUANG, MING T., and RANDALL VANDERMEY. *Genes and the Mind:The Inheritance of Mental Illness.* New York: Oxford University Press, 1980.

WALDHOLTZ, MICHAEL. "Probing the Cell: Help from a Handy 'Riflip.'" *Wall Street Journal,* February 3, 1986.

WALLIS, CLAUDIA. "Is Mental Illness Inherited?" *Time,* March 9, 1987.

WEISSMAN, MYRNA, et al. "Psychiatric Disorders in the Relatives of Probands with Affective Disorders." *Archives of General Psychiatry* 41 (January 1984):13–21.

WENDER, PAUL H., and DONALD F. KLEIN. *Mind, Mood, and Medicine.* New York: Farrar, Straus & Giroux, 1981.

CHAPTER 4

ALBERS, H. ELLIOT, RALPH LYDIC, PHILIPPA H. GANDER and MARTIN C. MOORE-EDE. "Role of the Suprachiasmatic Nuclei in the Circadian Timing System of the Squirrel Monkey. I. The Generation of Rhythmicity." *Brain Research* 300 (1984):275–84.

ATKINSON, MARTHA, DANIEL F. KRIPKE and SANFORD R. WOLF. "Autorhyth-mometry in Manic-Depressives." *Chronobiologia* 2 (1975):325–35.

BALDESSARINI, ROSS J. "An Overview of the Basis for the Amine Hypothesis in Affective Illness." *Archives of General Psychiatry* 32 (1975):1087–93.

BALDESSARINI, ROSS J. *Chemotherapy in Psychiatry,* rev. ed. Cambridge: Harvard University Press, 1985.

BANERJEE, SHAILESH P., LILY S. KUNG, STEPHEN J. RIGGI and SUBIR K. CHANDA. "Development of Beta-Adrenergic Receptor Subsensitivity by Antidepressants." *Nature* 268 (1977):455–56.

CHARNEY, DENNIS S., and DAVID B. MENKER. "Receptor Sensitivity and the Mechanism of Action of Antidepressant Treatment: Implications for the Etiology and Therapy of Depression." *Archives of General Psychiatry* 38 (1981): 1160–75.

COPPEN, ALEC. "Defects in Monoamine Metabolism and Their Possible Importance in the Pathogenesis of Depressive Syndromes." *Psychiatricet et Neurologic Scandinavia* 34 (1959):105–7.

CZEISLER, CHARLES A., JAMES S. ALLAN, STEVEN H. STROGATZ et al. "Bright Light Resets the Human Circadian Pacemaker Independent of the Timing of the Sleep-Wake Cycle." *Science* 233 (August 8, 1986):667–71.

DIVISH, MARGARET M., GUILIA SHEFTEL, VASUNDHARA D. KALASAPUDI, DEMITRI F. PAPOLOS and HERB M. LACHMAN. "Differential Effect of Lithium on fos Protooncogene Expression Mediated by Receptor and Postreceptor Activators of Protein Kinase C and Cyclic Adenosine Monophosphate: Model for Its Antimanic Action." *Journal of Neuroscience Research.* 28 (1991):40–48.

FARAVELLI, CARLO, GIAMPAOLO LA MALFA and SALVATORE ROMANO. "Circadian Rhythm in Primary Affective Disorder." *Comprehensive Psychiatry* 26 (July/August 1985):364–69.

FULLERTON, DONALD T., FREDERICK J. WENZEL, FRANCIS N. LORENZ and HAROLD FAHS. "Circadian Rhythm of Adrenal Cortical Activity in Depression." *Archives of General Psychiatry* 19 (December 1968):675–88.

GOODWIN, FREDERICK K. and KAY REDFIELD JAMISON. *Manic-Depressive Illness.* New York: Oxford University Press, 1990.

HAUGER, RICHARD L., and STEVEN M. PAUL. "Neurotransmitter Receptor Plasticity: Alterations by Antidepressants and Antipsychotics." *Psychiatric Annals* 13 (May 1983):399–407.

HAURI, PETER, DORIS CHERNIK and DAVID HAWKINS. "Sleep of Depressed Patients in Remission." *Archives of General Psychiatry* 1 (1974):386–91.

HOFFMAN, KLAUS. "The Role of the Pineal Gland in the Photoperiodic Control of Seasonal Cycles in Hamsters." In *Biological Clocks in Seasonal Reproductive Cycles,* ed. B. K. and D. E. Follet. Bristol: J. Wright, 1981.

ISAACSON, ROBERT L. *The Limbic System,* 2nd ed. New York: Plenum Press, 1982.

JACOBSON, LAUREN and ROBERT SAPOLSKY. "The Role of the Hippocampus in Feedback Regulation of the Hypothalamic–Pituitary–Adrenocortical Axis." *Endocrine Reviews* 12 (1991):118–34.

JANOWSKY, AARON, FUMIHKO OKADA, HAL D. MANIER et al. "Role of Serotinergic Input in the Regulation of the Beta-Adrenergic Receptor-coupled Adenylate Cyclase System." *Science* 218 (November 1982):900–1.

JOYCE, PETER R. "Neuroendocrine Changes in Depression." *Australian and New Zealand Journal of Psychiatry* 19 (1985):120–27.

KALASAPUDI, VASUNDHARA D., GIULIA SHEFTEL, MARGARET M. DIVISH, DEMITRI F. PAPOLOS and HERBERT M. LACHMAN. "Lithium Augments fos Protooncogene Expression in PC12 Pheochromocytoma Cells: Implications for Therapeutic Action of Lithium." *Brain Research* 521 (1990):47–54.

KANDEL, ERIC R., and JAMES H. SCHWARTZ. *Principles of Neural Science.* New York: Elsevier/North-Holland, 1981.

KAUFMAN, I. CHARLES, and LEONARD A. ROSENBLUM. "Depression in Infant Monkeys Separated from Their Mothers." *Science* 155 (1967):1030–31.

KETY, SEYMOUR S. "A Biologist Examines the Mind and Behavior." *Science* 132 (December 23, 1960):1861–70.

KRIEGER, DOROTHY T., and JOAN C. HUGHS, eds. *Neuroendocrinology.* Sunderland, MA: Sinauer Associates, Inc., 1980.

KRIPKE, DANIEL F., DANIEL J. MULLANEY, MARTHA ATKINSON and SANFORD WOLF. "Circadian Rhythm Disorders in Manic-Depressives." *Biological Psychiatry* 13 (1978):335–51.

KUPPER, DAVID J., and ELLEN FRANK. *Depression.* A "Current Concepts" publication, The Upjohn Company, 1981.

LACHMAN, HERBERT M., and DEMITRI F. PAPOLOS. "Abnormal Signal Transduction: A Hypothetical Model for Bipolar Affective Disorder." *Life Sciences* 45 (1989):1412–26.

LICKEY, MARVIN E., and BARBARA GORDON. *Drugs for Mental Illness.* New York: W. H. Freeman and Company, 1983.

LINGJAERDE, O. "The Biochemistry of Depression: A Survey of Monoaminergic Neuroendocrinological and Biorhythmic Disturbances in Endogenous

Depression." *Acta Psychiat Scanda, Supplement* 302 (1983):36–51.

LLINAS, RODOLFO, R., ed. *The Biology of the Brain: From Neurons to Networks.* New York: W. H. Freeman and Company, 1988.

MACCARI, STEFANIA, MICHAEL LE MOAL, LUCIANO ANGELUCCI and PIERRE MORMEDE. "Influence of 6-OHDA Lesion of Central Noradrenergic Systems on Corticosteroid Receptors and Neuroendocrine Response to Stress." *Brain Research* (1991):60–65.

MACCARI, STEFANIA, PIER VINCENZO PIAZZA, JEAN MARIE DEMINIERE et al. "Hippocampal Type I and Type II Corticosteroid Receptor Affinities Are Reduced in Rats Predisposed to Develop Amphetimine Self-Administration." *Brain Research* (1991) 305–9.

MENDLEWICZ, J., G. HOFFMAN, P. LINKOWSKI et al. "Chronobiology and Manic-Depression: Neuroendocrine and Sleep EEG Parameters." *Advanced Biological Psychiatry* 11 (1983):129–35.

MOORE-EDE, MARTIN C. "Physiology of the Circadian Timing System: Predictive Versus Reactive Homeostasis." *American Journal of Physiology* 250 (1986):735–52.

MOORE-EDE, MARTIN C., FRANK SULZMAN and CHARLES A. FULLER. *The Clocks That Time Us.* New York: Oxford University Press, 1982.

NAKAJIMA, TAKASHI, ROBERT M. POST, AGU PERT et al. "Perspectives on the Mechanism of Action of Electroconvulsive Therapy: Anticonvulsant, Peptidergic, and c-fos Protooncogene Effects." *Convulsive Therapy* 5 (1989):274–95.

PAPOLOS, DEMITRI F. "Serotonin, Seasonality, and Mood Disorders." in *The Role of Serotonin in Psychiatric Disorders.* Serena-Lynn Brown and Herman van Praag, eds. New York: Brunner/Mazel Publishers, 1991.

PAYKEL, E. S., ed. *Handbook of Affective Disorders.* New York: The Guilford Press, 1982.

PIHOKER, C. M. J. OWENS, et al. "Maternal Separation in Neonatal Rats Elicits Activation of the Hypothalamic–Pituitary–Adrenocortical Axis: A Putative Role for Corticotropin-Releasing Factor." *Psychoneuroendocrinology* 18 (7) (1993):485–93.

POST, ROBERT M., and JAMES C. BALLENGER, eds. *Neurobiology of Mood Disorders.* Baltimore: Williams & Wilkins, 1984.

SACHAR, EDWARD J., LEON HELLMAN, HOWARD P. ROFFWARG et al. "Disrupted 24-Hour Patterns of Cortisol Secretion in Psychotic Depression." *Archives of General Psychiatry* 28 (1973):19–26.

SAPOLSKY, ROBERT M. "Adrenocortical Function, Social Rank and Personality Among Wild Baboons." *Biological Psychiatry* (1990):937–52.

SAPOLSKY, ROBERT M. and PAUL M. PLOTSKY. "Hypercortisolism and Its Possible Neural Basis." *Biological Psychiatry* (1990):937–52.

SAPOLSKY, ROBERT M., LEWIS C. KREY and BRUCE S. MCEWEN. "Glucocorticoid-Sensitive Hippocampal Neurons Are Involved in Terminating the Adrenocortical Stress Response." *Proceedings of the National Academy of Science* 81 (October 1984):6174–77.

SCHILDKRAUT, JOSEPH. "Catecholamine Hypothesis of Affective Disorders." *American Journal of Psychiatry* 122 (1965):509–22.

SCHWARTZ, WILLIAM J., STEVEN M. REPPERT, SHARON M. EAGAN and MARTIN C. MOORE-EDE. "In Vivo Metabolic Activity of the Suprachiasmatic Nuclei: A Comparative Study." *Brain Research* 274 (1983):184-87.

SIEVER, LARRY, and FRIDOLIN SULSER. "Regulations of Amine Neurotransmitter Systems." *Psychopharmacology Bulletin* 20 (1984):500-4.

TEICHER, MARTIN A., JANET LAWRENCE, NATACHA BARBER et al. "Circadian Activity Rhythms in Geriatric Depression." Poster presented at the American Psychiatric Association Convention, 1986.

TRIMBLE, MICHAEL, R. and E. ZARIFIAN, eds. *Psychopharmacology of the Limbic System.* New York: Oxford University Press, 1985.

VAN PRAAG, HERMAN M. "Neurotransmitters and CNS Disease." *Lancet* 2 (December 1982):1259-63.

WEHR, THOMAS A., and FREDERICK K. GOODWIN. "Biological Rhythms and Psychiatry." In *American Handbook of Psychiatry,* Volume 7, 2nd ed. Boston: Basic Books, 1980.

WEHR, THOMAS A., and FREDERICK K. GOODWIN, eds. *Circadian Rhythms in Psychiatry.* Pacific Grove, CA: The Boxwood Press, 1983.

WEITZMAN, E. D. "Chronobiology of Man." *Human Neurobiology* 1 (1982): 173-83.

WEVER, RUTGER A. "Phase Shifts of Circadian Rhythms Due to Shifts of Artificial Zeitgebers." *Chronobiologia* 7 (1980):303-27.

WHITAKER-AZMITIA, PATRICIA M. and STEPHEN J. PEROUTKA, eds. *The Neuropharmacology of Serotonin.* New York: The New York Academy of Sciences, 1990.

WHYBROW, PETER C., HAGOP S. AKISKAL and WILLIAM T. McKINNEY, JR. *Mood Disorders: Toward a New Psychobiology.* New York: Plenum Press, 1984.

CHAPTER 5

AMERICAN PSYCHIATRIC ASSOCIATION. "Tardive Dyskinesia: Summary of a Task Force Report of the American Psychiatric Association." *American Journal of Psychiatry* 137 (October 1980):1163-72.

ANDREASEN, NANCY C. *The Broken Brain.* New York: Harper & Row, 1984.

AUSTIN, LINDA, GEORGE ARCANA and JAMES BALLENGER. "Rapid Response of Patients Simultaneously Treated with Lithium and Nortriptyline." *Journal of Clinical Psychiatry* 51 (1990):124-25.

BALDESSARINI, ROSS J. *Chemotherapy in Psychiatry,* rev. ed. Cambridge: Harvard University Press, 1985.

BALDESSARINI, ROSS J. "Fluoxetine and Side Effects." *Archives of General Psychiatry* 47 (1990):191-92.

BALDESSARINI, ROSS J. "Current Status of Antidepressants: Clinical Pharmacology Therapy." *Journal of Clinical Psychiatry* 50 (April 1989): 117-26.

BALDESSARINI, ROSS J., and M. TOHAN. "Is There a Long-Term Protective Effect of Mood-Altering Agents in Unipolar Depressive Disorder?" in *Psychopharmacology: Current Trends.* Berlin: Springer-Verlag, 1988.

BALLENGER, JAMES C., and ROBERT M. POST. "Carbamazepine in Manic-Depressive Illness: A New Treatment." *American Journal of Psychiatry* 137 (July 1980):782–90.

BLACKWELL, BARRY, "MAOI-Food Interactions (an interview)." *Currents in Affective Illness* VII (March 1988):5–12.

BRESSLER, RUBIN. "Treating Geriatric Depression." *Drug Therapy* (September 1984):35–50.

BUNNEY, WILLIAM E., and BLYNN L. GARLAND. "Lithium and Its Possible Modes of Action." In *The Neurobiology of Mood Disorders.* Baltimore: Williams & Wilkins, 1984.

BURTON, THOMAS M. "Anti-Depressant Drug of Eli Lilly Loses Sales After Attack by Sect." *The Wall Street Journal,* April 19, 1991.

CADE, JOHN F. "Lithium Salts in the Treatment of Psychotic Excitement." *Medical Journal of Australia* 1(195) (September 1949):349–52.

CAMMER, LEONARD. *Up from Depression.* New York: Pocket Books, 1969.

CHANEY, ERNIE, RUDI ANSBACKER, JAMES FRESTON et al. "Generic Drug Substitution: Implications for Patient Care." *Clinical Courier Special Edition,* January 1990.

CHARNEY, DENNIS S. "An Approach to the Treatment-Resistant Depressed Patient." Interview in *Currents in Affective Illness,* June 1990.

CHIU, E., B. DAVIES and R. WALKER. "Renal Findings After Thirty Years on Lithium (Letter to Editor)." *British Journal of Psychiatry* 143 (1983):424–25.

CHOUINARD, GUY. "The Use of Benzodiazepines in the Treatment of Manic-Depressive Illness." *Journal of Clinical Psychiatry* 49 (November 1988, Suppl.): 15–19.

COWLEY, GEOFFREY. "The Promise of Prozac." *Newsweek,* March 26, 1990, 38–41.

DAMLUJI, NAMIR F. and JAMES M. FERGUSON. "Paradoxical Worsening of Depressive Symptomatology Caused by Antidepressants." *Journal of Clinical Psychopharmacology* 8 (October 1988):347–49.

DAWBER, RODNEY, and PETER MORTIMER. "Hair Loss During Lithium Treatment." *British Journal of Dermatology* 125 (1982):124–25.

DEVANE, C. L. "Pharmacogenetics and Drug Metabolism of Newer Antidepressant Agents." *Journal of Clinical Psychiatry.* 55 (1994, Suppl.):38–45.

DOMINGUEZ, ROBERTO A. "Evaluating the Effectiveness of the New Antidepressants." *Hospital and Community Psychiatry* 34 (May 1983):405–7.

EMRICH, H. M., T. OKUMA and A. A. MULLER, eds. *Anticonvulsants in Affective Disorders.* Amsterdam: Elsevier Science Publishers, 1984.

FAEDDA, GIANNI, LEONARDO TONDO, TRICIA SUPPES, MAURICIO TOHEN and ROSS J. BALDESSARINI. "Outcome After Rapid vs. Gradual Discontinuation of Lithium Treatment in Bipolar Disorders." Presented at the Fifth Meeting of Biological Psychiatry in Florence, Italy, June 1991.

FAVA, MAURIZIO and JERROLD F. ROSENBAUM. "Suicidality and Fluoxetine: Is There a Relationship?" *Journal of Clinical Psychiatry* 52 (March 1991) 108–11.

FDA DRUG BULLETIN. "Safeguards Needed for Carbamazepine." 20 (1990).

"Foods Interacting with MAO Inhibitors." *Medical Letter of Drugs Therapy* 31 (1989):11–12.

FRANK, ELLEN, DAVID J. KUPFER et al. "Three Year Outcomes for Maintenance Therapies in Recurrent Depression." *Archives of General Psychiatry* 47 (December 1990):1093-99.

FREUD, SIGMUND. *Analysis Terminable and Interminable.* Volume 23, standard ed. London: Hogarth Press Ltd., 1937.

GOLDEN, ROBERT N., MATTHEW V. RUDORFER et al. "Buproprion in Depression." *Archives of General Psychiatry* 45 (February 1988):139-443.

GOODMAN, LOUIS S., and ALFRED GILMAN, eds. *The Pharmacological Basis of Therapeutics.* New York: Macmillan Publishing Company, 1975.

GOODWIN, FREDERICK K. and KAY REDFIELD JAMISON. *Manic-Depressive Illness.* New York: Oxford University Press, 1990.

GORMAN, JACK M. *The Essential Guide to Psychiatric Drugs.* New York: St. Martin's Press, 1990.

GREIST, JOHN H., and JAMES W. JEFFERSON. *Depression and Its Treatment.* Washington, DC: American Psychiatric Press, 1984.

HANNA, M.E., C.B. LOBEO and J.T. STEWART. "Severe Lithium Toxicity Associated with Indapamide Therapy." *Journal of Clinical Psychopharmacology* 10 (1990):379.

HENINGER, GEORGE, and DENNIS CHARNEY. "Research Issues and Models to Better Understand the Mechanism of Action of Treatments for Affective Illness: The Role of Lithium." Symposium presented at the American College of Neuropsychopharmacology, December 1986 Washington meeting.

HERMAN, JOHN B., ANDREW W. BROTMAN et al. "Fluoxetine-Induced Sexual Dysfunction." *Journal of Clinical Psychiatry* 51 (January 1990):25-27.

HUGHES, JENNIFER, B. BARRACLOUGH and W. REEVE. "Are Patients Shocked by ECT?" *Journal of the Royal College of Medicine* 74 (April 1981):283-85.

JAMISON, KAY R., ROBERT H. GERNER and FREDERICK K. GOODWIN. "Patient and Physician Attitudes Toward Lithium." *Archives of General Psychiatry* 36 (July 1979):866-69.

JAMISON, KAY R., et al. "Clouds and Silver Linings: Positive Experiences Associated with Primary Affective Disorders." *American Journal of Psychiatry* 137 (February 1980):198-202.

JEFFERSON, JAMES W. "Lithium Carbonate-Induced Hypothyroidism: Its Many Faces." *JAMA* 242 (July 1979):271-72.

JEFFERSON, JAMES W., and JOHN H. GREIST. *Primer of Lithium Therapy.* Baltimore: Williams & Wilkins, 1977.

JEFFERSON, JAMES W. and JOHN H. GREIST. *Valproate and Manic Depression: A Guide.* Madison: Lithium Information Center, 1991.

JEFFERSON, JAMES W., JOHN H. GREIST and DEBORAH L. ACKERMAN. *Lithium Encyclopedia for Clinical Practice.* Washington, DC: American Psychiatric Association Press, 1983.

JULIEN, ROBERT M. *A Primer of Drug Action,* 2nd ed. San Francisco: W. H. Freeman and Company, 1981.

KLINE, NATHAN S. *From Sad to Glad.* New York: G. P. Putnam Sons, 1974.

KLUG, JULIE. "Benefits of ECT Outweigh Risks in Most Patients." *Clinical Psychiatry News* 12 (June 1984).

KRIPKE, DANIEL L., LEWIS L. JUDD et al. "The Effect of Lithium Carbonate on the Circadian Rhythm of Sleep in Normal Human Subjects." *Biological Psychiatry* 14 (1979):545-48.

LACHMAN, H. M. and D. F. PAPOLOS. "Abnormal Signal Transduction: A Hypothetical Model for Bipolar Affective Disorder. *Life Sciences* (October 1989).

LAHR, M. B. "Hyponatremia During Carbamazepine Therapy." *Clinical Pharmacologic Therapies* 37 (1985):693-96.

LICKEY, MARVIN E., and BARBARA GORDON. *Drugs for Mental Illness.* New York: W. H. Freeman and Company, 1983.

LIPINSKI, JOSEPH F., and HARRISON G. POPE. "Possible Synergistic Action Between Carbamazepine and Lithium Carbonate in the Treatment of Three Acutely Manic Patients." *American Journal of Psychiatry* 139 (July 1982):948-49.

LIPINSKI, JOSEPH F., GEORGE S. ZUBENKO et al. "Propranolol in the Treatment of Neuroleptic-Induced Akathesia." *American Journal of Psychiatry* 141 (March 1984):412-15.

LITOVITZ, GARY L. "Contact Lenses and Antidepressants" (Letter to Editor). *Journal of Clinical Psychiatry* 45 (April 1984):188.

LOPPMAN, STEVEN. "A Comparison of Three Types of Lithium Release Preparations." *Hospital and Community Psychiatry* 34 (February 1983):113-14.

MONTGOMERY, STUART A. "Venlafaxine: A New Dimension in Antidepressant Pharmacotherapy." *Journal of Clinical Psychiatry* 54 (March 1993):119-26.

MUNIZ, CARLOS E., RONALD B. SALEM and KENNETH L. DIRECTOR. "Hair Loss in a Patient Receiving Lithium." *Psychosomatics* 23 (March 1982):312-13.

"Old Drug Offers Hope for Those with Depression." *The New York Times,* December 9, 1990.

PRIEN, ROBERT F. *Information on Lithium.* Rockville: U.S. Government Printing Office, 1981.

PRIEN, ROBERT F. and ALAN J. GELENBERG. "Alternatives to Lithium for Preventive Treatment of Bipolar Disorder." *American Journal of Psychiatry* 146 (1990):840-48.

PUZYNSKI, STANISLAW, and LUCJA KLOSIEWICZ. "Valproic Acid Amide in the Treatment of Affective and Schizoaffective Disorders." *Journal of Affective Disorders* 6 (1984):115-21.

QUITKIN, FREDERIC, ARTHUR RIFKIN and DONALD F. KLEIN. "Monoamine Oxidase Inhibitors." *Archives of General Psychiatry* 36 (July 1979):749-60.

SCHATZBERG, ALAN F., and JONATHAN O. COLE. *Manual of Clinical Psychopharmacology.* Washington, DC: American Psychiatric Press, 1986.

SCHOU, MOGENS. "Lithium Perspectives." *Neuropsychobiology* 10 (1983):7-12.

SCHOU, MOGENS. *Lithium Treatment of Manic-Depressive Illness,* 2nd ed. Basel: Karger, 1983.

SCHOU, MOGENS. "Practical Problems of Lithium Maintenance Treatment." In *Chronic Treatments in Neuropsychiatry,* ed. Dargut Kemali and Georgio Racagne. New York: Raven Press, 1985.

SCHUMER, FRAN. "Bye-Bye, Blues: A New Wonder Drug for Depression." *New York Magazine,* December 18, 1989, 46-53.

SUPPES, TRISHA, ROSS J. BALDESSARINI, GIANNI L. FAEDDA and MAURICIO TOHEN. "Risk of Recurrence Following Discontinuation of Lithium Treatment in Biopolar Disorder." Poster given at the May 1991 American Psychiatric Association Convention in New Orleans.

SWAZEY, JUDITH P. *Chlorpromazine in Psychiatry.* Cambridge: MIT Press, 1974.

TEICHER, MARTIN H., CAROL GLOD and JONATHAN O. COLE. "Emergence of Intense Suicidal Preoccupation During Fluoxetine Treatment." *American Journal of Psychiatry* 147 (February 1990):207-10.

TORREY, E. FULLER. *Surviving Schizophrenia.* New York: Harper & Row, 1983.

"Two Measures May Help Prevent Recurrent Depression, Study Shows." *Psychiatric News,* January 18, 1991.

VICTOR, BRUCE S., NAN A. LINK, RENEE L. BINDER and IRIS R. BELL. "Use of Clonazepam in Mania and Schizoaffective Disorders." *American Journal of Psychiatry* 141 (September 1984):111-12.

CHAPTER 6

ANDERSON, CAROL M., GERARD F. HOGARTY and DOUGLAS J. REISS. "Family Treatment of Schizophrenic Patients: A Psychoeducational Approach." *Schizophrenia Bulletin* 6 (1980):490-502.

BALINT, MICHAEL. *The Basic Fault.* London: Tavistock Publications Limited, 1968.

BECK, AARON T., STEVEN D. HOLLON, JEFFREY E. YOUNG et al. "Treatment of Depression with Cognitive Therapy and Amitriptyline." *Archives of General Psychiatry* 42 (February 1985):142-48.

BENSON, ROBERT. "The Forgotten Treatment Modality in Bipolar Illness: Psychotherapy." *American Journal of Psychiatry* (November 1975):634-37.

BOFFEY, PHILIP M. "Psychotherapy Is as Good as Drug in Curing Depression." *New York Times,* May 14, 1986.

BURNS, DAVID D. *Feeling Good.* New York: New American Library, 1980.

BURSTEN, BEN. "Medication Nonadherence Due to Feelings of Loss of Control in Biological Depression." *American Journal of Psychiatry* 142(2) (February 1985):244-46.

CONNELLY, CATHERINE ECOCK, YOLANDE B. DAVENPORT and JOHN I. NURNBERGER. "Adherence to Treatment Regimen in a Lithium Carbonate Clinic." *Archives of General Psychiatry* 39 (May 1982):585-88.

DAVENPORT, YOLANDE B., MARVIN L. ADLAND, PHILIP W. GOLD et al. "Manic-Depressive Illness: Psychodynamic Features of Multigenerational Families." *American Journal of Orthopsychiatry* 49 (January 1979):24-35.

DEPAOLO, J. RAYMOND and KEITH RUSSELL ABLOW. *How to Cope with Depression.* New York: McGraw-Hill, 1989.

FINK, PAUL J. "Response to the Presidential Address: Is 'Biopsychosocial' the Psychiatric Shibboleth?" *American Journal of Psychiatry* 145 (September 1988):1061-67.

FRANK, ELLEN, and DAVID J. KUPFER. "Maintenance Treatment of Recurrent Unipolar Depression: Pharmacology and Psychotherapy." In *Chronic Treat-*

ments in Neuropsychiatry, ed. D. Kemali and G. Racagni. New York: Raven Press, 1985.

FRANK, ELLEN, and DAVID J. KUPFER. "Psychotherapeutic Approaches to Treatment of Recurrent Unipolar Depression: Work in Progress." *Psychopharmacology Bulletin* 22 (1986):558–63.

GOODWIN, FREDERICK K., ROBERT H. GERNER and KAY R. JAMISON. "Patient and Physician Attitudes Toward Lithium." *Archives of General Psychiatry* 36 (July 1979):866–69.

KARASU, T. BYRUM. "Toward a Clinical Model of Psychotherapy for Depression, II: An Integrative and Selective Treatment Approach." *American Journal of Psychiatry* 147 (March 1990):269–78.

KLERMAN, GERALD L. Telephone conversation with Janice Papolos, May 20, 1986.

KLERMAN, GERALD L., MYRNA M. WEISSMAN, BRUCE J. ROUNSAVILLE and EVE S. CHEVRON. *Interpersonal Psychotherapy of Depression.* New York: Basic Books, 1984.

LEO, JOHN. "Talk Is as Good as a Pill." *Time Magazine,* May 26, 1986.

MAYO, JULIA A., RALPH A. O'CONNELL and JOHN D. O'BRIEN. "Families of Manic-Depressive Patients: Effects of Treatment." *American Journal of Psychiatry* 136 (December 1979):153–59.

MURPHY, GEORGE E., ANNE D. SIMONS, RICHARD D. WETZEL et al. "Cognitive Therapy and Pharmacotherapy." *Archives of General Psychiatry* 41 (January 1984):34–41.

PAPOLOS, DEMITRI F. "The Psychoeducational Approach to Major Affective Disorders." Presentation to the American Family Therapy Association, June 1984.

RUNCK, BETTY. "Conference Recommends Pharmacologic Prevention of Recurring Mood Disorders." *Hospital and Community Psychiatry* 35 (September 1984):871–73.

SCHAD-SOMERS, SUSANNE P. *On Mood Swings: The Psychobiology of Elation and Depression.* New York: Plenum Press, 1990.

WHYBROW, PETER C., HAGOP S. AKISKAL and WILLIAM T. MCKINNEY, JR. *Mood Disorders: Toward a New Psychobiology.* New York: Plenum Press, 1984.

YESS, JAMES P. "What Families of the Mentally Ill Want." *Community Support Service Journal* 2 (n.d.).

CHAPTER 7

FAEDDA, GIANNI L., ROSS J. BALDESSARINI, MAURICIO TOHEN, et al. "Episode Sequence in Bipolar Disorder and Response to Lithium Treatment." *American Journal of Psychiatry,* 148 (1991):1237–39.

KOUKOPOULOS, ATHANASIO, DANIELA REGINALDI et al. "Course of the Manic-Depressive Cycle and Changes Caused by Treatments." *Pharmakopsychiater* 13 (1980):156–67.

MAJ, MARIO, RAFFAELE PIROZZI and FABRIZIO STARACE. "Previous Pattern of Course of the Illness as a Predictor of Response to Lithium Prophylaxis in Biopolar Patients." *Journal of Affective Disorders* 17 (1989):237–41.

Post, Robert M., Peter P. Roy-Byrne and Thomas W. Uhde. "Graphic Representation of the Life Course of Illness in Patients with Affective Disorder." *American Journal of Psychiatry* 145 (July 1988):844–48.

Schou, Mogens. "Lithium as a Prophylactic Agent in Unipolar Affective Illness: Comparison with Cyclic Antidepressants." *Archives of General Psychiatry* 36 (1979):849–51.

Wehr, Thomas A., David A. Sack, and Norman E. Rosenthal. "Sleep Reduction as a Final Common Pathway in the Genesis of Depression." *American Journal of Psychiatry* 144 (1987):201–4.

CHAPTER 8

Seasonal Affective Disorders

Begley, Sharon, and William J. Cook. "The Sad Days of Winter." *Newsweek,* January 14, 1985.

Donaldson, Susan R. "The Dawn's Early Light: Remedy for Depression?" *Biological Therapies in Psychiatry* 7 (July 1984):25.

Donaldson, Susan R. "Seasonal Affective Disorder and Phototherapy: A Brief Review." *Psychiatric Times,* April 1985.

Faedda, Gianni L., Leonardo Tondo, Martin H. Teicher, Ross J. Baldessarini et al. "Seasonal Mood Disorders: Patterns of Seasonal Recurrence in Major Affective Disorders." *Archives of General Psychiatry* 50 (1991):17–23.

Kripke, Daniel F., S. Craig Risch and David S. Janowsky. "Lighting Up Depression." *Psychopharmacology Bulletin* 19 (1983):526–30.

"Light" (Talk of the Town). *New Yorker,* January 14, 1985.

Parker, Gordon, and Stephen Walter. "Seasonal Variation in Depressive Disorders and Suicidal Deaths in New South Wales." *British Journal of Psychiatry* 140 (1982):626–32.

Reiter, Russell J. "The Pineal Gland: An Intermediary Between the Environment and the Endocrine System." *Psychoneuroendocrinology* 8 (1983):31–40.

Rosenthal, Norman E., Alfred J. Lewy, Thomas A. Wehr et al. "Seasonal Cycling in a Bipolar Patient." *Psychiatry Research* 8 (1983):25–31.

Rosenthal, Norman E., David A. Sack, Christian Gillin et al. "Seasonal Affective Disorder: A Description of the Syndrome and Preliminary Findings with Light Therapy." *Archives of General Psychiatry* 41 (January 1984):72–79.

Wehr, Thomas A., and Frederick K. Goodwin. "Biological Rhythms and Psychiatry." In *American Handbook of Psychiatry,* 2nd ed. Vol. VII: *Advances and New Directions,* ed. Silvano Arieti and James Brodie. New York: Basic Books, 1981.

Wehr, Thomas A., Frederick K. Goodwin, Anna Wirz-Justice et al. "48-Hour Sleep-Wake Cycles in Manic-Depressive Illness." *Archives of General Psychiatry* 39 (May 1982):559–65.

WEHR, THOMAS A., DAVID A. SACK and NORMAN ROSENTHAL. "Seasonal Affective Disorder with Summer Depression and Winter Hypomania." *American Journal of Psychiatry* 144 (December 1987):1602-3.

Depression in Children and Adolescents

ANNELL, ANNA-LISA. "Lithium in the Treatment of Children and Adolescents." *Acta Psychiatrica Scandinavica* 207 (1969, Suppl.):19-33.

BASSUK, ELLEN L., STEPHEN C. SCHOONOVER and ALAN J. GELENBERG, eds. *The Practitioner's Guide to Psychoactive Drugs,* 2nd ed. New York: Plenum Medical Book Company, 1984.

BERG, IAN, ROY HULLIN, MICHAEL ALLSOP et al. "Bipolar Manic-Depressive Psychosis in Early Adolescence." *British Journal of Psychiatry* 125 (1974):416-17.

BIEDERMAN, JOSEPH, DAVID GASTFRIEND, MICHAEL S. JELLINEK and ALLAN GOLDBLATT. "Cardiovascular Effects of Desipramine in Children and Adolescents with Attention Deficit Disorder." *Journal of Pediatrics* 106 (June 1985):1017-20.

CANTWELL, DENNIS P., and GABRIELLE A. CARLSON, eds. *Affective Disorders in Childhood and Adolescence—an Update.* New York: Spectrum Publications, 1983.

CONNORS, C. KEITH, and THEODORE PETTI. "Imipramine Therapy of Depressed Children: Methodologic Considerations." *Psychopharmacology Bulletin* 19 (1983):65-69.

CYTRYN, LEON, DONALD H. MCKNEW, JR., and WILLIAM E. BUNNEY. "Diagnosis of Depression in Children: A Reassessment." *American Journal of Psychiatry* 137 (January 1980):22-25.

DSM-III: Diagnostic and Statistical Manual of Mental Disorders, 3rd ed. Washington, DC: American Psychiatric Association, 1980.

GELLER, BARBARA, JAMES M. PEREL, EDWARD F. KNITTER et al. "Nortriptyline in Major Depressive Disorder in Children: Response, Steady-State Plasma Levels, Predictive Kinetics, and Pharmacokinetics." *Psychopharmacology Bulletin* 19 (1983):62-65.

GREENBERG, ROSALIE. "Adolescent Suicide." *Fair Oaks Psychiatry Letter* 3 (12) (December 1985):67-70.

JEFFERSON, JAMES W., and JOHN H. GREIST. *Primer of Lithium Therapy.* Baltimore: Williams & Wilkins, 1977.

KASHANI, JAVAD, and JOHN F. SIMONDS. "The Incidence of Depression in Children." *American Journal of Psychiatry* 136 (September 1979):1203-5.

KASHANI, JAVAD, ARSHAD HUSAIN, WALID O. SHEKIM et al. "Current Perspectives on Childhood Depression: An Overview." *American Journal of Psychiatry* 138 (February 1981):143-53.

KESTENBAUM, CLARICE. "Children at Risk for Manic-Depressive Illness: Possible Predictors." *American Journal of Psychiatry* 136 (September 1979): 1206-8.

MALMQUIST, CARL P. "Depressions in Childhood and Adolescence (Part I)." *New England Journal of Medicine* 284 (April 1971):887-93.

PFEFFER, CYNTHIA R. "Suicidal Tendencies in Children and Adolescents." *Medical Aspects of Human Sexuality* 20 (February 1986):32-35.

STROBER, MICHAEL, JACQUELINE GREEN and GABRIELLE CARLSON. "Phenomenology and Subtypes of Major Depressive Disorder in Adolescence." *Journal of Affective Disorders* 3 (1981):281-90.

WELLER, ELIZABETH B., and RONALD A. WELLER, eds. *Major Depressive Disorders in Children.* Clinical Insights Series. Washington, DC: American Psychiatric Association, 1984.

YOUNGERMAN, JOSEPH, and IAN A. CANINO. "Lithium Carbonate Use in Children and Adolescents: A Survey of the Literature." *Archives of General Psychiatry* 35 (February 1978):216-24.

Affective Disorders in the Elderly

BASSUK, ELLEN L., STEPHEN C. SCHOONOVER and ALAN J. GELENBERG, eds. *The Practitioner's Guide to Psychoactive Drugs,* 2nd ed. New York: Plenum Medical Book Company, 1984.

BRESSLER, RUBIN. "Treating Geriatric Depression: Current Options." *Drug Therapy* (September 1984):35-50.

BUTLER, ROBERT N. "Psychiatry and the Elderly: An Overview." *American Journal of Psychiatry* 132 (September 1975):893-900.

GOODSTEIN, RICHARD K. "The Diagnosis and Treatment of Elderly Patients: Some Practical Guidelines." *Hospital and Community Psychiatry* 31 (January 1980):19-24.

PAYKEL, E. S., ed. *Handbook of Affective Disorders.* New York: The Guilford Press, 1982.

REIFLER, BURTON V., ERIC LARSON and RAY HANLEY. "Coexistence of Cognitive Impairment and Depression in Geriatric Outpatients." *American Journal of Psychiatry* 139 (May 1982):623-26.

ROOSE, STEVEN P., STANLEY BONE, CATHERINE HAIDORFER et al. "Lithium Treatment in Older Patients." *American Journal of Psychiatry* 136 (June 1979):843-44.

SCHATZBERG, ALAN F., BENJAMIN LIPTZIN, ANDREW SATLIN and JONATHAN O. COLE. "Diagnosis of Affective Disorders in the Elderly." *Psychosomatics* 25 (February 1985):126-31.

SCHATZBERG, ALAN F., ed. *Common Treatment Problems in Depression.* Washington, DC: American Psychiatric Press, 1985.

SHAMOIAN, CHARLES A., ed. *Treatment of Affective Disorders in the Elderly.* Washington, DC: American Psychiatric Press, 1985.

SHRABERG, DAVID. "The Myth of Pseudodementia: Depression and the Aging Brain." *American Journal of Psychiatry* 135 (May 1978):601-3.

TAYLOR, ROBERT L. *Mind or Body: Distinguishing Psychological from Organic Disorders.* New York: McGraw-Hill, 1982.

WELLS, CHARLES E. "Pseudodementia." *American Journal of Psychiatry* 136 (July 1979):895–900.

Pregnancy and Affective Disorders

ANATH, JAMBUR. "Side Effects in the Neonate from Psychotropic Agents Excreted Through Breast-Feeding." *American Journal of Psychiatry* 135 (July 1978):801–5.

BALDESSARINI, ROSS J. *Chemotherapy in Psychiatry,* rev. ed. Cambridge: Harvard University Press, 1985.

BASSUK, ELLEN L., STEPHEN C. SCHOONOVER and ALAN J. GELENBERG, eds. *The Practitioner's Guide to Psychoactive Drugs,* 2nd ed. New York: Plenum Medical Book Company, 1984.

GOLDFIELD, MICHAEL, and MORTON R. WEINSTEIN. "Lithium in Pregnancy: A Review with Recommendations." *American Journal of Psychiatry* 127 (January 1971):64–69.

JEFFERSON, JAMES W., and JOHN H. GREIST. *Primer of Lithium Therapy.* Baltimore: Williams & Wilkins, 1977.

NURNBERG, H. GEORGE. "Treatment of Mania in the Last Six Months of Pregnancy." *Hospital and Community Psychiatry* 31 (February 1980):122–26.

NURNBERG, H. GEORGE, and JOAN PRUDIC. "Guidelines for Treatment of Psychosis During Pregnancy." *Hospital and Community Psychiatry* 35 (January 1984):67–71.

REMICK, RONALD A., and WILLIAM L. MAURICE. "ECT in Pregnancy." *American Journal of Psychiatry* 135 (June 1978):761–62.

TARGUM, STEVEN D., YOLANDE B. DAVENPORT and MARIAN J. WEBSTER. "Postpartum Mania in Bipolar Manic-Depressive Patients Withdrawn from Lithium Carbonate." *Journal of Nervous and Mental Disease* 167 (1979):572–74.

WEINSTEIN, MORTON R., and MICHAEL D. GOLDFIELD. "Cardiovascular Malformation with Lithium Use During Pregnancy." *American Journal of Psychiatry* 132 (May 1975):529–31.

CHAPTER 9

Children

GREEN, WAYNE HUGO. *Child and Adolescent Clinical Psychopharmacology,* 2nd ed. Baltimore: Williams & Wilkins, 1995.

Pregnancy

COHEN, LEE S., J.M. FRIEDMAN et al. "A Reevaluation of Risk of In Utero Exposure to Lithium." *JAMA* 271 (January 1994):146–50.

PASTUSZAK, ANNE, BETSY SCHICK-BOSCHETTO et al. "Pregnancy Outcome Following First-Trimester Exposure to Fluoxetine (Prozac). *JAMA* 269 (May 1993): 2246–48.

Comorbidity

BRADY, KATHLEEN T., and SUSAN C. SONNE. "The Relationship Between Substance Abuse and Bipolar Disorder." *Journal of Clinical Psychiatry* 56 (1995): 19–24.

BRADY, KATHLEEN T., SUSAN S. SONNE et al. "Valproate in the Treatment of Acute Bipolar Affective Episodes Complicated by Substance Abuse: A Pilot Study." *Journal of Clinical Psychiatry* 56 (1995):118–21.

REGIER, DARRYL A., MARY FARMER et al. "Comordity of Mental Disorders with Alcohol and Other Drug Abuse, Results from the Epidemiologic Catchment Area (ECA) Study." *JAMA* 264 (1990):2511–18.

CHAPTER 10

BERNHEIM, KAYLA F., and ANTHONY F. LEHMAN. *Working with Families of the Mentally Ill.* New York: W. W. Norton and Company, 1985.

BOHAN, PATRICK. "A Call to Advocate." *Sibling Bond* 3 (Winter 1984).

BROWN, BERYL. "Growing Up." *Sibling Bond* 5 (Winter 1985).

JOHNSON, JULIE. "Great Expectations: A Sibling Experience." *Mental Health Advocate* 22 (April/May 1983).

TORREY, E. FULLER. *Surviving Schizophrenia.* New York: Harper & Row, 1983.

WALSH, MARYELLEN. *Schizophrenia: Straight Talk for Family and Friends.* New York: William Morrow, 1985.

CHAPTER 11

APPLEBAUM, PAUL S. "Civil Commitment: Is the Pendulum Changing Direction?" *Hospital and Community Psychiatry* 33 (September 1982): 703–4.

CAMMER, LEONARD. *Up from Depression.* New York: Pocket Books, 1969.

CHODOFF, PAUL. "The Case for Involuntary Hospitalization for the Mentally Ill." *American Journal of Psychiatry* 133 (May 1976):496–501.

DURAM, MARY L., HAROLD D. CARR and GLENN L. PIERCE. "Police Involvement and Influence in Involuntary Civil Commitment." *Hospital and Community Psychiatry* 35 (June 1984):580–84.

ENNIS, BRUCE J. *Prisoners of Psychiatry.* New York: Harcourt Brace Jovanovich, 1972.

ENNIS, BRUCE J., and RICHARD D. EMERY. *The Rights of Mental Patients.* New York: Avon Books, 1978.

GOLEMAN, DANIEL. "States Move to Ease Law Committing Mentally Ill." *New York Times,* December 9, 1986 (section C).

GOTS, RONALD, and ARTHUR KAUFMAN. *The People's Hospital Book.* New York: Avon, 1978.

HARBIN, HENRY T., ed. *The Psychiatric Hospital and the Family.* New York: Spectrum Publications, 1982.

HOSPITAL AND COMMUNITY PSYCHIATRY SERVICE. *Rights of the Mentally Disabled: Statements and Standards.* Washington, DC: American Psychiatric Press, 1983.

KORPELL, HERBERT S. *How You Can Help.* Washington, DC: American Psychiatric Press, 1984.

MCFARLANE, WILLIAM R. "Family Therapy in the Psychiatric Hospital." In *The Psychiatric Hospital and the Family,* ed. Henry T. Harbin. New York: Spectrum Publications, 1982.

MCPHEE, JOHN. "Family Doctors." *New Yorker,* July 23, 1984.

PARK, CLARA CLAIBORNE, with LEON N. SHAPIRO. *You Are Not Alone.* Boston: Little, Brown & Company, 1976.

ROSENBLATT, AARON. "Concepts of the Asylum in the Care of the Mentally Ill." *Hospital and Community Psychiatry* 35 (March 1984):244-50.

ROTH, LOREN H. "A Commitment Law for Patients, Doctors, and Lawyers." *American Journal of Psychiatry* 136 (September 1979):1121-26.

SADOFF, ROBERT L. *Legal Issues in the Care of Psychiatric Patients.* New York: Springer Publishing Company, 1982.

SCHWARTZ, HAROLD I., PAUL S. APPLEBAUM and RICHARD D. KAPLAN. "Clinical Judgments in the Decision to Commit." *Archives of General Psychiatry* 41 (August 1984):811-15.

SHEEHAN, SUSAN. *Is There No Place on Earth for Me?* New York: Vintage Books, 1983.

SKODOL, ANDREW E., ROBERT PLUTCHIK and TOKSOZ B. KARASU. "Expectations of Hospital Treatment." *Journal of Nervous and Mental Disease* 168 (March 1980):70-74.

STONE, ALAN A. "Recent Mental Health Litigation: A Critical Perspective." *American Journal of Psychiatry* 134 (March 1977):273-79.

SULLIVAN, RONALD. "Limits Ease on Committing the Mentally Ill." *New York Times,* July 15, 1985.

SZASZ, THOMAS S. *Psychiatric Slavery.* New York: The Free Press, 1977.

TORREY, E. FULLER. *Surviving Schizophrenia.* New York: Harper & Row, 1983.

TUCKER, GARY J., and JERROLD S. MAXMEN. "The Practice of Hospital Psychiatry: A Formulation." *American Journal of Psychiatry* 130 (August 1973): 887-91.

CHAPTER 12

AMMER, CHRISTINE, with NATHAN T. SIDLEY. *The Common Sense Guide to Mental Health Care.* Brattleboro, VT: The Lewis Publishing Company, 1982.

ANDRULIS, DENNIS P., and NOEL A. MAZADE. "American Mental Health Policy: Changing Directions in the 80's." *Hospital and Community Psychiatry* 34 (July 1983):601-6.

CENTER FOR HEALTH POLICY STUDIES. *Mandated Mental Health Benefits under Private Insurance: A Review of State Laws.* Prepared for the National Institute of Mental Health, December 1983.

GREENLEY, DIANNE. "Insurance and Other Third-Party Coverage for Persons Who Are Mentally Ill: Issues and Possibilities." Report written for the National Alliance for the Mentally Ill, February 1986.

HYMOWITZ, CAROL, and ELLEN JOAN POLLOCK. "The New Economics of Mental Health." *Wall Street Journal,* July 13, 1995.

MALLOY, MICHAEL. *Mental Illness and Managed Care: A Primer for Families and Consumers.* Arlington, VA: National Alliance for the Mentally Ill, 1995.

NATIONAL COMMITTEE FOR QUALITY ASSURANCE. "Draft Accreditation Standards for Managed Care Behavioral Healthcare Organizations." April 1996.

NERNEY, JOHN. "Fire." *AMI-NYS News,* November 1995.

SCHLACKMAN, NEIL. "The Quality Care Cycle." *Joint Commission Journal on Quality Improvement,* 17 (November 1991):360–64.

SCHLACKMAN, NEIL. "The Measurement of Physician Performance." *Quality Management in Health Care,* 4 (1995):1–12.

PEAR, ROBERT. "Conferees Agree on Bill to Revise U. S. Disability Law." *New York Times,* September 15, 1984.

PEAR, ROBERT. "Proposals for Mentally Disabled Ease Eligibility for U. S. Benefits." *New York Times,* December 8, 1984.

SHARFSTEIN, STEVEN, SAM MUSZYNSKI and EVELYN MYERS. *Health Insurance and Psychiatric Care: Update and Appraisal.* Washington, DC: American Psychiatric Press, 1984.

U.S. DEPARTMENT OF HEALTH AND HUMAN SERVICES. *Social Security Handbook.* SSA Publication No. 05-10135, July 1984.

CHAPTER 13

ARNSTEIN, HELENE S. *What to Tell Your Child about Birth, Death, Illness, Divorce and Other Family Crises,* rev. ed. Indianapolis: The Bobbs-Merrill Company, 1974.

FIEDLER, TOM. "Chiles Says Medicine Overcame Depression." *Miami Herald,* April 17, 1990.

HOLDEN, CONSTANCE. "Giving Mental Illness Its Research Due." *Science* 232 (May 30, 1986):1084–85.

RIMER, SARA. "Chiles Triumphs on Little Money." *The New York Times,* November 7, 1990.

INDEX

Note: Numbers followed by an *i* indicate illustrations; those followed by a *t* indicate tables.

Mental illness. *See also specific types, e.g.,* Depression.
diagnosis of, 31–55
medical model of, 32
public attitudes about, 352–9
Mental Illness and Managed Care (Malloy), 330
Mercury poisoning, 40*t*
Methylphenidate hydrochloride, 239
Millet, Kate, 15–6
Mixed state depression, 37, 38, 47–9
Monoamine oxidase, 78
Monoamine oxidase inhibitors (MAOIs), 82, 158–63
cautions with, 160–3
drug interactions with, 163*t*
foods to avoid with, 162*t*
"rapid cyclers" and, 46
side effects from, 160
Mononucleosis, 39*t*
Mood, diurnal variation of, 14, 252
Mood disorders. *See also specific types, e.g.,* Mania.
adolescents and, 225–31
alcohol and, 208–9
Amish study of, 58–67
children and, 225–31, 279–82
circadian rhythms and, 97, 102–11, 105*i*, 108*i*, 109*i*, 116
clinics for, 258–9
course of, 207–19
definition of, 3–4
eating disorders as, 53–4
elderly and, 234–40
epidemiology of, 67–9
genetic counseling for, 69–71
genetic markers for, 56–69
lability of, 24–7
questionnaire for, 364–7
recovery from, 343–59
subtypes of, 46–52
Mood Disorders: Major Depression and Manic-Depression (Papolos), 195

Mood Disorders: Toward a New Psychobiology (Whybrow, Akiskal, and McKinney), 25–7
Mood scale, for cycle charts, 216–27, 217*i*
Multiple sclerosis, 40*t*, 250

NAMI (National Alliance for the Mentally Ill), 195, 283, 328, 330, 350, 352–4, 368, 372
Nardil. *See* Phenelzine.
National Alliance for Research on Schizophrenia and Depression (NARSAD), 352–3
National Alliance for the Mentally Ill (NAMI), 195, 283, 328, 330, 350, 352–4, 368, 372
National Committee for Quality Assurance (NCQA), 328
National Depressive and Manic-Depressive Association, 247–8, 372
National Institute of Mental Health (NIMH), 49, 110, 111, 138, 172, 183, 204, 352, 356–7
National Mental Health Consumers' Association (NMHCA), 357
National Report Card (study), 329
Nefazadone, 169–70, 171*t*
Negri bodies, 76
Nemeroff, Charles, 100–1
Nemerov, Gertrude, 18–9
Neuroleptic drugs, 136*t*, 148–50
Neurological disorders, 40*t*
Neurontin. *See* Gabapentin.
Neuropeptide Y, 78
Neurotransmitters, 113
receptor sensitivity and, 83–4
types of, 77–8, 79*i*, 80*i*, 81*i*
Nihilistic delusions, 16–7
NIMH (National Institute of Mental Health), 49, 110, 111, 138, 172, 183, 204, 352, 356–7
Nimodipine, 47

COPYRIGHT
ACKNOWLEDGMENTS

ABOUT THE AUTHORS

Demitri F. Papolos, M.D., is Associate Professor of Psychiatry at the Albert Einstein College of Medicine and the Co-Director of the Program of Behavioral Genetics. Formerly the Director of Inpatient Psychiatry at Montefiore Medical Center, he is the coordinator of the teaching program on mood disorders for the psychiatric residency training program at the Albert Einstein College of Medicine. Dr. Papolos is currently involved in research that focuses on the molecular basis of manic-depressive illness and is a recipient of the Ruth Landau Wilkes Young Investigator Award granted by the National Alliance for Research in Schizophrenia and Depression (NARSAD), as well as an NIMH Physician/Scientist Career Development Award. Dr. Papolos developed the family psychoeducational approach to mood disorders. He is a diplomate in nerology and psychiatry and is in private practice in New York City and Westport, Connecticut.

Janice Papolos has written on a broad range of subjects for national magazines such as *Newsweek, McCall's, Self, High Fidelity,* and *Chamber Music Magazine.* Her first book, *The Performing Artist's Handbook,* has become a standard reference in the classical music field. *The Virgin Homeowner*, her newest book, was recently published by W. W. Norton. Janice Papolos is a member of the American Society of Journalists and Authors.